ABOUT THE AUTHORS

Bernard Gert, Ph.D., is the Eunice and Julian Cohen Professor of Ethics and Human Values at Dartmouth College.

Charles M. Culver, M.D., Ph.D., is Professor of Medical Education at Barry University in Miami, FL.

K. Danner Clouser, Ph.D., is Professor of Humanities at Pennsylvania State University College of Medicine, Hershey, PA.

Bioethics: A Return to Fundamentals

Bioethics: A Return to Fundamentals

BERNARD GERT, PH.D.
Eunice and Julian Cohen Professor of
Ethics and Human Values
Dartmouth College
Adjunct Professor of Psychiatry
Dartmouth Medical School

CHARLES M. CULVER, MD., PH.D.
Professor of Medical Education
Barry University

K. DANNER CLOUSER, B.D., PH.D.
University Professor of Humanities
Pennsylvania State University College of Medicine

New York   Oxford
OXFORD UNIVERSITY PRESS
1997

Oxford University Press

Oxford   New York
Athens   Auckland   Bangkok   Bogota   Bombay   Buenos Aires
Calcutta   Cape Town   Dar es Salaam   Delhi   Florence   Hong Kong
Istanbul   Karachi   Kuala Lumpur   Madras   Madrid   Melbourne
Mexico City   Nairobi   Paris   Singapore   Taipei   Tokyo   Toronto

and associated companies in
Berlin   Ibadan

Copyright © 1997 by Oxford University Press

Published by Oxford University Press, Inc.
198 Madison Avenue, New York, New York 10016

Oxford is a registered trademark of Oxford University Press

Library of Congress Cataloging-in-Publication Data
Gert, Bernard, 1934–
Bioethics. : a return to fundamentals /
Bernard Gert, Charles M. Culver, K. Danner Clouser.
p.   cm.   Includes bibliographical references and index.
ISBN 0-19-511430-2
1. Medical ethics.
I. Culver, Charles M.   II. Clouser, K. Danner.
III. Title.
R724.G46   1997   174'.2—dc21   96-40853

2 3 4 5 6 7 8 9

Printed in the United States of America
on acid-free paper

*To my wife Esther and
our children Heather and Joshua*

*To my wife Marta and
our son Martin*

*To my wife Mary Louise and
our children Charles and Mary Danner*

Preface

Our subtitle, *A Return to Fundamentals,* describes the book's content and speaks to a concern. The content deals with theory, concepts, and lines of reasoning that are basic to medical ethics and, for that matter, to all other branches of applied ethics. Our concern is provoked by numerous observations of the state of the field, chief among which is the tendency on the part of many to regard each area of applied ethics as an entity unto itself, that is, as independent of a general account of morality. Few, if any, systematic attempts are made to relate the applied ethics to a general account of morality. Correspondingly, there is a tendency for professionals coming into the field to be trained in the culture of medical ethics, in its classic cases and standard resolutions, but with no real understanding of common morality or of its relation to the various branches of applied ethics.

Witness the spate of medical ethics books being published. In the requisite sections of the books (usually the first chapter) dealing with theory, there is typically a gathering of various approaches to ethics with a brief description and, sometimes, a critique of each. But there is no systematic investigation of the different approaches, no attempt to discover or validate the foundations of these approaches, and no detailed attempt to relate these approaches to the systematic solving of medical ethics problems. Indeed, theory typically is never mentioned again in the rest of the book.

We acknowledge that medical ethics problems often can be satisfactorily resolved on the fly, citing ad hoc rules, cases, principles, or traditions, as they come to mind. In these instances, ordinary moral understanding provides those involved with an acceptable agreed-on resolution to the problem, and the subsequent citing of "proofs" or "principles" is generally nothing more than academic window dressing. However, ordinary moral understanding is often not sufficient to resolve more complex and difficult cases. Whenever a case provokes disagreement among different participants, something beyond shared moral intuitions is necessary.

Thus, in addition to its theoretical value, we believe that there is considerable practical value in discovering and validating the foundations of those moral beliefs that guide decisions and actions, and in relating them to fundamental concepts and problems in medical ethics. Indeed, we believe our exposition of the linkage between morality and its expression in medical ethics in particular is clear enough to be of conceptual help to all areas of applied ethics.

Although many themes and concepts in this book have been developed to some extent in other articles and books that we have individually or cooperatively written, this is a new book in almost every respect. For example, it contains themes that were addressed in *Philosophy of Medicine*,[1] but extensive changes, additions, and improvements have been made in the concepts of consent, competence, malady, paternalism, and death. Furthermore, it contains topics not discussed in that book: applications, morality, principlism, confidentiality, and euthanasia. Most significantly, the current book integrates all of these themes and concepts, grounding them in a systematic account of morality. The connections between bioethics and morality are explored and made explicit.

We are aware that talk of a "systematic account" may connote something monolithic and presumptuous. That is unfortunate, since misunderstanding of this matter has had a considerable negative impact on bioethics. Our systematic account of ethics is not monolithic; it does not claim that there is a unique right answer to every moral question. Indeed, one of its virtues is that it provides an explanation of why some legitimate moral disagreement is inevitable. It is also not presumptuous, for it includes as morally acceptable all views that any impartial rational person might put forward.

To be systematic means that each part of the account of morality has implications for every other part. There must be consistency throughout the moral system. If a feature is judged to be morally relevant in one case, that same feature must be judged to be morally relevant in every other case. Not only must there be consistency within the moral system, but there must be consistency with regard to those to whom the rules, ideals, and lines of reasoning apply. If a violation of a moral rule is justified in one case, it must be justified in all cases with the same morally relevant features. The emphasis on system is in direct opposition to the ad hoc approach characteristic of much of bioethics.

Furthermore, we emphasize morality as a *public* system; for example, in

considering whether a moral rule violation is justified, the decisive consideration is not the consequences of the particular violation in question, but the
consequences of everyone knowing that these kinds of violations are allowed.
Breaking a moral rule when one would not be willing to have everyone know
that such violations are allowed is contrary to the very essence of morality,
namely, its requirement of impartiality. That morality is a public system that
applies to all rational persons explains why everyone knows what morality forbids, requires, encourages, and allows. Our recognition of this is why our account of morality does not lead to the kinds of counterexamples that have led so
many in bioethics and in other areas of applied ethics to oppose moral theory
or, what amounts to the same thing, to adopt the anthology approach to ethical
theory, that is, to advocate different theories for different problems.

The foregoing gives a brief hint about why we prefer to refer to our approach
to ethics as "morality as a public system." The appropriateness of that descriptive name for our account of ethics will become clearer as the reader progresses
through the book. Meanwhile, in this context, we wish to make the point that
the way our approach has often been described, namely, as "rule-based ethics,"
is simply wrong. Although rules are one aspect of our account of morality, there
are other essential components of the moral system: ideals, specification of the
morally relevant features of situations that help focus the search for and the
comparison of facts, and an explicit procedure for dealing with conflicts among
rules and ideals. "Morality as a public system" comes closest to encompassing
all the elements and as such is a more adequate description of our approach.

Notes

1. Charles M. Culver and Bernard Gert, *Philosophy in Medicine* (New York: Oxford
University Press, 1982).

Acknowledgments

We wish to acknowledge the encouragement and help that we have received from our colleagues and students. In particular, we want to acknowledge the help of several people and institutions who played a special role. We gratefully acknowledge the financial help provided by funds associated with Professor Clouser's University Professorship in Humanities at The Penn State University College of Medicine. On several occasions these funds brought the authors to Hershey and permitted the three of us to meet together to produce a genuinely collaborative book. Ken Goodman of the University of Miami Medical School arranged for workshops that enabled the three of us to work together and facilitated discussion of several of the topics included in this book.

We are particularly grateful to Professor Maria Julia Bertomeu, who arranged for Charles M. Culver and Bernard Gert to teach at Nacional Universidad de La Plata in La Plata, Argentina. Professor Bertomeu also provided a Fulbright teaching position at La Plata that allowed Bernard Gert to teach both at the Nacional Universidad de La Plata and the Universidad de Buenos Aires in the fall of 1995. Teaching in Argentina provided an opportunity and an incentive to improve both the clarity and universality of the views expressed in this book. It is a pleasure to be able to acknowledge the help of Maria Victoria Costa, an outstanding philosophy graduate student, who served as translator for Bernard Gert and without whom he would have been unable to participate in the many discussions of bioethics that took place during his stay there. As suggested above, we are also grateful for the Fulbright award that enabled Bernard Gert to teach in Argentina, and for an earlier Fulbright award to Charles M. Culver to teach in Uruguay.

All three of us are grateful to the students of Dartmouth College where, at one time or another, all of us have taught philosophy of medicine. We are also grateful to our colleagues at Dartmouth, especially James L. Bernat of the Dartmouth Medical School for his advice and counsel. Bernard Gert is especially grateful to Eunice and Julian Cohen for their friendship and support. Danner Clouser is indebted to his students and colleagues at The Penn State University College of Medicine and The Hershey Medical Center who for 28 years interactively honed his understanding of medicine and ethics.

B.G.
C.M.C.
K.D.C.

Contents

Bioethics: A Return to Fundamentals

1

Introduction

The Rationale

Background

Our goal is to present an account of morality that is systematic, accessible, and usable. We hope the reader will understand the moral system, appreciate its foundations, and see it in action. The relationship of common morality to bioethics will be explained and clarified; core concepts of bioethics will be explicated and grounded in common morality.

An important emphasis in our work is the centrality of common morality. Common morality is the foundation on which we build: first by explicating how morality works, then by justifying the practice as a public system for everyone, and finally by showing how it is manifested in different cultures, including subcultures like professions, all the while remaining one integrated morality. In knowing what one already knows about common morality, a person knows a great deal about bioethics. Morality is all one, though within particular contexts it is accordingly and appropriately modified. That is why one is able to have sophisticated discussions about moral problems within biomedicine without ever having had a course in ethics or moral theory.

Ours is a deliberate effort to counteract the generally ad hoc character of biomedical ethics since its birth (or rebirth) in the 1960s. Bioethics has often been derisively referred to as "quandary ethics" or "dilemma ethics," implying thereby that it consists of puzzles which, though they may fascinate or entertain, are not amenable to systematic analysis and resolution, and hence almost any answer will, and usually does, suffice. This implies a lack of system, in that the answer to any one puzzle is unrelated to the answer to any other, and this in turn implies that there is no way to show whether the answers to two distinct dilemmas are consistent with each other.

The any-answer-will-suffice (or, all-answers-are-unique) mindset has been perpetuated by the way medical ethics is usually taught. We call it the "anthology" method. Typically, several different ethical theories are presented with no attempt to reconcile them. Kant would say this, Mill would say that, and Rawls would say something else. The student naturally concludes that moral theory is either confused, irrelevant, or completely relativistic.

Often the anthologies suggest using one theory to solve a particular kind of problem and another theory for a different kind of problem. Yet there is neither unification among the different theories nor a clue as to how problems are to be assigned to which theory. There is certainly nothing wrong with assimilating the best from every theory, but these insights must be unified in a comprehensive theory and not left at odds with each other. Our own theory is significantly informed by the importance of consequences for the Utilitarians and by the importance of impartiality and publicity for Kant. Yet we blend these insights into a single coherent and comprehensive framework within which *all* moral problems can be considered.[1]

The irrelevance of moral theory is the theme of a movement growing out of the last decade of applied ethics. Not seeing how the abstractions and high-level generalizations of moral theory could ever be used specifically with respect to the particulars of moral experience, many have concluded that moral theory is irrelevant to practical moral decisions.[2] Others believe that "one morality," especially one that is justified by a moral theory, must be wrong. They believe that such a morality must be seen as an axiomatic system that works by deduction from assumed first principles, and consequently cannot be sensitive to different cultures and practices.[3] We think that both these critiques apply only to inadequate theories. The critics who argue that moral theories do not connect with the particulars of moral experience consider only theories that are, in fact, inadequate. Therefore we understand why they reach those conclusions.

We agree with much of the criticism of moral theories as not really usable or guiding in particular circumstances. But we consider this to be a criticism of particular theories rather than a criticism of moral theory itself or its role. The critics of moral theory seem to share an unspoken assumption that a moral theory should be simple, that it should be statable as a one-liner, and that it should provide a quick fix or decision procedure.[4] Although morality must be understandable and able to be followed by everyone, morality, like grammar, need not be simple. For an adequate account of morality one must be prepared to consider a theory sufficiently complex to deal with its complicated subject matter.

Moral System and Moral Theory

It is important not only to distinguish the moral system from the moral theory that describes and justifies it, but to make this distinction correctly. The moral system is common morality at work; it comprises the considered moral judgments everyone commonly makes. For us, the moral system comes first; the moral theory is a systematic description and justification of that moral system. Many philosophers mistakenly use a moral theory to generate a moral system. We recognize that common morality does not provide unique answers to all moral questions, whereas the moral systems that are generated by moral theories are supposed to provide a unique answer to every moral problem. The moral system described by our moral theory simply provides a common framework for working through moral problems.

We believe that an adequate moral theory, especially an adequate description of the common moral system, is not only possible but that it is also important for doing applied and professional ethics. Moral theory should be firmly based on and tested by clear moral intuitions. Inasmuch as a description of morality is a central feature of a moral theory the accuracy of that description must be continually examined by seeing if it accords with considered moral judgments. Thus the theory remains strongly related to moral experience. It is the philosophical analysis of this database that leads to the explicit formulation of the moral system, which in turn gives guidance in circumstances that are not intuitively morally clear.

Moral theory should also give an account of the demarcation of the moral realm from the nonmoral realm; it should be able to distinguish a moral matter from a nonmoral matter. It should give an account of the scope of morality: why, whether, and how morality gets extended to nonrational beings. It should help in distinguishing morality from many of its look-alikes, such as philosophies of life, which can significantly mislead if they are viewed as moral systems. Moral theory should identify what situations give rise to moral concern as well as what aspects of those circumstances are morally relevant. Identifying the facts or features about a situation that are morally relevant is crucial. Failure to provide such a list of features (and defend it) is typical of all the standard moral theories. However, without a list of morally relevant features, a determination of the morality of an action or correctness of a moral judgment by appeal to the theory is impossible, since there would be no way to consistently determine if two cases are of the same kind.

Moral theory should be able to distinguish morally acceptable from morally unacceptable solutions in particular circumstances and to help in identifying relevant factors in deciding among the morally acceptable alternatives. Moral theory should explain why there is often more than one morally acceptable alternative and why equally informed impartial rational persons can sometimes disagree. Similarly, in irresolvable situations, the theory should make clear precisely why they are irresolvable and what it would take to arrive at a unique morally acceptable solution to the problem. Moral theory should be unifying in the sense not only of conceptually holding together in a single framework all the strands of emphasis which individually form the basis for one or another moral theory (consequentialism, deontology, rights theory, virtue theory), but also in showing what is necessary and sufficient in order for a violation of a moral rule to be justified. And finally, moral theory should give an account of morality's universality as well as its sensitivity to cultural, professional, and local practices.

In this book we provide a framework for making bioethical decisions. This framework includes an account of morality grounded in certain universal features of humankind. It also includes analyses of basic concepts, such as rationality, malady, competence, consent, confidentiality, paternalism, death, and euthanasia, which are explicated and integrated with the moral theory. This framework by no means provides a decision procedure for moral reasoning. It does not provide a conceptual machinery for churning out moral conclusions. Rather it guides one in determining what is and is not relevant in moral decision making; it shows the strengths and the limitations of moral theory; it shows where and why moral disagreements occur and why some cannot be resolved. We do not attempt to deal with the complete array of medical ethics problems; rather we provide a sound, rigorous, and adequate conceptual foundation for dealing with such problems.

The Nature of Morality: An Overview

Our account of morality is central to all that we do, and to the novice it can seem complicated. Therefore the point of the following overview is to present an easy introduction, a helpful gestalt. We want to assure readers that they already know most of what we are going to say and that we are only making this knowledge explicit and more precise. What follows is only a sketch of our view, accurate but not complete, and with only hints of arguments. Its purpose is to describe an overall framework within which to understand the details that will emerge, particularly in Chapters 2, 3, and 4.

On Demarcating Morality

Consider for a moment what you would do if you were just setting out to describe the phenomenon of morality. Where would you look? What phenomena would you describe? How would you know what was within the moral realm and what was outside it? That is, how would you distinguish the moral from the nonmoral (as opposed to the immoral)? What is it that marks something as distinctively within the realm of morality? Though commonly claimed by philosophers, it is not the language used, e.g., such words as "ought," "should," "bad," "good." (Only a small minority of the uses of these terms have anything to do with morality.) The point, almost universally overlooked, is that one must already know the essential features of morality (at least in some rough, preliminary way) before setting out to study the phenomenon of morality or else one would not know what in the world to focus upon.

This work of demarcation is an important first step for us. We argue that the existence of certain kinds of considerations, such as various rules, ideals, and procedures, constitutes the clearest indication of morality at work. The specific rules we take as a component of the core of morality are those usually categorized as "moral rules." They are such rules as "Don't deceive," "Don't cheat," "Don't kill," "Keep your promises," and so on. Of course, these rules are only part of what constitutes a system of morality, but they are absolutely crucial parts of the raw material of morality on which a philosopher of ethics must work. It is a philosopher's job to explicate, clarify, and organize these rules. More importantly, a philosopher must show how these rules fit within a system, so that conflicts between the rules can be resolved. As deeper understanding develops, some preanalytically selected rules may even be excluded because they fail to meet the developing body of criteria for a moral rule. These conceptual maneuvers, accomplishing the systematization, are dictated by the underlying rationales discovered as the philosopher analyzes these moral phenomena.

We do not claim that the moral rules (whose essential role is to proscribe certain actions which commonly cause harm) are all there is to morality, or even that they are the foundation for the rest of morality. Very significant also are the moral ideals, which are what many consider to be the heart of morality, because the moral ideals encourage people not just to avoid causing some harm, but instead to go out of their way to prevent or relieve harm to others. Morality is even more than rules and ideals. It also encompasses a list of the features of situations that are morally relevant and that must be used to describe situations which are to be subjected to moral reasoning and analysis. And, lastly, morality must have a procedure for dealing with rules as they conflict with each other and with ideals. We have been described as having a "rule-based" morality, but that is misleading. A more accurate characterization is that we regard morality as a public system. It is a complex system known to all to whom it applies and it has those four main components: moral rules, moral ideals, the morally relevant features of situations, and a detailed procedure for dealing with conflicts. Thus the system is not "rule based"; rather, rules are only one component of the system and can be properly understood only as functioning within that system.

Our demarcation of moral phenomena is a significant starting point for "doing ethics." It recognizes that morality is an ongoing human enterprise that long predates the attempts of any philosopher to understand it. It also means that the philosopher's systematic and explicit account of morality will be grounded in the ordinary practice of morality. This system of morality must not go against the firm and basic intuitions expressed in ordinary morality. In that sense, the philosopher "discovers" (or, perhaps, "uncovers") morality rather than invents it. It makes no sense to speak or think of "inventing" morality. Such a morality would have no purchase on human behavior, no authority, no basis in the experience of human purposes, interactions, and emotions. Morality is a phenomenon that has existed from the beginning of human history, a phenomenon that we must try to understand more thoroughly. Any result of reasoning that goes against basic moral intuitions throws great suspicion on that line of reasoning or on the theory that embodies it. Beginning, as we do, with the ordinary understanding and practice of morality, insures that our account of morality will ring true to the human experience of morality. There will be no problem of "principles" or "axioms" so abstract or so general that their application to real problems turns out to be nearly impossible.

As indicated above, ordinary moral rules and ideals are not one's only points of departure for understanding morality. There are other commonly accepted features of morality, such as that it is rational, beneficial, impartial, and applicable to all persons, all of the time, in all times and places. This is not to say that it is universally agreed that there is a universal code of behavior that answers all questions, but only that everyone who is not a moral skeptic believes that these features are essential characteristics of morality.

The system of morality must be a public system; that is part of the very meaning of morality. It is a public system in that it is known to all to whom it applies. It also applies to everyone impartially; to say that morality requires this or encourages that is to say that it requires this or encourages that for everyone in those same morally relevant circumstances. In being systematic, one dare not be content with the commonly employed *ceteris paribus* clauses ("all other things being equal"), which effectively hide the problem of having to determine precisely what those other things are that have to be equal. It is crucial that what counts as "the same morally relevant circumstances" be specified. Because humans do not and cannot have complete knowledge and because they are fallible and narrowly focused on their own concerns, they need a public system to guide them. In order to avoid bias, to gain perspective beyond their own self-serving interests, and to regularize their behavior in the face of inadequate knowledge about the present and the future, this public system must apply impartially to all. God does not need rules or a public system. He or She can foresee the total consequences of all actions (and thus could unerringly choose in every instance an action which has the best consequences, insofar as there are "best consequences," for all time) and would need no public system to avoid partiality, witting or unwitting.

The Content of Morality

An important conclusion, based on our systematic and explicit account of morality (referred to above) is that the purpose of morality is to minimize the amount of evil or harm suffered by those protected by morality. (We use "evil" and "harm" interchangeably.) Given the finitude of human beings, this requires a set of moral rules which, the more they are followed, the more the amount of evil or harm in the world will be reduced. The evils humans care about avoiding comprise a specifiable and finite list. These are harms that all rational persons want to avoid unless they have an adequate reason not to. Therefore a rational person has a strong self-interest in having others act in accord with the moral rules, namely, in order to avoid having harm caused to himself and those he cares about. These evils are death, pain, disability, loss of freedom, and loss of pleasure. They are not ranked in the same way by everyone. Although everyone agrees that some harms are worse than others, rationality does not require that any one kind of evil *always* be considered greater than some other kind of evil. This fact lies at the source of many moral disputes, in which the participants fail to understand that, although there will be some rational limit on what counts as an acceptable ranking, there is no objective ranking of the various harms to be avoided that will resolve all controversies.

Each general moral rule takes the form of a prohibition; each either proscribes the causing of one of the evils on that finite list of evils on which all rational persons would agree or proscribes kinds of actions that generally increase the amount of harm. Acting in accord with these moral rules is what is required by morality. Because they are in the form of prohibitions (don't kill, don't cheat, don't cause pain, and so on) anyone can follow them, all the time, toward everyone, equally (thus satisfying several key features of morality.) Meeting these basic requirements of morality does not usually involve great dedication, inner strength, outstanding character, or noble virtues; it simply involves abstaining from causing harm. Anyone can do it, although admittedly occasions often arise in which it is very tempting to act immorally.

As we have stressed, however, the moral rules are not all there is to morality. To be sure, obedience to the moral rules is required of everyone, but since the moral rules are basically proscribing specific actions, one could conceivably be perfectly moral by staying home in bed. However, the aspect of morality that most people generally associate with being moral, namely, going out of one's way for others to prevent or relieve harm, sacrificing for them, or running risks for them is what we call "following moral ideals." It is not simply not causing harms directly or indirectly but it is positively engaging in some action to prevent or relieve such harms. On our account these kinds of actions are an essential part of morality. The exhortations to prevent those very harms that the moral rules require us not to cause, we call "moral ideals."

There are crucial conceptual differences between moral rules and moral ideals. It is praiseworthy to follow moral ideals, whereas it is simply expected that everyone obey moral rules (indeed, in many cases, punishment seems appropriate if one violates a moral rule). The key difference is that morality requires that the moral rules be obeyed toward everyone, impartially, all the time. Clearly the moral rules can be obeyed toward everyone, impartially, all the time, but that is not true of the moral ideals. Even if one spent a significant part of one's life preventing evil, it would not be humanly possible to be doing it for everyone, impartially, all the time.

There is another perspective from which to grasp the orientation of our approach to morality. This begins with the fundamental realization that there is a finite core of evils that all rational persons would avoid unless they had an adequate reason not to. These harms (the deliberate nonavoidance of which constitutes the very meaning of irrational action—as discussed in Chapter 2) would naturally form the basis of a morality wherein not causing these harms to each other is required and helping each other avoid these harms is encouraged. It would be irrational not to agree with such a public policy.

Traditionally, philosophers sought "the greatest good," believing that once that was discovered, all the rest would fall neatly into place.

From the dawn of philosophy, the question concerning the summum bonum, or, what is the same thing, concerning the foundation of morality, has been accounted the main problem in speculative thought . . .[5]

Whatever action would bring about the greatest amount of that greatest good would be the moral act for that occasion. But there is no agreement on what that greatest good is; rationality requires that certain evils be avoided, but there is no universally agreed upon ranking of the evils, nor is there any agreed-upon ranking of the various goods. All rational persons would agree on what the goods are (freedom, pleasure, and abilities) insofar as they are the "opposites" of the evils. Further, no rational person would avoid these goods unless he or she had an adequate reason to do so. Nonetheless, gaining these goods is far less important than avoiding the evils, in the development of a moral system that rational persons advocate as a guide for the behavior of everyone. Consequently, the hard-core foundation of morality is what all rational persons can agree they would want to avoid (unless they had an adequate reason not to), namely those specifiable evils: death, pain, disability, loss of freedom, and loss of pleasure. Humans do not want to suffer such harms, so keeping others from causing them becomes the consensual core of morality (the moral rules) along with the exhortations actually to prevent or relieve those evils (the moral ideals).

It would be dangerous to urge everyone simply to "promote good," if that precept were believed to give moral authority for everyone to impose on others whatever he thinks is good. It would be giving license for universal paternalism. There is wisdom in the old expression "Don't do me any favors" as well as in the ancient medical imperative "Most importantly, do no harm." Common morality adopts the safer policy of urging others never to cause harms and, if and when possible, to prevent harms. The danger in adopting "Promote good" as a basic moral precept is that it gives moral justification for imposing one's own view of what is best on others. Of course, if no moral rules were violated in fulfilling that directive, promoting good would be morally acceptable, and often even praiseworthy. Moral rules prohibiting the causing of harms are not only a safer option, but also far more important; humans are far more certain of and concerned with what they want to avoid than with what they wish to gain. The world's great literature has often described in exquisite detail the tortures of hell, but very seldom the pleasures of heaven, for it is very easy to describe what all people want to avoid, but much harder to describe what they all want to have. Exhorting humans to prevent evils is morally preferable to encouraging them to promote goods; acting on moral ideals is not only morally praiseworthy, doing so often provides a justification for violating a moral rule.

Particular Moral Rules

The moral rules that individually proscribe causing each of the listed evils and that proscribe certain kinds of actions known to cause those harms we call "the general moral rules." These are considered general because they apply to all rational persons, at all times, and in all places. What might constitute pain, disability, loss of freedom or pleasure may differ in fine detail from one culture to another, but whatever the details, the causing of the basic harms to another person is always proscribed.

In order for these rules to be general, that is, applicable to all persons in all times and places, there can be no reference to anything that might not have existed in all times and places, such as cars, legislatures, marriage, alcohol, contracts, guns, and so on. Yet many moral rules in every culture are formed around these various objects, technologies, institutions, and practices that differ from one culture to another. Those moral rules, in effect, are proscribing the causing of the same list of harms that are proscribed by the general moral rules. If a culture has both deadly chemicals and streams of pure water, they will very likely have the "particular" moral rule, "Do not pollute the streams." If a culture has family units and an education of sorts available, there well might be a "particular" moral rule, "Do not deprive your children of an education." These rules are referred to as "particular" because they are formed by a relevant general moral rule in conjunction with a cultural behavior which might lead to the harm in question. In our examples, the general moral rule "Do not kill" was conjoined with the existence of chemicals and streams, and the general moral rule "Do not deprive of freedom" plus "Do your duty" was conjoined with the existence of family responsibilities and liberation provided by educational opportunities for children.

The general moral rules provide the universal strands that unify all the various formulations of particular moral rules throughout various cultures, times, and places. That is because the harms that are proscribed by the general moral rules are universally recognized as harms to be avoided. Thus, particular moral rules are formulated to discourage whatever idiosyncratic cultural institutions and practices are apt to perpetuate such harms.

Professional Ethics

One hears constantly of many "ethics": business ethics, medical ethics, environmental ethics, legal ethics, military ethics, administrative ethics, and many more. Are these all different? Are they each making up their own ethics? Are they each distinctive? It would certainly make a multi-ring circus of ethics if they were. Ethics would be without form or content and refer only to rules of behavior which could totally differ from one realm of activity to another. That view would be contrary to our sense of ethics as well as contrary to our empirical knowledge of these various specialty ethics.

Our view of professional ethics is roughly analogous to our account of particular moral rules. In the case of medicine, for example, professional ethics would be the general moral system in combination with the various institutions, practices, and relationships indigenous to the "culture" of medicine. Interacting with the structures of medical practice, "Do not deprive of freedom" would yield the moral requirement "Obtain valid consent." Similarly "Do not cause pain or suffering" would lead to the particular medical moral rule "Do not breach confidentiality."

Thus professional ethics should not be seen as a unique and distinctive enterprise nor even as a different kind of ethics. Ethics is one basic and universal moral system which can take different forms in different contexts, but only in order to accomplish the same purposes. The circumstances, the concepts, the relationships, the actions, and the goals of a practice, profession, or enterprise certainly differ from each other. Nevertheless, the basic moral system will be expressed in the terms of that activity so as to avoid causing those harms acknowledged as such by all rational persons.

Professional ethics has an additional and significant aspect by our account.

One of the basic moral rules is "Do your duty," so that what constitutes one's duty in a particular profession is crucial to the ethics of that profession. The determinants of that duty are considered in Chapter 3, where we discuss professional ethics more extensively.

A Preview of the Book

Our intention is to provide the moral framework and the conceptual tools that are sufficient to allow those with adequate knowledge of the relevant biomedical practices and of the facts of particular cases to determine the morally acceptable alternatives open to them. We present our view of the moral enterprise (including the need for theory), a description of morality, an account of key concepts integrally related to morality and to moral matters within medicine, and proposed solutions to some of medicine's central ethical issues (as illustrative of a theory at work).

Chapters 2, 3, and 4 focus on moral theory as such. Chapter 2 describes our account of the moral system as it works in its complex ways. As grammar underlies ordinary speaking, whether the speakers know it or not, so the moral system underlies ordinary moral deliberations, whether the deliberaters know it or not. Our mission is to describe that moral system. As part of the moral system, Chapter 2 describes moral rules, moral ideals, morally relevant features, and a procedure for handling moral conflicts. It also discusses such related matters as the scope of morality and why there are unresolvable moral disputes. Additionally, it shows that it is moral theory that comprises the justification of the moral system. Thus Chapter 2 provides the theoretical framework for our analysis and our application of basic concepts.

Chapter 3 demonstrates how morality is manifested in many areas of life, consistent with our account of morality. In different societies and professions the same morality is found, though changed in a systematic and predictable way. We explore the system underlying those different faces of morality, showing that they are variations of one morality. We pay particular attention to the relationship of professional ethics to ordinary morality. The concept of duty is developed: its grounding in roles and relationships, its relation to professions, and its moral significance.

In Chapter 4, in order to sharpen the distinctiveness and adequacy of our approach, we contrast it with the most popular "theory" being used in bioethics. We coined the term "principlism" to describe that approach because it appeals to certain "principles" such as those of beneficence, nonmaleficence, autonomy, and justice.[6] Principlism's popularity and familiarity make it a convenient vehicle through which to make crucial points concerning moral theory. It is instructive to see in what way principlism is flawed; it enables us to highlight important features necessary for an adequate account of morality.

The first three chapters constitute our account of morality and chapter 4 presents the major alternative, while the remaining chapters present a mixture of concepts and approaches to problem solving. These concepts are ones we regard as fundamental for dealing with the moral problems of biomedicine. Chapter 5 presents our concept of "malady," which is an explication of the common concept of disease. However, malady is broader and more systematic, though it builds on and does not distort the ordinary concept of disease. Chapter 6 deals with competence, its task-specific nature, and its relationship to rationality, irrationality, and the emotions. The importance of a thorough analysis of competence becomes clear in Chapter 7, wherein we discuss in detail the elements of consent. For example, we explore the effects of how the risks are thought about (relative risks versus absolute risks) and told about (the effects of framing). Chapter 8 presents an analysis of confidentiality, exploring its relationship to privacy and emphasizing the role of consent and duty in relation to confidentiality.

Chapters 9 and 10 analyze paternalism and its justification. Paternalism, in our view, is a rich, crucial, and helpful concept. As a syndrome label assists in pulling together what were previously thought to be disparate signs and symptoms, thereby enabling them to be seen as an organized, identifiable process, so the concept of paternalism leads one to see many facets of the doctor-patient relationship in a kind of paradigmatic way. Drawing in issues of consent, competence, self-determination, and duty, the concept of paternalism helps one focus on the real moral issues involved. Having narrowed in on the fundamental moral issues, one knows more precisely what actions need to be morally justified. Paternalistic behavior always needs to be justified, because it always involves violating a moral rule. Because we regard the procedure for justifying a violation of a moral rule to be essential in moral reasoning, we discuss that procedure in detail in the context of paternalistic behavior. That also provides the occasion for us to contrast how the utilitarians, casuists, and virtue theorists would deal with this "essential in moral reasoning" and how they fall short on such a fundamental moral maneuver.

Chapter 11 deals with the definition of death, and, in light of some new considerations, arrives at a more basic and encompassing definition than what we and others have previously offered. It enables us to reach a reconciliation with certain other accounts of death. Chapter 12 discusses euthanasia. Like our analyses of the other concepts, it utilizes many of the insights, maneuvers, and distinctions that are embedded in our account of morality. We focus on the moral relevance of the various means of "helping to die," and of withdrawing food and fluids in particular. We also stress the important difference between patient refusals and patient requests: the former generally must be obeyed, but not the latter.

Our aim is to demonstrate the unity, adequacy, and necessity of theory for understanding and resolving some of the moral problems of biomedicine. The concepts, the maneuvers, the distinctions, and the exceptions should all be consistent with and unified through theory. The fact that equally informed, impartial, and rational persons often disagree also must be accounted for by moral theory. Theory, in other words, should give a unified account of all the bits and pieces of moral experience. We realize that such claims about theory are controversial, but our intention in this book is to make good on those very claims.

Although it is clear that we take moral theory seriously, this does not conflict with the seriousness with which we take common morality. Nor does it conflict with our belief in the natural ability of human beings to deliberate insightfully and successfully about moral problems. On the contrary, our moral theory rests upon these foundations. We intend this book to encourage people to have more trust in their basic moral intuitions. It is ironic that it can be so difficult to supply the grounds for that encouragement. As we said, moral theory needs to be complex to account for the complexity of morality, but morality need not be any more difficult than speaking and understanding one's native language. Complexity is not the same as difficulty.

Notes

1. There are many examples of the anthology method. Most do not even seem aware that they are offering several theories and leaving the reader in a quandary over what to make of such a variety. Even one of the most self-aware books in this regard nevertheless concludes that all we can do is look for insights from each of the various theories, but the book provides no clues as to which insight to apply when, nor which insight outweighs which. In Chapter 3 of that book, *Health Care Ethics Committees,* by Judith Wilson Roth, John W. Glaser, Dorothy Rasinski-Gregory, Joan McIver, Corrine Bayley (Chicago: American Hospital Publishing Company, 1993), "Ethics for Committees: Understanding Ethics and Methodology," at least raises the question of how one is to choose among the many favorite theories—feminist ethics, care ethics, clinical ethics, narrative ethics, casuistry, and virtue ethics. She suggests, in addition to using some insights from each, that we focus on reasons for making one choice rather than another (p. 18). Of course, this suggested method is also completely eclectic, since what constitutes a "good reason" will depend on the particular theory chosen. It is still "pick and choose" without any clues as to which and why.

2. S. G. Clarke and Evan Simpson, *Anti-Theory in Ethics and Moral Conservatism,* (Albany: SUNY Press, 1989).

3. For example, Arthur Caplan, *If I Were a Rich Man, Could I Buy a Pancreas?* (Bloomington: Indiana University Press, 1992), pp. xii–xvii.

4. We have in mind the many articles, usually in medical journals and usually dealing with practical moral problems, that all too often give a passing, obligatory nod to a phrase of a moral theory which the authors seem to believe justifies whatever conclusions they have reached. The phrase might simply be "the justice principle"—not stating it nor arguing for it, but simply mentioning it as though its name alone furnished sufficient backing for the authors' position. Often it is the "autonomy principle" that is named as the "theory" that proves the author's conclusion. Sometimes it is slightly more elabo-

rate, e.g., "the greatest good for the greatest number," or "Always treat a human being as an end in himself and never as a means." At best, these are overly simplistic slogans, but they are frequently presented by authors as a sophisticated theoretical validation of the points they are making.

5. John Stuart Mill, *Utilitarianism,* first paragraph.

6. See K. Danner Clouser and Bernard Gert, "A Critique of Principlism," *The Journal of Medicine and Philosophy,* 15 (1990), pp. 219–236.

2

Morality

We are aware that many people believe there is no substantial agreement on moral matters. We are also aware that there is even less agreement on the adequacy of any account of morality. We believe that these views are due to the understandable, but mistaken, concentration on such controversial moral issues as abortion and euthanasia, without realizing that such controversial matters form only a very small part of those matters on which people make moral decisions and judgments. Indeed, most moral matters are so uncontroversial that people do not even make any conscious decision concerning them. The uncontroversial nature of these matters is shown by almost everyone's lack of hesitancy in making negative moral judgments about those who decide to harm others simply because they do not like them. It is shown by the same lack of hesitancy in making moral judgments condemning unjustified deception, breaking of promises, cheating, disobeying the law, and not doing one's duty.

We believe that an explicit, clear, and comprehensive account of morality helps to make clear the uncontroversial nature of many medical decisions. We also believe that such an account helps in understanding some of the controversial moral problems that arise in the practice of medicine. Our account provides a common framework on which all of the disputing parties can agree, thus making clear what is responsible for the disagreements, and what might be done to manage that disagreement. It is intended to be an account of the moral system that is already implicitly used by people when dealing with everyday moral problems. We want to make the moral system explicit so it can be used by people when they are confronted with new, difficult, or controversial moral decisions[1]

Those who deny the possibility of a comprehensive account of morality may in actuality be denying that any systematic account of morality provides an answer to every moral problem. We acknowledge that the common moral system does not provide a unique solution to every moral problem. Readers should not expect that every moral problem will have a single best solution, one that all fully informed, impartial, rational persons will prefer to every other solution. In many cases, however, common morality does provide a unique answer. Although most of these cases are not interesting, in a very few situations an explicit account of morality does settle what initially seemed to be a controversial matter, for example, some aspects of euthanasia. Most controversial cases do not have a unique answer, but even in these cases morality is often quite useful. It places significant limits on legitimate moral disagreement; that is, it always provides a method for distinguishing between morally acceptable answers and morally unacceptable answers. That there is not always agreement on the best solution does not mean that there is not agreement on the boundaries of what is morally acceptable.

Most people, including most physicians and philosophers, tend to be interested more in what is controversial than in what is uncontroversial. It is routine to start with a very prominent example of unresolvable moral disagreement, such as abortion, and then treat it as if it were typical of the kinds of issues on which one must make moral judgments. The fact that moral disagreement on some issues is compatible with complete agreement on many other issues seems to be almost universally overlooked. Many philosophers seem to hold that if equally informed impartial rational persons can disagree on some moral matters, they can disagree on all of them. Thus many philosophers hold either that there is no unique right answer to any moral question or that there is a unique right answer to every moral question. The unexciting, but correct, view is that some moral questions have unique right answers and some do not. Our view is that the matters on which there is moral agreement far outnumber the matters on which there is moral disagreement, although the areas of moral disagreement are more interesting to discuss.

Common Morality

The existence of a common morality is shown by the widespread agreement on most moral matters. Everyone agrees that such actions as killing, causing pain or disability, and depriving of freedom or pleasure are immoral unless one has an adequate justification for doing them. Similarly, everyone agrees that deceiving, breaking a promise, cheating, breaking the law, and neglecting one's duties also need justification in order not to be immoral.[2] No one has any real doubts about this. People do disagree about the scope of morality, for example, whether animals or embryos are protected by morality; however, everyone agrees that moral agents—those whose actions are themselves subject to moral judgment—are protected. Thus doubt about whether killing animals or embryos needs to be justified does not lead to any doubt that killing moral agents needs justification. Similarly, people disagree about what counts as an adequate moral justification for some particular act of killing or deceiving and on some features of an adequate justification, but everyone agrees that what counts as an adequate justification for one person must be an adequate justification for anyone else in the same situation, that is, when all of the morally relevant features of the two situations are the same. This is part of what is meant by saying that morality requires impartiality.

Everyone also agrees that people, for example the severely retarded, should not be subject to moral judgment if they do not comprehend the nature of the general kinds of behavior morality prohibits (such as deceiving), requires (such as keeping one's promise), encourages (relieving someone's pain), and allows (going to a movie). Although it is difficult even for philosophers to provide an explicit, clear, and comprehensive account of morality, most cases are clear enough that everyone knows whether some particular act is morally acceptable. No one engages in a moral discussion of questions like "Is it morally acceptable to deceive patients in order to get them to participate in an experimental treatment that has no hope of benefiting them but that one happens to be curious about?" because everyone knows that such deception is not justified. The prevalence of hypocrisy shows that people do not always behave in the way that morality requires or encourages. It also shows that people know the general kind of behavior that morality does require and encourage even if they sometimes have difficulty applying this knowledge to particular cases, especially those in which they are emotionally involved. That everyone who is subject to moral judgment knows what morality prohibits, requires, encourages, and allows is part of what is meant by saying that morality is a public system.

Morality as a Public System

A public system is a system that has the following two characteristics: (1) All persons to whom it applies (those whose behavior is to be guided and judged by that system) understand it (they know what behavior the system prohibits, requires, encourages, and allows). (2) It is not irrational for any of these persons to accept being guided and judged by that system. The clearest example of a public system is a game. A game has an inherent goal and a set of rules that form a system that is understood by all of the players, and it is not irrational for all players to use the goal and the rules of the game to guide their own behavior and to judge the behavior of other players by them. Although a game is a public system, it applies only to those playing the game. Morality is a public system that applies to all moral agents; all people are subject to morality simply by virtue of being rational persons who are responsible for their actions. This may explain Kant's claim that the demands of morality are categorical, not hypothetical.

In order for all rational persons to know what morality requires, prohibits, allows, and encourages, such knowledge of morality cannot involve beliefs that are not held by all rational persons. Only facts that are known to all moral agents can be necessary for knowing what morality requires. Thus no facts discovered by modern science are necessary, for none of these facts are known by all moral agents. The same is true of any religious belief, for no particular religious belief is held by all rational persons. Only those beliefs which it would be irrational for any moral agent to doubt, are essential for knowledge of morality. We call such beliefs *rationally required* beliefs. Beliefs that it would be irrational for any moral agent not to doubt, we call *rationally prohibited* beliefs. Beliefs which are neither rationally required nor rationally prohibited, we call *rationally allowed* beliefs.

Rationally required beliefs include general factual beliefs such as: people are mortal, can suffer pain, can be disabled, and can be deprived of freedom or pleasure, and that people are fallible. Having these beliefs is necessary in order to be a moral agent. On the other hand, not all moral agents share the same scientific and religious beliefs, so that *rationally allowed* beliefs such as scientific or religious beliefs cannot be necessary to be a moral agent; however, such beliefs may be necessary for making particular moral decisions or judgments. Some rationally allowed beliefs, for instance beliefs about the facts of the particular case, are often necessary for making particular moral decisions or moral judgments. In addition to the rationally required *general* beliefs, there are rationally required *personal* beliefs. These are beliefs that all moral agents have about themselves, such as beliefs that they themselves can be killed and suffer pain, and so on. These differ from the rationally allowed general beliefs only in that they are about a particular person not known to all.[3] All personal beliefs about one's race, gender, religion, abilities, and so on are excluded as part of what is required for knowledge of morality, because not all moral agents share these same beliefs about themselves.

Although morality is a public system that is known by all those who are held responsible for their actions, it is not a simple system. A useful analogy is the grammatical system used by all competent speakers of a language. Almost no competent speaker can explicitly describe this system, yet they all know it in the sense that they use it when speaking and in interpreting the speech of others. If presented with an explicit account of the grammatical system, competent speakers have the final word on its accuracy. It would be a mistake to accept any description of a grammatical system that rules out speaking in a way that they know is commonly regarded as acceptable or allows speaking in a way that they know is commonly regarded as completely unacceptable.

A *moral theory* is an attempt to make explicit, explain, and, if possible, justify morality. By morality we mean the *moral system* that people use, not necessarily consciously, in deciding how to act when confronting moral problems and in making their moral judgments. An adequate moral theory must present an account of morality that uses concepts or principles that are understood by everyone who is subject to moral judgment.[4] Although we realize that most moral decisions are not made by explicitly employing any account of morality, we hope that the account of morality that we present will accomplish three tasks: (1) reassure health care professionals who have made correct decisions, but who still feel uneasy because they cannot make their moral reasoning explicit; (2) provide a framework that can be used for understanding disputes among health care professionals or between health care professionals and patients, making clear why there may be no unique best solution; and (3) provide a framework for explicitly dealing with those rare cases in which health care professionals do not know what to do.

We also hope it will be used to teach those entering the health care professions that the moral framework that is used in medicine is the same moral framework that they have always used. Although doctors, nurses, and other health care professionals have specific duties that cannot be deduced from common morality, these duties cannot be incompatible with it either. The difficult moral problems that health care professionals commonly face require knowledge of both common morality and of the specific duties and ideals of medicine. These specific duties and ideals may sometimes seem to conflict with the requirements of common morality, but a proper understanding of both will show that the moral system provides a method for dealing with those conflicts in the same way that it deals with conflicts within common morality.

Mistaken Accounts of Morality

Most moral theories, like those of Kant and Mill, no matter how complex they are themselves, unfortunately present an incomplete account of morality.[5] Indeed, many philosophers seem to regard their moral theories as generating a new and improved morality, rather than as describing and justifying common morality. Some philosophers seem to value simplicity more than agreement with commonly accepted moral judgments. This may be because normally they do not use the systems generated by their theories to help resolve specific moral problems, although almost all of them hold that every moral problem has a unique right answer. These philosophers seem as if they would rather put forward theories which lead to obviously counterintuitive moral judgments than to make their theories complex enough to account for many of the actual agreed-upon moral judgments.

In reaction to this oversimplification of morality, many in applied ethics, particularly medical ethics, claim to be against moral theory. They quite rightly regard these overly simple theories as worse than useless. Unfortunately, they seem to accept the false claim that an ethical theory must be simple. One of the legitimate attractions of principlism (see Chapter 4) is that it correctly denies that there is a unique solution to every moral problem. Unfortunately, principlism also accepts the false view that there cannot be a single unified moral system which provides a framework for dealing with all moral problems. The antitheory view sometimes leads those in bioethics to accept the incorrect and damaging view that all moral reasoning is ad hoc or completely relative to the situation. Casuistry is often taken as if it were against theory and did not presuppose a common moral system for which casuistry was a method of interpretation and application.

Careful reflection on what is normally considered to be morality makes it clear that morality is best conceived as a guide to behavior that rational persons put forward to govern the behavior of others, whether or not they plan to follow that guide themselves. Many philosophical accounts of morality, however, present morality as if it were primarily a personal matter. The dominant philosophical view of morality now, and perhaps as far back as Socrates, seems to be that morality is primarily intended to provide a guide for the individual person who adopts it.[6] In order to reconcile this personal-guide view of morality with the acknowledged view that morality applies to everyone, many philosophers have tried to show that all rational persons would adopt the guide to conduct that they were proposing.

Regarding morality as providing a personal guide also results in a far wider account of morality than is appropriate, as if any judgment about how a person ought to act (that he ought to brush his teeth, for example) is part of a moral guide. Morality is about how one ought to act, but that is not a definition of morality; rather it is a claim that morality is primarily about actions. It corrects another widespread but mistaken philosophical view that morality is primarily about what is the best state of affairs. From the moral point of view, the only reason for wanting to know what is the best state of affairs is because it may have some bearing on what actions ought to be done. Sometimes, of course, it will not have any bearing on this, as that state of affairs cannot be brought about. The reason why it is dangerous to view morality as being concerned with the best state of affairs is that often what is regarded as the best state of affairs can be brought about only in a morally unacceptable way, such as deceiving patients in order to get them to consent to a beneficial treatment. Of course, whether or not one' s behavior counts as morally unacceptable will sometimes be determined by the end to be achieved; saving a patient's life, for instance, may justify deception. We discuss these kinds of problems in more detail later, for example in the chapters on paternalism and its justification.

Morality as an Informal Public System

Although morality always distinguishes between the set of morally acceptable answers and those that are morally unacceptable, it does not provide a unique answer to every question. One of the tasks of a moral theory is to explain why, sometimes, even when there is complete agreement on the facts, genuine moral disagreement cannot be eliminated, but the theory must also explain why all moral disagreement has legitimate limits. It is very easy, as noted above, to overlook that unresolvable moral disagreement on some important issues, like abortion, is compatible with total agreement in the overwhelming number of cases in which moral judgments are made. This agreement is based on agreement about the nature of morality, that it is a public system with the goal of reducing the amount of harm suffered by those protected by it. Everyone agrees that morality prohibits some kinds of actions (such as killing and breaking promises), and encourages certain kinds of actions (such as relieving pain). But it is acknowledged that a prohibited kind of action is sometimes morally justified even when it does not conflict with another prohibition, such as when it conflicts with what is morally encouraged. Breaking a trivial promise in order to aid an injured person is regarded by all as morally acceptable.

Sometimes, however, people disagree about whether a particular act counts as a prohibited kind of action like killing or deceiving.[7] People sometimes disagree on when not feeding counts as killing, or when not telling counts as deceiving. Although these disagreements in interpretation are occasionally unresolvable, once it is agreed that an action is of a certain prohibited kind (such as killing or deceiving), all impartial rational persons agree that it needs moral justification. Further, everyone agrees that intentionally killing or deceiving needs moral justification. Similarly, everyone agrees that actions of a certain kind (for instance relieving pain and suffering) should be encouraged unless they involve a prohibited kind of action. The prohibitions of the former kinds of actions we call moral rules; the encouragement of the latter kind we call moral ideals. They are part of the common moral system.

The most divisive and significant kind of moral disagreement concerns the scope of morality, that is, who should be included in the group toward which morality requires impartial treatment. This unresolvable disagreement about who is impartially protected by morality leads to the great controversies concerning abortion and the treatment of animals. Some maintain that morality is only, or primarily, concerned with the suffering of harm by moral agents, while others maintain that the death and pain of those who are not moral agents is as important, or almost as important, as the harms suffered by moral agents.[8] All agree that morality prohibits killing moral agents, but there is disagreement about whether it also prohibits killing fetuses and at least the higher animals such as primates and dolphins. However, even if fetuses and animals are not included in the group impartially protected by morality, they might still have some protection. Killing them or causing them pain might require some justification, even if does not require as strong a justification as killing or causing pain to moral agents.

Another source of unresolvable disagreement in moral judgment is due to differences in the rankings of harms, including differences in how one ranks probabilities of harms. Disagreement on the proper speed limit is a disagreement on whether the certain deprivation of some freedom to millions, namely, the freedom to drive between 55 and 70 miles an hour, is justified by the probability that some lives will be saved. Indeed, many political disagreements seem to be about this kind of difference in rankings and can be regarded as a conflict between freedom and welfare (for example, disagreement over how strict pollution regulations should be). However, the difference in rankings can also be between death and pain, which is one important issue involved in the euthanasia debate. The presence of these kinds of unresolvable moral disagreements must be reflected in an adequate account of morality.

Although morality is a public system, one which all rational persons know and understand, and which it is not irrational for any of them to follow, we have now shown that this does not mean that there are no unresolvable moral disagreements. Morality is an informal public system, a system that has no authoritative judges or procedures for determining the correct answer. A formal system such as law, or a formal public system, such as a game of a professional sport, does have ways of arriving at a unique correct answer within that system.[9] But most games, including sports, are informal public systems. When people get together to play a game of cards, or backyard basketball, they are involved in an informal public system. For the game even to get started, there must be overwhelming agreement on most aspects of the game, but disagreements can arise which have no agreed upon way to be resolved. These unresolvable disagreements either are resolved in an ad hoc fashion (such as flipping a coin or asking a passerby) or are not resolved at all, in which case the game may be disbanded.

Morality, like all informal public systems, presupposes overwhelming agreement on most matters that are likely to arise. However, like all informal public systems, it has no established procedures or authorities that can resolve every moral disagreement. There is no equivalent in morality to the United States Supreme Court in deciding legal disputes, or the pope in deciding some religious matters for Roman Catholics. When there is no unique right answer within morality and a decision has to be made, the decision is often made in an ad hoc fashion; people may ask a friend for advice. If the moral disagreement is on some important social issue like abortion, the problem is transferred from the moral system to the political or legal system. Abortion is an unresolvable moral question; since it has to be decided whether or not abortions are to be allowed and in what circumstances, the question is transferred to the legal and political system. They resolve the question on a practical level, but they do not resolve the moral question, as is shown by the continuing intense moral debate on the matter.

Failure to appreciate that morality is an informal public system has caused considerable confusion when talking about public policies, not only with regard to health care, but also in many other areas. It is assumed that if morality does not directly provide a solution to the problem, it can always provide an indirect solution by means of an appropriate voting procedure. It is sometime mistakenly said that a just solution, that is, a morally acceptable solution, is one that is arrived at by a democratic voting procedure. The justness or moral acceptability of a solution to a problem cannot be determined by any voting procedure, for a majority can vote to unjustifiably deprive members of a minority group of some freedom. The moral acceptability of a solution is determined by the moral system; all that the voting procedure determines is which solution will be adopted. This democratic voting procedure may be the morally best way to determine which solution will be adopted, but it does not *make* that solution either morally acceptable or the morally best solution.

Justice

Justice has become a very important topic in medicine, partly because of the realization that the necessity for changing the allocation of health care has, and will have, a dramatic effect on the practice of medicine. Everyone agrees that the present allocation of health care in the United States is not just, but there is considerable disagreement on what is necessary to make it just. In this section we shall talk about justice only with regard to the actions of government. A government that acts in a morally acceptable way, acts justly. But what is required for a government to act in a morally acceptable way? A full answer to this question would require a whole book in political theory; we shall not try to provide even an outline of an answer. We think, however, that showing the relationship between our account of morality and some issues of justice in health care may help achieve a better understanding of these issues. The recognition that morality is an informal public system suggests the most important point; it is extremely unlikely that there is a unique right answer to how the government should act with regard to the allocation of health care. There is so much disagreement on the factual matters, that it may almost be secondary to point out that there is also disagreement in the ranking of the harms and benefits involved, as well as significant ideological disagreements about human nature.

Since we have no special expertise with regard to the economic and political facts, and do not wish to enter into any ideological disputes about human nature, we shall limit our discussion to what we take to be fairly uncontroversial points. One of the primary responsibilities, if not the primary responsibility, of government is to lessen the amount of harm suffered by its citizens. Diseases, injuries, and so on, all of which we classify as maladies (see Chapter 5), are among the primary sources of harm. Thus it is one of the duties of government to lessen the harm caused by maladies. Other things being equal, it would be far better to prevent maladies than to treat them once they have occurred, for prevention will result in far less harm being suffered. Thus if the costs are equal, it is far better to engage in preventive medicine, primarily public health measures, than to spend the same amount of money to cure or treat maladies after they occur.[10] If it costs less to prevent a specified number of maladies than to cure a smaller number of those same maladies, it becomes clearly irrational for any impartial person not to prefer prevention. Thus, spending a given amount of money to cure a specified number of maladies when that same amount could be used to prevent a far great number of equally serious maladies, is clearly unjust.

The previous paragraph assumes that the government is spending some money to prevent the harms caused by maladies. We think it is appropriate for it to do so, but there may be some controversy on this matter. Any money the government spends it must collect from its citizens. Some may want to claim that taking money from its citizens deprives them of freedom and that this loss of freedom is so significant that preventing the harms caused by maladies does not justify causing this massive loss of freedom. We do not think many would agree with this ranking; indeed, when considering some public health measures, for example vaccinations for children, we know of no one who accepts it. However, we accept that after a certain amount of money is spent on health care, including public health, it is appropriate to question whether more ought to be spent. And there are also questions, without uniquely correct moral answers, about how much ought to be spent on health care compared to education, public defense, the criminal justice system, and so on.

Assuming a fixed amount of government spending on health care, what would count as a morally acceptable way of spending that money, that is, what would count as a just health care delivery system? A formal, but not very useful answer to that question is whatever system a fully informed impartial rational person could advocate adopting. What kind of system could such a person advocate adopting? The answer to this is somewhat more informative; any system which such a person could regard as resulting in the least amount of harm being suffered due to maladies. If no fully informed person could regard a particular health care delivery system as resulting in the least amount of harm being suffered, then such a system cannot be regarded as just. The present health care delivery system is not regarded by anyone as resulting in the least amount of harm being suffered, which explains why no one regards the present health care delivery system as just.

Note that this account of a just health care delivery system says nothing about equality, nor about providing the most aid to those who are worst off. This is not because equality and aiding the worst off are irrelevant, rather it is because insofar as they are relevant they are included within the more encompassing goal of lessening the amount of harm suffered. Unlike the utilitarian account of justice, which has a goal of increasing the amount of net benefits and so would allow massive inequality, the moral goal of lessening the amount of harm suffered sets strict limits on inequality. It also necessarily results in great concern for those who are worst off, for they are suffering greater harm than others, and so relieving their suffering will almost always be included in the overarching goal of lessening harm. The goal of justice does not, however, require that the government spend a given amount of money in order to aid 1,000 who are worst off, if that same amount of money will prevent more harm for 100,000 who are not as badly off. It is not required that the government spend a given amount of money on treating 1,000 children with a serious genetic malady rather than spending that same amount on preventing 100,000 children from suffering some lesser malady. It is also not required that they not spend the money on the 1,000 who are worst off, for impartial rational persons can disagree on which alternative most lessens the amount of harm suffered. But keeping the cost the same, if the number of the worst off gets smaller and the number who can be prevented from suffering some lesser disease gets greater, it is quite likely that a point will be reached where it will be unjust to spend that amount of money on the worst off.

Since a government that acts in a morally acceptable way acts justly, and since there is usually more than one morally acceptable way for a government to act, it is very likely that there will not a unique right answer to the question of how health care should be allocated. Even if there is agreement that the goal of health care allocation is to minimize the amount of harm suffered due to maladies, there will be unresolvable disagreement about what counts as the lesser amount of harm suffered. Some may claim that what is most important is minimizing the suffering of the worst off, those suffering great harm, whereas others may maintain that it is irrelevant whose suffering is minimized, as long as the total amount of harm suffered is minimized. Since there is no agreed upon way to weigh and balance different evils, there is no way to resolve any plausible disagreement. Further, even if there were agreement on a more specific goal, there would still be disagreement about the best way to achieve that goal, for example, can the government, and if so how best can it, regulate and constrain medical practice to achieve that goal. But, even with all of this disagreement, there is universal agreement that the present allocation of health care is not just.[11]

Rationality and Morality

To justify morality is to show that morality is the kind of public system that all rational persons would favor as a guide for everyone to follow. Everyone admits that if a certain way of acting has been shown to be irrational, that is, not even rationally allowed, no one ought to act in that way. But just because an action is rationally allowed does not mean that everyone agrees that one ought to act in that way. On the contrary, it is often rationally allowed, that is, not irrational, to act immorally. That an action is rationally allowed does not entail that one ought to act that way. However, everyone agrees that no one ever ought to act irrationally. An adequate moral theory must provide an account of rationality that explains why it has this kind of force.[12]

Although everyone agrees that they ought never act irrationally, people often do act irrationally. Acting on one's emotions is usually acting rationally, but people sometimes act on their emotions without considering that their actions will have harmful consequences. Sometimes even when they do consider these consequences, their emotions impel them to act irrationally. People who have a mental disorder, a phobia for instance, often act irrationally. But regardless of how they actually act, people acknowledge that they should not act irrationally. An adequate account of rationality must be such that it explains why, even though people do sometimes act irrationally, no one thinks that he ought to act irrationally.

Rationality is very intimately related to harms and benefits. Everyone agrees that unless one has an adequate reason for doing so, it would be irrational to avoid any benefit or not to avoid any harm for oneself or for those for whom one cares. Our account of rationality, although it accurately describes the way in which the concept of rationality is ordinarily used, differs radically from the accounts normally provided by philosophers in two important ways. First, it makes irrationality rather than rationality the basic concept; second, it defines irrationality by means of a list rather than a formula. The basic definition is as follows: *To act irrationally is to act in a way that one knows (justifiably believes), or should know, will significantly increase the probability that oneself, or those one cares for, will suffer death, pain, disability, loss of freedom or loss of pleasure; and one does not have an adequate reason for so acting.*[13] Any intentional action that is not irrational is rational.

The close relationship between irrationality and harm is made explicit by this definition, for this list also defines what counts as a basic harm or an evil.

Everything that anyone counts as a harm or an evil—thwarted desires, maladies, punishments—necessarily involves at least a significant increase in the probability of death, pain, disability, loss of freedom, or loss of pleasure. However, complete agreement on what are the basic harms is compatible with considerable disagreement on the ranking of these harms. Especially since all of the harms except death have degrees, and even death occurs at very different ages, there can be no agreement that any one of these harms is always worse than the others. Some people rank dying several months earlier as worse than a specified amount of pain and suffering while other people rank that same amount of pain and suffering as worse. Thus, it is rationally allowed for most terminally ill patients either to refuse death-delaying treatments or to consent to them.

Our experience on ethics committees is that most moral disagreements (such as whether to treat an incompetent patient) are based on disagreements on the facts of the case (such as on how painful the treatment will be and how long it will relieve the painful symptoms of the patient's disease). Differences in the rankings of the harms accounts for most of the remaining disagreements, for example, how much pain and suffering is it worth to prevent a patient from dying? Often the factual disagreements about prognoses are so closely combined with different rankings of the harms involved that they cannot be disentangled. Further complicating the matter, the probability of suffering any of the harms can vary from insignificant to almost certain, and people can differ in the way that they rank a given probability of one harm against a different probability of another harm.

Involuntary commitment of people with mental disorders that make them dangerous to themselves often involves two kinds of disagreement. The first is a disagreement about what percent of these people would commit suicide if not committed. The second is a disagreement about whether a certain probability (for example a 5% risk of death within one week for one person) compensates for the certainty of three to five days of a very serious loss of freedom and a significant probability of long-term mental suffering, secondary to that loss of freedom (for example a 30% risk for twenty persons). Actual cases usually involve much more uncertainty about outcomes as well as the rankings of more harms. (Chapter 10, "Justification of Paternalism," discusses these issues in more detail.) Considerable disagreement on what counts as the lesser evil or greater harm in any particular case is compatible with complete agreement on what counts as a harm or evil.

A decision that involves an increase in the probability of oneself suffering some harm will be irrational unless one has an adequate reason for that decision. Thus, not only what counts as a reason, but also what makes a reason adequate must be clarified. We realize that in its normal use, "a reason" refers both to (1) a conscious rational belief that can make an otherwise irrational action rational, and to (2) a conscious belief that explains one's actions, whether the belief is rational or not. We do not use "a reason" to refer to (2); that is what we call a motive. We use "a reason" to refer only to (1). Although most beliefs that are reasons are also motives for most people, some reasons, such as a belief that those unknown to one will benefit from one's action, may never serve as a motive for some people. But this belief is a reason for everyone in an appropriate situation, whether or not it serves as a motive for them.

A reason is a conscious rational belief that one's action will help anyone, not merely oneself or those one cares about, avoid one of the harms, or gain some good, namely, ability, freedom, or pleasure, and this belief is not seen to be inconsistent with one's other beliefs by almost everyone with similar knowledge and intelligence.[14] What was said about evils or harms in the last paragraph also holds for the goods or benefits mentioned in this definition of a reason. Everything that people count as a benefit or a good—health, love, friends—is related to one or more of the items on this list or to the absence of one or more of the items on the list of harms. Complete agreement on what counts as a good is compatible with considerable disagreement on whether one good is better than another, or whether gaining a given good or benefit adequately compensates for suffering a given harm or evil.

A reason is adequate if any significant group of otherwise rational people regard the harm avoided or benefit gained as at least as important as the harm suffered. People count as otherwise rational if they almost never knowingly act so as to suffer any harm without some reason. No rankings that are held by any significant religious, national, or cultural group count as irrational. The ranking by Jehovah's Witnesses of the harms that would be suffered in an afterlife as worse than dying decades earlier than one would if one accepted a transfusion, is not an irrational ranking. Similarly, psychiatrists do not regard any beliefs held by any significant religious, national, or cultural group as delusions or irrational beliefs. The belief by Jehovah's Witnesses that accepting blood transfusions will have bad consequences for one's afterlife is not regarded as an irrational belief or delusion. If a belief is a reason, we count it as an adequate reason for an action if any significant group regards it as an adequate reason for that action. Irrationality would not be the fundamental normative concept, if there were not complete agreement (among all those whose views are taken seriously) that no one ever ought to act irrationally. Thus we are required to count as irrational only those actions on which there is almost universal agreement that they should not be done.

Counting any action that is not irrational as rational results in two categories of rational actions; those that are *rationally required* and those that are merely *rationally allowed.* If no religious beliefs are involved, an example of a rationally required action (an action that it would be irrational not to do) would be an otherwise healthy person taking a proven and safe antibiotic for a life-threatening infection. However, refusing a death-delaying treatment for a painful terminal disease, even if no religious beliefs are involved, will be rationally allowed (will not be irrational either to do or not to do). These two categories share no common feature except that they are both not irrational. This account of rationality has the desired result that everyone who is regarded as rational always wants himself and his friends to act rationally. Certainly, on this account of rationality, no one would ever want himself or anyone for whom he is concerned to act irrationally.

Although an action counts as rational when it is rationally allowed for a person to act in that way, it may be *unreasonable* for a particular person to act in that way, given her particular rankings of the harms and benefits involved. *An unreasonable action is a rationally allowed action that conflicts with the rankings of harms and benefits of the person acting.* For example, it may be rationally allowed to choose either of two alternative treatments, both equally effective, but with a different mix of harms and benefits. Suppose, however, that the first treatment involves the risk of a harm that the patient ranks as very serious, such as impotence, whereas the second involves the risk of causing allergies to certain kinds of foods, which the patient has no particular desire to eat. Unless he has an adequate reason, it would be unreasonable for that patient to choose the first alternative. For another patient with different rankings, one who liked the foods to which the treatment might cause an allergy and who had no interest in sexual activity, it would be unreasonable to choose the second treatment.[15]

Although this account of rationality may sound obvious, it is in conflict with the most common account of rationality, where rationality is limited to an instrumental role. A rational action is often defined as one that maximizes the satisfaction of all of one's desires, but without putting any limit on the content of those desires. This definition results in an irrational action being defined as any action that is inconsistent with such maximization.[16] Unless desires for any of the harms on the list are ruled out, however, it turns out that people would not always want those for whom they are concerned to act rationally. Consider a young person who becomes extremely depressed and desires to kill himself. No one concerned with him would encourage him to satisfy that desire even if doing so would maximize the satisfaction of his present desires. Rather, everyone concerned with him would encourage him to seek psychiatric help. They would all hope that he would be cured of his depression and then come to see that he has no adequate reason to kill himself.[17] The fact that rationality has a definite content and is not limited to a purely instrumental role conflicts with most philosophical accounts of rational actions, as well as those offered by most of the social sciences, including economics.[18]

Some may claim that both of these accounts of rationality are misconceived. Following Hume, they may claim that the basic account of rationality is not primarily related to actions at all, but rather to obtaining true beliefs. Scientific rationality consists of using those scientific methods best suited for discovering truth. We do not deny that there is a concept of rationality related to belief, but we think that rationality related to belief cannot be taken as the fundamental sense of rationality. The account of rationality as avoiding harms is more basic than that of rationality related to belief or of reasoning correctly. Scientific rationality cannot explain why it is irrational not to avoid suffering avoidable harms when no one benefits in any way. The avoiding-harm account of rationality does explain why it is rational to reason correctly and to discover new truth; because doing so helps people to avoid harms and to gain benefits.[19]

The avoiding-harm account of rationality makes clear that in a conflict between morality and self-interest, it is not irrational to act in either way. It is neither irrational to act contrary to one's own best interests in order to act morally, nor is it irrational to act immorally if it is in one's own best interest to do so. It may even be rationally allowed to act contrary to both self-interest and morality, if others—friends, family, colleagues—benefit. Morality and self-interest do not always oppose each other, indeed they are usually quite compatible. Many people, including some physicians and scientists, mistakenly believe that they cannot be acting immorally if they act for the benefit of others and contrary to their own self-interest. They do not recognize that they are acting immorally in helping to cover up the mistakes of their colleagues, because they believe that since they, themselves, have nothing to gain and are even putting themselves at risk, they must be acting morally. Those who hold a virtue theory of ethics may have difficulty in explaining why self-sacrifice for others is sometimes immoral. That altruism and morality are not the same is also shown by the phenomenon of sincere but unjustified paternalism.

Although some philosophers have tried to show that it is irrational to act immorally, this conflicts with the ordinary understanding of the matter. Everyone agrees, for example, that if a physician is certain that he will not be discovered, it may not be irrational—that is, it may be rationally allowed—for him to deceive a patient about a mistake that he has made, even if this is acting immorally. Although we favor people acting morally, in this book we are not attempting to provide motivation for acting morally. That motivation comes from family, or religion, or whatever leads one to be concerned for others.

However a concern for others must be tempered by the realization that it is arrogant to think that morality does not apply to oneself and one's colleagues in the same way that it applies to everyone else. Morality is a public system, and with regard to obeying the moral rules, it requires impartiality. It is morally unacceptable to violate a moral rule if one could not publicly allow that violation, that is, if one could not will that everyone know that they are allowed to violate that moral rule when all of the morally relevant features are the same.

Failure to appreciate the significance of impartiality leads to misguided loyalty and unjustified paternalism.

Impartiality

Impartiality is a more complex concept than is generally recognized. Even the dictionary defines it simply as not favoring one more than another and regards impartiality as equivalent to fairness, as if one could not impartially enforce laws which one knew to be unfair. Impartiality does not, by itself, guarantee moral behavior, if one is impartial with regard to an inappropriate group, or in an inappropriate respect. In fact, it cannot even be determined if A is impartial, until the group with regard to which A is impartial and the respect in which A is impartial are specified. The following analysis of the basic concept of impartiality shows that to understand fully what it means to say that a person is impartial involves knowing both the group with regard to which her impartiality is being judged and the respect in which her actions are supposed to be impartial with regard to that group. *A is impartial in respect R with regard to group G if and only if A's actions in respect R are not influenced at all by which members of G benefit or are harmed by these actions.*

It is also not generally made clear that morality does not always require impartiality. Morality requires impartiality only when one is considering violating a moral rule. It does not require impartiality when deciding which people to help, for example when deciding which charity to give to. One reason most philosophical accounts of morality are correctly regarded as having little practical value is that they do not recognize that morality requires impartiality only in very limited circumstances, namely, when considering violating a moral rule.

Just as an adequate general account of impartiality must relate impartiality to some group, such as a father being impartial with regard to his own children, so an adequate account of the impartiality required by morality must relate it to some group. People differ concerning who is included in the group with regard to which morality requires impartiality. The minimal group toward which morality requires impartiality consists of (1) all moral agents and (2) former moral agents who are still persons (incompetent but not permanently unconscious patients). This group is the minimal group because all rational persons would favor impartial obedience to the moral rules,—"Do not kill," "Do not deceive"—with regard to a group including at least all of these people. Further, in the United States and the rest of the industrialized world, almost everyone would include in the group toward whom the moral rules require impartiality, all children, including infants, who will become moral agents. However, the claim that moral rules require impartiality with regard to any more extended group quickly becomes more controversial.

Many hold that the impartially protected group should include only moral agents, former moral agents, and children who will become moral agents, while many others hold that this group should include all potential moral agents, even nonsentient ones like a fetus from the time of conception. Still others hold that this group should include all sentient beings, that is, all beings who can feel pleasure or pain, whether potential moral agents or not, for example horses and pigs. Since fully informed rational persons disagree about who is included in the group toward which morality requires impartiality, there is no way to resolve the issue philosophically. This is why discussions of abortion and animal rights are so emotionally charged and often involve violence. We do not think there are conclusive arguments for any of these competing views, which is why we regard the morality of abortion as an unresolvable issue. Morality, however, does set limits to the morally allowable ways of settling unresolvable moral disagreements. These ways cannot involve violence or other unjustified violations of the moral rules, but must be settled peacefully. One of the often neglected functions of a moral theory is to determine what counts as a genuinely unresolvable moral disagreement. Once this is determined, one of the proper functions of a democratic government is to settle these genuinely unresolvable moral disagreements by peaceful means.

As noted, the respect in which one must be impartial toward the minimal group (or any larger group) concerns violating a moral rule, for instance killing or deceiving. Since all of the moral rules can be regarded as prohibitions, it is fairly easy to obey them impartially. Impartiality is not required in following the moral ideals, such as relieving pain and suffering, for it is humanly impossible to follow the ideals impartially even with regard to the minimal group toward which morality requires impartiality. One of the more obvious flaws of almost all forms of consequentialism, such as utilitarianism, is that they make no distinction between moral rules and ideals and so seem to require impartiality in all of one's actions. Failure to understand that morality requires impartiality only with respect to obeying the moral rules has even caused some to deny that morality requires impartiality.[20] The kind of impartiality required by morality involves allowing a violation of a moral rule with regard to one member of the protected group, such as a stranger, only when the same kind of violation would be allowed with regard to everyone else in the group, such as friends.

Acting impartially with respect to the moral rules is analogous to a referee impartially officiating a basketball game, except that the referee is not part of the group toward which he is required to be impartial and the moral agent is. The referee judges all participants impartially if he makes the same decision regardless of which player or team is benefited or harmed by that decision. All impartial referees need not prefer the same style of basketball; one referee might prefer a game with less bodily contact, hence calling somewhat more fouls, while another may prefer a more physical game, hence calling fewer fouls. Impartiality allows these differences as long as the referee does not favor any particular team or player over any other. In the same way, moral impartiality allows for differences in the ranking of various harms and benefits as long as one would be willing to make these rankings public and one does not favor any particular person or group, including oneself or one's friends, over any others when one decides to violate a moral rule or judges whether a violation is justified.

Common Morality as a Justified Moral System

A justified moral system is a public system that all rational persons could advocate as a guide for everyone to follow. But there is no way to guarantee that all rational persons will agree unless they use only beliefs that all of them share, namely, rationally required beliefs. This limitation to rationally required beliefs is not an arbitrary limitation, for since morality is a public system that applies to all rational persons, it can involve only those factual beliefs which are shared by all rational persons. Both morality itself and the justification of morality can make use only of rationally required beliefs. But this is true only of the moral framework that is shared by all moral systems; societal moral systems can also use beliefs that are shared only by all those to whom that system applies, the members of the society.[21]

Further, particular moral decisions and judgments depend not only on knowledge of the moral system, but also on beliefs about the particular situation. As noted above, our experience on ethics committees and in doing ethics consultations has been that most actual moral disagreements are based on disagreements about the facts of the case, including especially, disagreements about prognoses. However, we have noted that particular moral decisions and judgments may also depend on how different harms and benefits are ranked. A decision about whether to withhold a genetic diagnosis from a patient (for example a diagnosis of Huntington disease) involves a belief about the *magnitude* of the risk of telling (for example, the probability of the information leading the patient to kill himself or to suffer a severe lengthy depression) and the *ranking* of that degree of risk against the certain loss of freedom to act on the information that would result from not providing that information. Equally informed impartial rational persons may differ not only in their beliefs about the degree of risk, but also in their rankings of the harms involved, and either of these differences may result in their disagreeing on what morally ought to be done.

Common morality, which is a justified moral system, is for vulnerable and fallible people. Its goal is to lessen the amount of harm suffered by those protected by it; it must recognize and accomodate the fallibility of people and the need for the system to be understood by everyone to whom it applies. It includes (1) *rules* prohibiting acting in ways that cause, or significantly increase the probability of causing, any of the five harms that all rational persons want to avoid; and (2) *ideals* encouraging the prevention of any of these harms. It is useful to provide a clear, comprehensive, and explicit account of the justified moral system that is common morality. It is not useful but dangerous to provide a system that can be applied mechanically to arrive at the correct solution to a moral problem; not all moral problems have unique correct solutions. Common morality only provides a framework for dealing with moral problems in a way that will be acceptable to all who are involved; this justified moral system does not provide a unique right answer to every moral question. We claim that all impartial rational persons would accept common morality as a public system that applies to all moral agents; we do not claim that it eliminates all moral disagreement. In what follows we shall attempt to make explicit the details of the common moral system. We do not think that anyone will find anything surprising in our explication.

The Moral Rules

The first five moral rules prohibit directly causing the five harms.

Do not kill. (We also include causing permanent loss of consciousness.)
Do not cause pain. (Includes causing mental pain, for example, sadness or anxiety.)
Do not disable. (More precisely, do not cause loss of physical, mental, or volitional abilities.)
Do not deprive of freedom. (Includes freedom from being acted upon as well as depriving of opportunity to act.)
Do not deprive of pleasure. (Includes future as well as present pleasure.)

The second five moral rules include those rules which when not followed in particular cases usually, but not always, cause harm, and which always result in harm being suffered when they are not generally followed.

Do not deceive. (Includes more than lying.)
Keep your promise. (Equivalent to Do not break your promise.)
Do not cheat. (Primarily involves violating rules of a voluntary activity, such as a game.)
Obey the law. (Equivalent to Do not break the law.)
Do your duty. (Equivalent to Do not neglect your duty.)

The term "duty" is being used in its everyday sense, to refer to what is required by one's role in society, primarily one's job, not as philosophers customarily use it, namely simply as a synonym for "what one morally ought to do."

What Counts as a Violation of a Moral Rule?

As mentioned earlier, there is often a difference in interpretation about what counts as breaking the rule. Not every action that results in someone suffering a harm or an evil counts as breaking one of the first five rules. It is sometimes important to determine whether an action is a justified violation of a moral rule or is not even a violation of a rule at all. A scientist who discovers that another scientist's apparently important new discovery was plagiarized, may know that reporting this will result in harm to the plagiarist. Reporting her findings, however, is not a violation of any rule against causing harm. Almost no one would say that it is, but determining whether it is depends upon the practices and conventions of the society (see Chapter 3, "Application").

On the other hand, a doctor who, after receiving valid consent from a patient, causes pain to that patient in order to prevent greater pain in the future, is breaking the rule against causing pain, even though this violation is strongly justified. Now consider a physician who responds to a couple's question and informs them that their fetus has some serious genetic problem, for example cystic fibrosis, when she knows that this will result in their suffering considerable grief. If she has verified the information and told them in an appropriately considerate way, then many would say that she did not break the rule against causing pain and her action requires no justification. Indeed, not responding truthfully to their question would be an unjustified violation of the rule against deception. On this interpretation, the physician is acting like the scientist reporting a mistake by another scientist. However, one might interpret the situation to be like the doctor justifiably breaking the rule against causing pain with the valid consent of the patient. On either interpretation, it is at least a moral ideal to be as kind and gentle in telling that truth as she can. Indeed, we claim it is part of the duty of doctors not to cause more suffering than necessary when giving information about any serious malady.

It is quite clear that lying (making a false statement with the intent to deceive) counts as a violation of the rule prohibiting deception, as does any other action which is intentionally done in order to deceive others. But it is not always clear when withholding information counts as deception. Thus it not always clear that one needs a justification for withholding some information, for instance that the husband of the woman whose fetus is being tested did not father that fetus.

In scientific research, what counts as deceptive is determined in large part by the conventions and practices of the field or area of research. If it is a standard scientific practice to smooth curves depicting data or not to report unsuccessful experiments, then doing so is not deceptive, even if some people, especially those who are not expected to read the reports, are deceived. However, when a practice results in many people being deceived, especially if it is known they will read the results, it is a deceptive practice even if it is a common practice within the field or area. An example would be releasing to the public press a premature and overly optimistic account of a "cure," which would create false hope for many of those suffering from the related malady. Recognition that one's action is deceptive is important, for then one realizes that without an adequate justification, one is acting immorally.

Justifying Violations of the Moral Rules

Almost everyone agrees that the moral rules have justified exceptions; most agree that even killing is justified in self-defense. Further, there is widespread agreement on several features that all justified exceptions have. The first of these involves impartiality. Everyone agrees that all justified violations of the rules are such that *if they are justified for any person, they are justified for every person when all of the morally relevant features are the same.* The major value of simple slogans like the Golden Rule, "Do unto others as you would have them do unto you," and Kant's Categorical Imperative, "Act only on that maxim whereby you can at the same time will that it be a universal law of nature," are as devices to persuade people to act impartially when they are contemplating violating a moral rule. However, given that these slogans are often misleading, a better way to achieve impartiality is to consider whether one would be prepared for everyone to know that this kind of violation is allowed.

The next feature on which there is almost complete agreement is that *it has to be rational to favor everyone being allowed to violate the rule in these circumstances.* Suppose that someone suffering from a mental disorder both wants to inflict pain on others and wants pain inflicted on himself. He is in favor of allowing any person who wants others to cause pain to himself, to cause pain to others, whether or not they want pain inflicted on themselves. This is not sufficient to justify that kind of violation. No impartial rational person would favor allowing anyone who wants pain caused to himself to cause pain to everyone else whether or not these others want pain caused to themselves. The result of allowing that kind of violation would be an increase in the amount of pain suffered with no benefit to anyone. That is clearly irrational.

Finally, there is general agreement that a violation is justified only if *it is rational to favor allowing that violation even if everyone knows that this kind of violation is allowed.* A violation is not justified simply if it would be rational to favor allowing everyone to violate the rule in the same circumstances when almost no one knows that it is allowable to violate the rule in those circumstances. What counts as the same kind of violation, or the same circumstances, is determined by the morally relevant features of the situation. We will discuss these features in the next section, but we can provide a simple example now. It might be rational to favor allowing a physician to deceive a patient about his diagnosis if that patient were likely to be upset by knowing the truth, when almost no one knows that this kind of deception is allowed. In order to make this kind of deception justified, however, it has to be rational to favor allowing this kind of deception when everyone knows that deception is allowed in these circumstances. Only the requirement that the violation be publicly allowed guarantees the kind of impartiality required by morality. (see Chapter 10, "Justification," for further discussion.)

Not everyone agrees about which violations satisfy these three conditions, but there is general agreement that no violation is justified unless it satisfies all three of these conditions. Recognizing the significant agreement concerning justified violations of the moral rules, while acknowledging that people can sometimes disagree, results in all impartial rational persons accepting the following attitude toward violations of the moral rules: *Everyone is always to obey the rule unless an impartial rational person can advocate that violating it be publicly allowed. Anyone who violates the rule when no impartial rational person can advocate that such a violation be publicly allowed may be punished.* (The "unless" clause only means that when an impartial rational person can advocate that such a violation be publicly allowed, impartial rational persons may disagree on whether one should obey the rule. It does not mean that they agree one should not obey the rule.)

Morally Relevant Features

When deciding whether or not an impartial rational person can advocate that a violation of a moral rule be publicly allowed, the kind of violation must be described using only morally relevant features. Since the morally relevant features are part of the moral system, they must be understood by all moral agents. This means that any description of the violation must be such that it can be reformulated in a way that all moral agents can understand it. Limiting the way in which a violation must be described makes it easier for people to discover that their decision or judgment is biased by some consideration which is not morally relevant. All of the morally relevant features that we have discovered so far are answers to the following questions (It is quite likely that other morally relevant features will be discovered, but we think that we have discovered the major features. Of course, in any actual situation, it is the particular facts of the situation that determine the answers to these questions, but all of these answers can be given in a way that can be understood by all moral agents):

1. What moral rules would be violated?
2. What harms would be (a) avoided (not caused), (b) prevented, and (c) caused? (This means foreseeable harms and includes probabilities as well as kind and extent.)
3. What are the relevant beliefs and desires of the people toward whom the rule is being violated? (This explains why physicians must provide adequate information about treatment and obtain their patients' consent before treating.)
4. Does one have a relationship with the person(s) toward whom the rule is being violated such that one sometimes has a duty to violate moral rules with regard to the person(s) without their consent? (This explains why a parent or guardian may be morally allowed to make a decision about treatment that the health care team is not morally allowed to make.)
5. What benefits would be caused? (This means foreseeable benefits and also includes probabilities, as well as kind and extent.)
6. Is an unjustified or weakly justified violation of a moral rule being prevented? (Usually not relevant in medical contexts, applies more to police work and national security.)
7. Is an unjustified or weakly justified violation of a moral rule being punished? (Not relevant in medical contexts, applies more to the legal system.)
8. Are there any alternative actions that would be preferable?[22]
9. Is the violation being done intentionally or only knowingly?[23]
10. Is it an emergency situation that no person is likely to plan to be in?[24]

It may be worthwhile to illustrate this general account of the morally relevant features by using standard medical situations.

1. Among the moral rules that might be violated are those against causing pain, depriving of freedom, deceiving (including withholding information), breaking promises, for instance, of confidentiality, and breaking the law.
2. The harms that might be prevented by deceiving are the anxiety suffered by the patient and a 25% risk of a heart attack. The harm caused might be the loss of freedom to make decisions based on the facts. In another example, the harm that might be prevented by refusing to abide by a patient's decision to stop life-sustaining treatment would be the patient's death; the harms caused would be suffering and the loss of freedom.
3. In medical situations the relevant beliefs and desires are normally those that lead a competent patient to validly consent to, or refuse, a suggested

treatment, such as beliefs about the consequences of accepting and refusing treatment, and desires or aversions to those consequences.

4. Except in emergency situations doctors do not normally have a relationship with the patient that requires them to break moral rules with regard to patients without their consent. Parents and guardians do have such a relationship. This explains why guardians must be appointed if it is regarded as medically necessary to treat a patient without his consent.

5. Benefits include only the conferring of positive goods, not the prevention or relief of harms, and normally medical situations are concerned only with the prevention or relief of harms. Cosmetic plastic surgery for someone who is not disfigured would be an example of providing benefits. This can almost never be done without the valid consent of the person who is to be benefited.

6. Preventing the violation of a moral rule does not normally apply in medical situations, but it can occur when a doctor considers violating confidentiality in order to prevent an AIDS patient from having unprotected sex with his wife who is unaware of his HIV + status.

7. Punishment should never be relevant in a medical situation.

8. This is perhaps the most overlooked feature. Many actions that would be morally acceptable if there were not a better alternative, become morally unacceptable if there is. Persuading a husband to tell his wife that he is HIV + is a better alternative than simply violating confidentiality and the doctor telling her himself, even though, if the husband is not persuaded, it may be morally acceptable for the doctor to tell her himself.

9. It is uncontroversially morally acceptable to provide adequate pain medication to a terminally ill patient even though one knows that this medication may hasten his death. It is, at least, controversial to provide pain medication in order to hasten the patient's death.

10. It may be morally acceptable to overrule a patient's refusal of life-preserving treatment in an emergency situation when it is not morally acceptable to overrule the same refusal in a nonemergency situation.

When considering the harms being avoided (not caused), prevented, and caused, and the benefits being promoted, one must consider not only the kind of benefits or harms involved, one must also consider their seriousness, duration, and probability. If more than one person is affected, one must consider not only how many people will be affected, but also the distribution of the harms and benefits. Two violations that do not differ in any of their morally relevant features count as the same kind of violation. Anyone who claims to be acting or judging as an impartial rational person who holds that one of the two violations be publicly allowed must hold that the other also be publicly allowed. Impartiality requires this.

However, two people, both fully informed impartial and rational, who agree that two actions count as the same kind of violation, need not always agree on whether to advocate that this kind of violation be publicly allowed. They may rank the benefits and harms involved differently or they may differ in their estimate of the consequences of publicly allowing that kind of violation. For example, two persons may agree on the increase in the probability that a post-stroke patient will discontinue his physical therapy if his therapist does not harass him. They may also agree on the amount of pain that harassment will cause and on the amount of disability that will result if the therapy is discontinued. But they may disagree in their rankings of the pain caused by harassment, and the probability of the increase in disability that results from discontinuing therapy. They may also disagree about the consequences of publicly allowing that kind of violation, one holding that everyone knowing that this kind of violation is allowed will result in a very large increase in the amount of pain inflicted, and the other holding that it will result in only a small increase, which will be more than justified by the extra amount of disability lessened.

To act or judge as an impartial rational person is to estimate what effect this kind of violation, one with all of the same morally relevant features, would have if publicly allowed. If all informed, impartial, rational persons would estimate that less harm would be suffered if this kind of violation were publicly allowed, then all impartial rational persons would advocate that this kind of violation be publicly allowed and the violation is strongly justified; if all informed impartial rational persons would estimate that more harm would be suffered, then no impartial rational person would advocate that this kind of violation be publicly allowed and the violation is unjustified. However, impartial rational persons, even if equally informed, may disagree in their estimate of whether more or less harm will result from this kind of violation being publicly allowed. When there is such disagreement, even if all parties are rational and impartial, they will disagree on whether to advocate that this kind of violation be publicly allowed, and the violation counts as weakly justified.

Disagreements about whether the same kind of violation being publicly allowed will result in more or less harm stem from two distinct sources. The first source is differences in the rankings of the various kinds of harms. If someone ranks a specified amount of pain and suffering as worse than a specified amount of loss of freedom, and someone else ranks them in the opposite way, then although they agree that a given action is the same kind of violation, they may disagree on whether or not to advocate that this kind of violation be publicly allowed. The second source is differences in estimates of how much harm would result from everyone knowing that a given kind of violation is allowed, even when there seem to be no differences in the rankings of the different kinds of harms. These differences may stem from differences in beliefs about human nature or about the nature of human societies. For example, different views on

(1) how many people would violate the rule against deceiving in these circumstances if they knew such a violation was allowed; and on (2) what effect this number of violations would have upon the society. Insofar as these differences cannot be settled by any universally agreed upon empirical method, they are best regarded as ideological.

The disagreement about whether physicians should assist the suicides of terminally ill patients, is an example of such a dispute. People disagree on whether publicly allowing physician-assisted suicide will result in more bad consequences (significantly more people dying sooner than they really want to) than good consequences (many more people being relieved of pain and suffering). However, it is quite likely that most ideological differences also involve differences in the rankings of different kinds of harms, such as whether the suffering prevented by physician-assisted suicide ranks higher or lower than the earlier deaths that might be caused. This issue will be discussed in more detail in Chapter 12, "Euthanasia."

Moral Ideals

In contrast with the moral rules, which prohibit doing those kinds of actions which cause people to suffer some harm or increase the risk of their suffering some harm, the moral ideals encourage one to do those kinds of actions which lessen the amount of harm suffered (including providing goods for those who are deprived) or decrease the risk of people suffering harm. As long as one is not violating a moral rule, common morality encourages following any moral ideal. In particular circumstances, it may be worthwhile to talk of specific moral ideals; for instance one can claim that there are five specific moral ideals involved in preventing harm, one for each of the five harms. Physicians seem primarily devoted to the moral ideals of preventing death, pain, and disability. Genetic counselors may have as their primary ideal preventing the loss of freedom of their clients. One can also specify particular moral ideals that involve preventing unjustified violations of the moral rules. Insofar as lack of a proper understanding of morality leads to unjustified violations of the moral rules, providing a proper understanding of morality is also following a moral ideal.

It is not important to decide how specific to make the moral ideals, for, normally, following any moral ideal is praiseworthy. It is, however, important to distinguish moral ideals from other ideals, for except in very special circumstances, only moral ideals can justify violating a moral rule with regard to someone without her consent. Utilitarian ideals, which involve promoting goods, such as abilities and pleasure, for those who are not deprived, do not justify individuals in violating moral rules without consent.[25] Those who train athletes, engage in much historical or scientific research, or create delicious new recipes, are following utilitarian ideals. Religious ideals involve promoting activities, spirituality, traits of character, and so on which are idiosyncratic to a particular religion or group of religions. Personal ideals involve promoting some traits of character, which are idiosyncratic to particular persons, for instance, ambition, about whose value people disagree.

The moral ideals differ from the moral rules in that only for the latter is there a possibility of their being impartially obeyed all of the time. No one can impartially follow moral ideals all of the time; indeed, it is humanly impossible to follow them all of the time, impartially or not, because everyone needs to sleep sometimes. Of course, everyone favors people following the moral ideals, but most do not favor everyone following them as much as possible. Most people believe that everyone is entitled to spend some time relaxing and having fun. It is only failure to obey a moral rule that always needs an excuse or justification. None of this should be surprising at all. All that we claim is that everyone counts certain kinds of actions—killing, causing pain, deceiving, breaking promises—as immoral unless one can justify doing that kind of act; and that everyone agrees that acting to relieve pain and suffering is encouraged by morality, but doing so is not required unless one has a duty to do so. This distinction between moral rules and moral ideals should not be taken as simply an alternative formulation of the common distinction between negative and positive duties, for it is a moral rule that one keep one's promise and do one's duty, and keeping one's promise or doing one's duty may require positive action.[26]

That two moral rules can conflict, that, for example, doing one's duty may require causing pain, makes it clear that it would be a mistake to conclude that one should always avoid breaking a moral rule. Sometimes breaking one of these rules is so strongly justified that not only is there nothing immoral about breaking it, it would be immoral not to break the rule. A physician who, with the rational informed consent of a competent patient, performs some painful procedure in order to prevent much more serious pain or death, breaks the moral rule against causing pain, but is not doing anything that is immoral in the slightest. In fact, refusing to do the necessary painful procedure, given the conditions specified, would itself be a violation of her duty as a doctor and thus would need some stronger justification in order not to be immoral. Two moral rules need not conflict for it to be strongly justified to break a moral rule. Sometimes acting on a moral ideal, like stopping to help an accident victim, may involve breaking a moral rule, like breaking a promise to meet someone at the movies, and yet everyone would publicly allow breaking the rule. It is clear, therefore, that to say that someone has broken a moral rule is not, by itself, to say that anything morally unacceptable has been done, it is only to say that some justification is needed. Normally, most medically indicated treatments which involve causing harm to the patient, including most medical operations, are completely morally unproblematic because valid consent has been given.

Applying Morality to a Particular Case

Sometimes there seems to be an unresolvable difference when a careful exam-ination of the issue shows that there is actually a correct answer. For example, a physician may claim that deceiving a patient about a diagnosis, for example of multiple sclerosis, to avoid causing a specified degree of anxiety and other mental suffering is justified. He may claim that withholding these unpleasant findings in this case will result in less overall harm being suffered than if he did not deceive. He may claim that this patient does not deal well with bad news and also is unlikely to find out about the deception. Thus he may claim that his deception, at least for a limited time, actually results in his patient suffering less harm than if he were told the truth.

Another physician, however, may claim that this deception, no matter how difficult it will be for the person to accept the facts now or how confident the physician is that the deception will not be discovered, is not justified. The latter may hold that this deception will actually increase the amount of harm suffered because the patient will be deprived of the opportunity to make decisions based upon the facts and that if he does find out about the deception he will not only have less faith in statements made by the physician, he will also have less faith in statements made by other health care providers, thus increasing his anxiety and suffering. This is a genuine empirical dispute about whether withholding bad news from this patient is likely to increase or decrease the amount of harm he suffers. Which of these hypotheses about the actual effects of deception in this particular case is correct, we do not know, but if one is concerned with the moral justifiability of such deception the consequences of the particular case are not decisive.

The morally decisive question is, What would be the consequences if this kind of deception were publicly allowed? The former physician has not taken into account that a justifiable violation against deception must be one that is publicly allowed, that is, one that everyone knows is allowed. Once the physi-cian realizes that everyone knows that it is allowable to deceive in certain circumstances, for instance to withhold bad news in order to avoid anxiety and other mental suffering, then the loss of trust involved will obviously have a worse result than if everyone knew that such deception was not allowed. It is only by concentrating on the results of one's own deception, without recogniz-ing that morally allowed violations for oneself must be such that everyone knows that they are morally allowed for everyone, that one could be led to think that such deception was justified. Consciously holding that it is morally allowable for oneself to deceive others in this way when one would not want everyone to know that everyone is morally allowed to deceive others in the same circumstances, is what is meant by "arrogance." It is arrogating exceptions to the moral rules for oneself which one would not want everyone to know are allowed for all. This arrogance is clearly incompatible with the kind of impartiality that morality requires with regard to obeying the moral rules.

This does not mean that it is never morally justified to deceive patients. Sometimes the consequences of being told the truth may be so serious, such as a significant increase in the chances of a fatal heart attack, that a physician would be willing to publicly allow everyone to deceive in this kind of case, at least for a period of time. What is important is that one must think of one's decision as if it were setting a public policy, one that everyone could act on when the morally relevant features were the same. Indeed, actually formulating a public policy is probably the best way to deal with controversial cases.

The Importance of Having Public Policies

Should physicians inform parents of young teenagers (13 to 15) if their children are sexually active or taking drugs? We do not claim to have the answer to this question, for there are good arguments both in favor of informing parents and against informing them. However, we do claim that having an explicit public policy stating that parents will be informed, or that they will not, is preferable to not having any public policy at all. In the absence of any public policy, whether parents will be informed is a matter of chance, based solely on which doctor happens to examine their child, and perhaps even on how that doctor happens to feel that day. Further, neither parents nor children know what to expect. If parents are not told, they can justifiably complain that they should have been told, so that they would have been able to talk with their children. If parents are told, the children can justifiably complain that their confidentiality has been violated and that if they had known that their parents would be informed, they would never have confided in the doctor.

Not having a public policy makes it impossible for either parents or children to give informed valid consent. Both are deprived of the opportunity to make an important decision because neither knows the consequences of the teenager being examined. Further, it is quite likely that both believe what they want to believe; parents, that they will be informed, and children, that their parents will not be informed. Neither will have any evidence for their belief. This means that it is quite likely that someone will feel betrayed by what actually happens. If there is a public policy, then both parents and children will know what is going to happen, so that neither will be misled. If the policy is that parents will be notified, then children will know that their confidentiality is limited and can decide what they are prepared to tell the doctor. If the policy is that parents will not be notified, then parents will know that they cannot count on the physician to inform them of any problems and that they must seek to find out about any problems directly from their child. But even if the policy is that parents will not be notified, that does not prohibit doctors from trying to persuade the child to talk to his parents.[27]

Further, the policy does not have to be and should not be stated in some simple way that prohibits a physician from exercising her judgment in a particular case, contrary to the general policy. Thus, if the general policy is not to inform, it should have exceptions in several cases, such as those which threaten the child's life. If the policy is to inform, it should also have exceptions, for example, if the child provides evidence that informing his parents would have serious bad consequences. A public policy is an informal public system and, like morality itself, allows for cases in which people can disagree about what should be done. It would be worse than naive to think that one could formulate an acceptable public policy that would never allow the physician to exercise his considered judgment. The point of having a public policy is not to eliminate judgment, but to provide a context so that everyone involved has a better idea of what to expect.

Another advantage of having a public policy is that it needs to be preceded by discussion among all those involved. Once it is agreed that it is better to have some public policy rather than none, all of those involved must cooperate to formulate such a policy. This discussion is quite likely to result in everyone becoming better informed and learning about alternatives and arguments that they had not considered. This is quite likely to result in better decisions, for everyone will now be aware of the complexities of the issue. Indeed, many may become aware for the first time that what they have been doing is not the same as what others have been doing. They also may become aware of consequences that had previously escaped their attention.

Perhaps most important, the discussion should make everyone aware that fully informed rational persons can disagree, even on moral matters, without anyone being mistaken. That one can compromise one's position without any loss of moral integrity is a valuable lesson. Having a public policy, rather than each person making her own judgment, has sufficient value that as an impartial person one should see that it outweighs the fact that the public policy may limit her freedom to make her own judgment. Being guided by a public policy that one has contributed to and about which one can claim that it is not irrational for anyone to follow, is a wonderful preparation for the kind of moral reasoning that is required for all moral problems. Indeed, if the public policy is in accord with the common moral system, it always will involve the kind of moral reasoning that we have been trying to make explicit in this chapter.

Contrasts with Other Systems for Guiding Conduct

For those who are concerned with the philosophical foundations of bioethics, it may clarify our account of the justified moral system to compare it with the views put forward by many contemporary followers of Immanuel Kant (1724–1804) and John Stuart Mill (1806–1873). The Kantian Categorical Imperative, "Act only on that maxim whereby can at the same time will that it be a universal law of nature," and an imperative form of Mill's Utilitarian Greatest Happiness Principle, "Act so as to bring about the greatest happiness for the greatest number," are two of the most popular and influential moral philosophical slogans. But these slogans, though often cited, are inadequate by themselves to provide a useful moral guide to conduct. It is not fair to Kant and Mill to compare these slogans with our account of the moral system sketched in this chapter, for Kant and Mill have far more to say than simply working out the consequences of these slogans. However, neither Kant nor Mill nor their contemporary followers discuss the morally relevant features and so they provide no plausible account of how one determines whether two violations count as violations of the same kind for the purpose of moral decision making.

In a Kantian deontological system one should never act in any way that one cannot will to be a universal law. If it would be impossible for everyone always to do a specific kind of action, then everyone is prohibited from doing that same kind of action. For example, what makes it morally prohibited to make lying promises is that, if everyone always made lying promises, it would be impossible for there to be a practice of promising. In the common moral system, one is prohibited from doing a kind of action only if, given the morally relevant facts, no impartial rational person would publicly allow that kind of action. A Kantian system seems to rule out ever making lying promises, whereas our morality allows the making of lying promises in some circumstances, such as when making the lying promise is necessary to prevent a harm sufficiently great that it is rational to believe that less overall harm would be suffered even if everyone knew that such lying promises were allowed in these kinds of circumstances.

In a consequentialist system one not only may, but should, violate any common moral rule if the foreseeable consequences of that particular violation (including the effects on future obedience to the rule) are better than the consequences of not violating the rule.[28] A consequentialist system is concerned only with the foreseeable consequences of the particular violation, not with the foreseeable consequences of that kind of violation being publicly allowed.[29] On the moral system, however, it is precisely the foreseeable consequences of that kind of violation being publicly allowed that are decisive in determining whether or not it is morally allowed. The importance of the consequences of the particular violation are in determining the kind of violation. A consequentialist system favors cheating on an exam if it were extremely unlikely that the student would get caught, no harm would result from that particular violation of the rule against cheating, and the student would benefit from cheating. On the assumption that the exams are not pointless, the moral system would not allow this kind of violation of the rule against cheating, for if this kind of violation were publicly allowed, it would not be possible for exams to perform the functions they are supposed to perform.

According to classical Utilitarianism (Bentham and Mill), the only relevant consequences are pleasure and pain. Later consequentialists allow for the relevance of other consequences, such as death and disability. They claim that the act which is morally best is that which produces the greatest balance of benefits over harms. It is, paradoxically, the kind of moral theory usually held by people who claim that they have no moral theory. Their view is often expressed in phrases like the following: "It is all right to do anything as long as no one gets hurt," "It is the actual consequences that count, not some silly rules," or "What is important is that things turn out for the best, not how one goes about making that happen." On the moral system, it is not the consequences of the particular violation that are decisive in determining its justifiability, but rather the consequences of publicly allowing such a violation.

As we have described the common moral system, it is dependent on certain features of human nature, namely, that people are vulnerable and fallible, and it also regards rationality as involving the avoidance of harms. Kant thinks of morality as completely independent of human nature and he has a very different account of rationality. Thus common morality differs from a Kantian system and resembles a consequentialist system in that it has a purpose, and consequences are explicitly taken into consideration. It resembles a Kantian system and differs from a consequentialist system in that common morality is a public system in which rules are essential.

The Kantian system requires all of one's actions to be impartial, and consequentialist systems require one to regard the interests of everyone impartially. Morality does not require impartiality with respect to all of one's actions, it requires impartiality only with respect to obeying the moral rules. Nor does morality require one to regard the interests of everyone impartially, it requires that one act impartially only when considering violating a moral rule. Indeed, it is humanly impossible to regard the interests of everyone impartially, even when concerned only with those in the minimal group (moral agents). Impartiality with respect to the moral ideals (Kant's imperfect duties) is also humanly impossible. That all the moral rules are, or can be taken as, prohibitions, is what makes it humanly possible for them to be followed impartially. The public nature of morality and the limited knowledge of rational persons help to explain why impartial obedience to the moral rules is required to achieve the point of morality, which is lessening the suffering of harm. Morality also differs from both systems in that it does not require all moral questions to have unique answers, but explicitly allows for a limited area of disagreement among equally informed impartial rational persons.

Notes

1. A more extended account of morality, and of the moral theory that justifies it, is contained in Bernard Gert, *Morality: A New Justification of the Moral Rules* (New York: Oxford University Press, 1988).

2. It may seem that some people think that breaking laws such as tax laws need no justification. But this is only when they are considering their own breaking of these laws, not when they are considering their being broken by someone else. For a more detailed discussion of why all rational persons would regard "Obey the law" as a moral rule, see Gert, *Morality*, especially pages 135–153.

3. Perhaps one would need only the single personal belief, I am a moral agent, and then all of the other rationally required personal beliefs could be inferred from the rationally required general beliefs.

4. For example, although the principle of respecting autonomy has become exceedingly popular in bioethics, autonomy is an extremely difficult concept that is not clearly understood by philosophers, let alone by those patients to whom it is applied. (See Chapter 4 for a further critique of autonomy.)

5. For example, none of them provide anything that is even comparable to the list of morally relevant features discussed below.

6. This is Plato's and Aristotle's view and also seems to be Kant's. It is explicitly the view of R. M. Hare in all of his earlier books. It is held by all those who hold that the question Why be moral? is answered by referring to the benefits to the person who asks the question, or who regard the question as nonsensical. Those who do not view morality in this way are those for whom morality and political theory are regarded as very closely related, such as Hobbes, the Utilitarians, and Rawls.

7. There are clear paradigms or prototypes of killing, like stabbing or shooting a person, but other cases are not so clear. This topic is very important in the discussion of euthanasia and is discussed in more detail in Chapter 12.

8. Kant seems to hold that morality is only concerned with protecting moral agents, whereas Bentham clearly holds that morality protects all those who can suffer.

9. Law is not a public system for it applies to people who are ignorant of what the law requires. This is illustrated by the saying, "Ignorance of the law is no excuse."

10. However, since preventive measures may involve many people who do not need them, the costs of prevention per person benefited may be significantly greater than the costs of treatment.

11. In the world's richest nation, no one can provide a sound argument with the conclusion that it is morally acceptable to have millions of children with little or no access to even minimally acceptable pediatric care.

12. We are aware that the terms "rational" and "irrational" are sometimes used in such a way that a person might favor acting irrationally, as when irrational means "spontaneous." However, we think that philosophers as diverse as Plato, Hobbes, and Kant agree that no one ever ought to act irrationally. We are attempting to provide the descriptive content of the concept of rationality which is compatible with its fundamental normative character.

13. When we talk about increasing the probability of death, we mean increasing the probability of dying earlier than one would if the action had not been performed, for nothing can increase the probability of death; it is already 100% certain.

14. A belief that is seen to be inconsistent with one's other beliefs by almost everyone with similar knowledge and intelligence, is an irrational belief. Psychiatrists regard such beliefs as delusions. Irrational beliefs cannot serve as reasons.

15. The importance of the concept of unreasonable decisions is explored further in Chapter 7, "Consent."

16. This is no minor definitional squabble. Accepting such a definition of an irrational action makes it impossible for irrationality to play its role as the fundamental normative concept.

17. See Bernard Gert, "Irrationality and the *DSM-III-R* Definition of Mental Disorder," *Analyze & Kritik,* 12 (1990), pp. 34–46.

18. See Bernard Gert, "Rationality, Human Nature, and Lists," *Ethics,* Vol. 100, No. 2 (January 1990), pp. 279–300, and Gert, "Defending Irrationality and Lists," *Ethics,* Vol. 103, No. 2 (January 1993), pp. 329–336.

19. See *The Journal of Medicine and Philosophy,* 11 (1986), Rationality and Medicine, co-edited by K. Danner Clouser and Bernard Gert.

20. See Bernard Gert, "Moral Impartiality," *Midwestern Studies in Philosophy* (Notre Dame, Ind.: Notre Dame Press, 1996), pp. 102–128.

21. See Chapter 3, "Application."

22. This involves trying to find out if there are any alternative actions such that they would either not involve a violation of a moral rule, or that the violations would differ in some morally relevant features, especially, but not limited to, the amount of evil caused, avoided, or prevented.

23. There are many other questions whose answers will affect the moral judgment that some people will make. For example, Is the violation being done (a) voluntarily or because of a volitional disability? (see Bernard Gert and Timothy Duggan, "Free Will as the Ability to Will," *Nous,* Vol. 13, No. 2 (May 1979), pp. 197–217; reprinted in *Moral Responsibility,* edited by John Martin Fisher (Ithaca, NY: Cornell University Press, 1986) (b) freely or because of coercion? (c) knowingly or without knowledge of what is being done? (d) Is the lack of knowledge excusable or the result of negligence? The primary reason for not including answers to these questions as morally relevant features is that they apply to completed actions, and our goal in listing morally relevant features is to help those who are deciding whether or not to commit a given kind of violation. Thus we do not include those features that are solely of value in judging violations that have already been committed, and cannot be used in deciding how to act. For questions (a), (b), (c), and (d) one cannot decide whether or not to commit one rather than another of these kinds of violations, hence they are not useful in deciding how to act.

Although one does not usually decide whether or not to commit a violation intentionally or only knowingly, sometimes that is possible. For violations that are alike in all of their other morally relevant features, a person might not publicly allow a violation that was done intentionally, but might publicly allow a violation that was not done intentionally, even though it was done knowingly. For example, many people would publicly allow nurses to administer sufficient morphine to terminally ill patients to relieve their pain even though everyone knows it may hasten the death of some patients. However, even with no other morally relevant changes in the situation, they would not allow nurses to administer morphine with the intention of hastening the death of a patient. This distinction explains what seems correct in the views of those who endorse the doctrine of double effect. We think that such a distinction may also account for what many regard as a morally significant difference between lying and other forms of deception, especially some instances of withholding information. Lying is always intentional deception; although withholding information is sometimes intentionally deceptive, it is sometimes only knowingly deceptive. Nonetheless, it is important to remember that most violations that are morally unacceptable when done intentionally are also morally unacceptable when done only knowingly.

24. We are talking about the kind of emergency situation that is sufficiently rare that no person is likely to plan or prepare for being in it. This is a feature that is necessary to account for the fact that certain kinds of emergency situations seem to change the moral judgments that many would make even when all of the other morally relevant features are the same. For example, in an emergency when a large number of people have been seriously injured, doctors are morally allowed to abandon patients who have a very small chance of survival in order to take care of those with a better chance, in order that more people will survive. However, in the ordinary practice of medicine doctors are not morally allowed to abandon their patients with poor prognoses in order to treat those with better prognoses. Patients' knowledge that they could be abandoned by their doctor in common non-emergency situations would cause so much anxiety that it would outweigh the benefits that might be gained by publicly allowing doctors to do so.

25. Utilitarian ideals may sometimes justify governments in violating moral rules, but that is due to morally relevant feature four, that governments have special relationships with their citizens. See Chapter 12 of *Morality* for a more detailed discussion of this issue.

26. As we discuss in more detail in the following chapter, there is a common misuse of the term "duty" such that all of the moral rules are taken as describing duties, rather than duties arising from specific roles and circumstances.

27. See Chapter 8, "Confidentiality," for further discussion of confidentiality and the usefulness of promulgating public policies concerning it.

28. By a consequentialist system we mean an act consequentialist system, for rule consequentialism, regarded as a system for guiding behavior, is a deontological system. Rules are an essential feature of the system, not merely a useful device for calculating the consequences of the particular act.

29. Some consequentialists claim that their systems use actual consequences, not merely foreseeable ones, but this has such counterintuitive results that it cannot be taken seriously.

3

Application

In the preceding chapter we described the basic structure of morality. In this chapter we show how that basic framework is related to everyday moral practices and to professional ethics. Morality at its core is a universal system of conduct, though it is manifested variously in different societies and segments within societies. There are moral codes in business, in various health professions, in sports, in law, in government, in the many different occupations, and so on. Properly understood, these are all expressions of the ordinary morality incumbent on all rational persons, outcroppings of the same underlying rock formation. How this is so and what gives them their different forms is the focus of this chapter. In everyday life it is these outcroppings that are mostly confronted, so it is important to demonstrate how these manifestations are grounded in a common morality. Otherwise, these multitudinous pockets of "moral practices" are seen as just so many diverse, unrelated, free-floating enterprises with rules, customs, and practices peculiar to themselves. Revealing their close ties with the basic structure of morality constitutes a major argument against such a random view of moral conduct.

Moral Theory and the Moral System

In Chapter 2 we provided a systematic account of morality, beginning with the way people make moral decisions and judgments, and then describing the moral system that underlies those decisions and judgments. Morality in practice is not always clear or consistent, so at times we have had to clarify, distinguish, and sharpen in order to nurture consistency. What emerged was a moral system that is free of the aberrations and ambiguities that are inevitably introduced by local beliefs and practices that have not been reflectively integrated into the moral system. We then provided a rational justification of that clarified moral system. That justification, based on the nature of morality as a public system, on rationality, and on universal features of human nature, is what is most properly referred to as "moral theory." In short, we first described the moral system as it functions in ordinary life, and then we showed by argument that it was a valid, rationally justified moral system.

It is important to emphasize that we have started with morality as it is and has been practiced. We have not invented a new morality nor have we derived a morality from some abstract theory or principles. We have analyzed ordinary morality in order to uncover the conceptual structure that underlies it. We are neither modifying the old structure nor creating a new one; rather, we are clarifying and making explicit the common moral system in order to make our moral decisions and judgments more consistent. Our moral theory, then, is our account of how that moral system, presented in an idealized form, is rationally justified. We showed how and why rational persons who know they are vulnerable and have limited knowledge would espouse morality as a public system known to and binding upon all rational persons.

Particular Moral Rules

In Chapter 2 we asserted that the *general* moral rules were integrally connected with human nature and with rationality. Rationality requires all persons to avoid certain harms unless they have an adequate reason not to. These harms, listed individually, are those which the first five moral rules admonish everyone not to cause to each other. (Do not kill, Do not cause pain, Do not disable, Do not deprive of freedom, and Do not deprive of pleasure.) The second five rules admonish humans not to do those things that usually result in someone suffering those harms. (Do not deceive, Do not break your promise, Do not cheat, Do not break the law, and Do not neglect your duty.) In short, all rational persons want to avoid suffering harm and the moral system directs everyone to behave in ways that avoid causing harm to others. Thus rationality requires that persons espouse morality as a public system to be taught to everyone. Furthermore, the very close relation of morality to universal features of human nature, especially limited knowledge and the vulnerability to harm, means that these general moral rules would be endorsed by all people in all times and in all places.

Yet it is clear that the particular moral rules which people work with in myriad settings, scattered widely in time and place, are far more diverse and context-sensitive than these ten general moral rules. What follows is our explanation of how these more specific, particular moral rules are related to the general moral rules that we have described. Examples of these myriad particular moral rules are "Do not drink and drive," "Do not commit adultery," "Keep confidences," "Obtain informed consent." Our account provides an analysis of these ever-present particular rules, showing how they are fundamentally related to the general moral rules. Seeing the integral relationship of particular moral rules to the common moral system leads to understanding a great deal about what is important for working through moral problems. One develops a standard against which to measure rules claiming moral status and comes to see where, how, and to what extent cultural variables enter into moral deliberations. One also comes to understand the necessary ingredients for formulating new particular moral rules, which is an ongoing need in society.

Looking closely at particular moral rules in a wide variety of contexts, such as in various professions, occupations, practices, and organizations, shows that many particular rules are expressions of the general moral rules adapted to a special context. It is as if the beliefs, practices, customs, expectations, and traditions within various communities and subcommunities have combined with the general moral rules to produce rules more specifically designed for the community or culture or profession in question. (Later we focus more explicitly on various professional contexts within which general moral rules become specific and moral ideals become duties.) Only the general moral rules are universal because only they involve no beliefs which are not universally held and no practices which are not universal. The rules generated by blending the general moral rules with characteristics of a particular culture are not universal, for they involve beliefs held by those in that culture and practices which may be limited to that particular culture. Thus particular moral rules are the manifestation of the general moral rules as they are expressed within a particular culture or subculture.

General moral rule + a cultural institution or practice ↔ a particular moral rule.

For example,

"Do not kill, cause pain, or disability," + the practice of drinking alcoholic beverages and the practice of driving cars ↔ "Do not drink and drive."

And also,

"Do not cheat" + the institution of marriage ↔ "Do not commit adultery." (depending, of course, on the specific rules and practices governing the institution of marriage in that culture.)

Although "Do not kill" is a universally valid moral rule, not every society drinks alcoholic beverages and drives automobiles, so "Do not drink and drive" cannot be a universal moral rule. But in any society that imbibes intoxicating substances and has vehicles that can cause death, pain, and disability when not used properly, it is a particular moral rule. Similarly for the institution of marriage: "Do not cheat" is the general, universally valid moral rule, but within a society that has a practice of marriage that includes the expectation of sexual exclusivity, that general moral rule is expressed in the particular moral rule "Do not commit adultery." So particular moral rules are the expression of general moral rules in and through the nature, practices, and beliefs of a particular context. Thus morality is universal but responsive to the nuances of culture. Furthermore, even general moral rules take on special meanings and interpretations in light of various beliefs, customs, and practices within society and within professions. Indeed, the role of cultural context (including professional contexts) for interpreting the moral rules is very significant. We expand more explicitly on this notion later.

The beliefs prevalent in one culture might have the result that certain actions cause suffering, actions which in another culture cause no suffering whatsoever. Knowing that administering a blood transfusion to a devout Jehovah's Witness would cause him lifelong anguish (in his estimation perhaps worse than the death which otherwise probably would occur) entails that giving that transfusion is a violation of the general moral rule "Do not cause pain," as well as the rule "Do not deprive of freedom."

Even conventions of etiquette in a culture are related to the general moral rules. In anything like normal circumstances, a gratuitous breach of good manners that offends another person would, however minor, be an instance of morally unacceptable behavior. Examples might be anything from foul language to surly behavior to extremely casual dress at a formal occasion. Although the general moral rules relate to that which concerns all rational persons in every place and time, through features or aspects of particular cultures these general moral rules take on more particular content and interpretation. General moral rules admonish everyone not to cause pain and not to deprive of freedom, but it is the cultural setting that in part determines what is considered painful or offensive and what counts as depriving a person of freedom. In short, the moral rules are interpreted in light of the cultural context of beliefs and practices.

This interpretation is not a wide-open, free-for-all interpretation; the limits are rather tightly drawn. Disagreement on what counts as death, pain, disability, loss of freedom, and loss of pleasure is limited to unusual cases. Disagreement on what counts as causing these harms or on what counts as deceiving, breaking a promise, cheating, disobeying a law, or neglecting a duty, although not quite so limited, is not indefinitely malleable. The rules cannot be given just any interpretation one wants; every culture knows their function and finds the consequences of their unjustified violation destructive.

Particular Moral Ideals

It should be noted that there is an analogous culturally sensitive specification that takes place with respect to the moral ideals. Earlier we portrayed the particularization of the general moral rule as:

General moral rule + a cultural institution or practice ↔ a particular moral rule

One would expect that the same formulation could work with respect to the particularization of the moral ideals. The parallel formulation would be:

General moral ideal + a cultural institution or practice ↔ a particular moral ideal

Recall that the moral ideals encourage positive actions to prevent or relieve harms, but following them is not morally required. A general moral ideal mentions the general categories of harms, as in "Prevent or relieve pain," "Prevent disabilities"; a particular moral ideal would specify the particular harm to be prevented, for example, "Prevent drug addiction." What is odd about this is that moral ideals do not tend to be formulated in precise ways, not even the general moral ideals. The general moral rules require not causing harms and classifying the harms in precise categories makes it less likely for someone to be unjustifiably punished. Since preventing harm is not morally required, there is no need to have specific ideals that tell one precisely what to prevent or relieve. The moral ideals encourage preventing or relieving all harms, so there is no need to pick out certain categories of harms to be prevented or relieved. However, in certain contexts, more precise moral ideals are expressed, as in "Defend freedom," "Create equal opportunity," "Relieve pain," "Work for world peace," and "Feed the hungry." Obviously, whatever particular harm a society regards as serious, it encourages action to relieve or to prevent it. So the harms with which the society is most concerned strongly influences their formulation of particular moral ideals.

An interesting aspect to the moral ideals as they are expressed in different cultures, including professions, is that the prevention of a specific harm often becomes the duty of an individual or a group of individuals, by virtue of role, profession, occupation, or circumstance. All "citizens" might even acquire a common duty if a particular prevention of harm were seen as crucial to everyone. For example, in the context of the vast expanses of the western United States where being stranded in the desert can be life-threatening, everyone has the mutually beneficial and agreed-on duty to assist stranded motorists, providing it does not subject one to undue risk or burden.

The contextual specification of the moral ideals often results in positive duties, that is, duties incumbent on certain individuals or groups to take action, for example, the duty of nurses to relieve pain of patients, whereas the contextual specification of the moral rules usually results in prohibition of particular actions incumbent on everyone, for example, the prohibition of doctors from causing unnecessary pain. Thus many codified professional duties are contextual specifications of the ideals of preventing specific harms, rather than simply avoiding causing specific harms. Within the profession these ideals become duties, and as such they are morally required; they apply to all members of the profession just as the moral rules apply to everyone in society at large. Later in this chapter when we discuss the duties of those in the health care professions, it becomes clear that the scope of the duties in time and place are limited by the practices and purposes of the professions.

Interpretation of the Moral Rules

The influence of cultural or professional settings on the understanding of moral rules and ideals needs to be probed in more detail. In the preceding sections we provided a variety of examples of how cultural settings yield particular moral rules; in this section we show how they may result in some apparently immoral behavior not being considered as a violation of any moral rule. We first examine kinds of actions that are not violations of the moral rules, even though on the surface they might appear to be because the actions result in someone becoming stressed, annoyed, unhappy, or misled. Although this kind of action, wearing an orange necktie with a fuchsia shirt, for example, results in someone being annoyed, it does not need moral justification unless one intentionally wears this clothing in order to annoy someone. Even if one knows that someone will be annoyed by what he is wearing, he violates no moral rule with respect to that person although his action results in the other person being annoyed. However, it might be following a moral ideal not to wear those clothes after discovering that person's psychological distress.

These kinds of actions typically include one's choice of clothing, hairstyle, office decor, and so on. They could also include life-styles, such as whether one rides motorcycles or goes mountain climbing. In the medical context, examples of such actions would be a patient rationally deciding whether the particular burdens of his life make it not worth living, or a patient rationally deciding whether to have a less disfiguring procedure even though it decreases the probability of her long-term survival. These kinds of actions or decisions may cause psychological distress to others, but they need not violate any moral rules. What all these actions and decisions have in common is that the harm that would result from taking away a person's freedom to engage in such activities or make such decisions is greater than the harm that results from their not being morally prohibited.

Part of what underlies this line of reasoning is the realization that no matter what choices one makes in the above personal kinds of situations, there is probably someone somewhere who will be upset, misled, or, at the very least, annoyed. It is as if humans intuitively and mutually understand that if *my* objections are sufficient to prohibit *your* choice of neckties (because your neckties are aesthetically painful to me), then *your* objections are sufficient to prohibit *my* hairstyle. Similarly, if morality prohibited your dangerous (to yourself) hobbies (because they cause me stress), then morality could prohibit my selection of friends (because they annoy you). Thus all of these kinds of actions that are not intentional violations of the moral rules (that is, actions done for the purpose of causing others pain, and so on) are, under normal circumstances, allowed even if others suffer as a result, because the annoyances are, on balance, lesser harms than the deprivation of freedom involved in prohibiting them. It is certainly a matter of mutual accommodation, but it is also and especially a matter of contextual interpretation of the moral rule and of what counts as a violation.[1]

Furthermore, and more basically, these actions are interpreted as not being violations of the moral rules by a procedure analogous to the procedure for justifying violations of moral rules discussed in Chapter 2. For example, if one knows he will offend someone in his office by wearing his hair in a ponytail, he can consider whether this violation of a moral rule is allowed. Or, rather than consider if this violation of the moral rule proscribing the causing of pain is allowed, he can consider whether his action should even be interpreted as a violation of that moral rule. After looking at all the morally relevant features of the case, essentially he is determining how he, as an impartial rational person, would judge the consequences of everyone knowing that this kind of act is interpreted as a violation of a moral rule that has to be justified. In effect he is judging whether these consequences are significantly better or significantly worse than the consequences of everyone knowing that this kind of act is not interpreted as a violation of a moral rule.

For some personal actions, such as choosing a hairstyle, it seems clear that interpreting them as "violations" would result in more harm than not interpreting them as violations. These kinds of actions include (1) actions involving matters so personally important, affecting primarily oneself, that each person wants to make his or her own decision and not have it imposed by someone else, like deciding when one's suffering outweighs the value of life, (2) actions whose effects are so variable that there is always someone somewhere who finds it objectionable, like a man wearing earrings, and (3) actions that are too trivial to worry about, like using a toothpick in a public place. In all these kinds of cases surely most rational persons would find it preferable not to interpret the moral rules so as to declare these kinds of actions immoral, even if some people sometimes suffer or are offended as the result of such actions.

As stated above, the ultimate justification for these interpretations of general and particular moral rules is determined by a procedure similar to the procedure for justifying moral rule violations described in Chapter 2. The essence of that procedure is to identify the morally relevant features of the particular circumstances, to calculate the balance of harms caused by interpreting that kind of act as a violation versus not so interpreting it, and to consider what impartial rational persons would find acceptable as a public policy incumbent on everyone in these same morally relevant circumstances. This is to say that the interpretation of moral rules is ultimately justified in the same way that any intentional violations of moral rules are justified, so there are not two different standards at work.

There are several reasons why it is important to clarify the matter of the interpretation of moral rules. Such clarification explains a large variety of actions, such as personal actions, all of which, under normal conditions, have roughly the same interpretation. It is handy and efficient simply to refer to "the matter of interpretation." Behind that phrase lies a line of reasoning based on our moral theory. The theory explains why the interpretation of moral rules that should be chosen is the interpretation which produces a public system resulting in less harm than any alternative interpretations.

Highlighting the matter of rule interpretation also helps one to see that interpretations can change in different settings. The changes are not ad hoc and whimsical; they are appropriate and systematic, explained by the concept of morality as a public system. With regard to interpretations of general and particular moral rules, this theory explains why the domain of actions not covered by a moral rule can contract or expand in different groups and subgroups. Depending on the nature of the group of persons who are interacting and the intensity and frequency of their interaction, an interpretation of a moral rule may be more or less inclusive of particular actions. For example, within a family there might be a more expansive interpretation, that is, an interpretation such that more actions would need justification than is true for actions in the public at large. Thus fewer actions might be completely up to the individual's own discretion. A style of dress or of haircut, a personal habit, or a linguistic expression that in the public at large is interpreted as not needing justification might well need justification within a family setting. That is because the family is living in such close quarters that small annoyances can really become major irritants for others. In that microcosm (or, micro public system) the harms that result from the behavior may outweigh the harms that result from prohibiting that kind of behavior. But, of course, impartial rational persons may disagree about these different interpretations.

Similarly, within a club, a congregation, or a business office, the interpretation of moral rules might be broader, meaning that more actions need moral justification—actions which in the public at large would not be interpreted as moral rule violations. Among the reasons for the differences of interpretation are duties of certain individuals within the group, such as a parent's duty to set standards of behavior and self-expression, and the fact that the family is living in such close quarters that one's irritating behavior can result in significantly more harm than would result from restraining that behavior. Also the fact that some of these groupings have a voluntary membership indicates that the member has accepted the broader (more inclusive) interpretation and will refrain from certain behaviors that ordinarily (outside the "club" membership) are allowed by the standard interpretation of the rule.

In discussing the interpretation of moral rules, we have used the qualifying expression "in normal circumstances." This expression served as a reminder that actions which normally are not interpreted as violations of moral rules (even though they result in irritation or discomfort or offense) nevertheless might in unusual circumstances be considered violations. Of course, doing any action with the intention that it result in harm to another, for instance wearing a necktie known to be offensive to a particular person specifically to annoy that person, is a moral rule violation. However, using language known, or that should be known, to be offensive to a person who is currently confined to bed and in severe pain is also regarded as a moral rule violation and is usually morally unacceptable. This kind of behavior is usually termed thoughtless or callous, and unlike most actions that are not intentional violations of moral rules, there is a low cost in avoiding this hurtful behavior and a high cost to the individuals hurt.

This crucial matter of interpretation is another area where moral disagreement can take place. Facts and the ranking of harms were previously acknowledged as sources for much of moral disagreement, but there also can be genuine disagreement about how a moral rule should be interpreted in a particular context. Should it be narrowly or broadly interpreted? Is it a standard interpretation of a rule of one's profession, or is it a newer and more questionable one? Is it an interpretation significant to an ethnic subculture but not to the hospital culture in which the person finds himself?

Cautions Concerning the Interpretation of Moral Rules

Our examples have generally been instances of behavior considered acceptable by virtue of being of a special kind (namely, those unintentionally harmful actions whose prohibition in a public system would cause more harm than if they were not interpreted as violations of moral rules). However, there are many unintentionally harmful actions that offend so many people that they are regarded as morally unacceptable behavior. For example, public nudity or public displays of sexual intimacy are deemed offensive to so many people that such behavior is interpreted as a violation of the moral rule "Do not cause pain or suffering." It might be argued as a matter of taste, of religion, or of the public good, but in any case the balance of harm caused and harm avoided shifts, so that it seems more harm is prevented by prohibiting such actions than is caused by having the prohibitions.[2]

We have been discussing actions that are usually not interpreted as violations even though sometimes they result in harm. Similarly, there are activities, practices, or policies that often result in someone being offended or upset or disappointed even though it was never intended that any particular person be hurt in any way. A lottery has a lot of losers; a sporting event not only has to have losers if it is to have winners but its venue necessarily has limited capacity for spectators (so someone may fail to get in); an art show can award only a limited number of prizes (so the first-prize winner may be regarded as having "harmed" the second-prize winner by keeping her from first place.) These and many other such activities are instances where, by the nature of the activity, someone inevitably suffers, though there was never any intention that any particular identifiable individual or group suffer.

These instances of resulting harm are not interpreted as violations of moral rules because to do so would eliminate desired activities. The resulting harms are not only not intentionally caused, they may not be "caused" by the action at all; they are simply the natural consequences of the "rules of the game." No moral blame is attached to these practices. They are not interpreted as violations because to do so would eliminate desired activities which, viewed from the perspective of a public system, significantly outweigh any resulting harms. Of course these policies, practices, games, and social arrangements that result in someone suffering (though not intentionally) could (if in doubt) be examined from a moral point of view, that is, by seeing if these practices could be justified by consideration of the variables detailed in Chapter 2.

If, for example, the activity involved serious harm or deceit or deprivation of freedom against a particular group, it might well be judged immoral. Boxing is an activity that now and again comes up for this kind of moral review. Though boxers voluntarily subject themselves to the pain and risks of injury and are not supposed to try intentionally to seriously injure each other (but only to win points or render the other unable to get up before a count of ten), the fact that serious injuries often do occur can offend the sensitivities of the public sufficiently for them to consider boxing immoral. One important lesson one learns from all these examples is that there is no simple identity between a harm resulting from one's actions on the one hand and "causing a harm" (or breaking a moral rule) on the other. Thus there is no simple inference from "harm resulted from his action" to "he caused harm" or "he broke a moral rule." And given that many violations of moral rules are justified, it is even more clearly false to infer, from the fact that "harm resulted from his action," that he acted immorally.

How Many Moralities?

Readers may be confused by the apparent conflict between their own awareness that there are many moral codes or "moralities" and our continuing treatment of morality as though it were one. We are, of course, aware that there are many domains with their own explicit or implicit moral codes: business ethics, environmental ethics, medical ethics, computer ethics, military ethics, government ethics, and many others. Our discussion of interpretation in this current chapter should explain, at least partially, why it appears that there are so many moralities, even though we maintain that there is but one general morality which holds for everyone in all times and places. As shown in Chapter 2, morality is an informal public system that applies to all rational persons and is grounded in universal features of human nature (vulnerability, fallibility, the desire to avoid harm). The different interpretations of the moral rules, allowed by the informal nature of morality, explain how it seems that there are so many moralities.

Part of our task in this chapter is to show how common morality relates to all these various manifestations. It has been shown how the general moral rules, in combination with institutions, beliefs, and practices of various cultures, yield particular moral rules. That phenomenon illustrates the universality of morality, while accounting for its protean manifestations in various cultures and settings. Morality, properly understood, is culture-sensitive; it is expressed through the practices, beliefs, and institutions of a culture. As we have emphasized, this does not mean that anything goes, for the general moral rules establish ranges of morally permissible and morally required actions. The various cultures provide the shading and nuances that weigh the various harms differently or even add some harms as a result of particular beliefs held by a significant number of people in the culture. For example, in some cultures there might be such a strong belief in a desirable afterlife that loss of life is not ranked as worse than any significant pain or disability. Even in a certain age group, maybe octogenarians, death is generally more welcome than enduring significant pain. In one culture, failure to provide a dowry is considered a terrible offense, whereas in another it is a matter of relative indifference.

Professional Ethics

Professional ethics is just another "culture" in which the general moral rules yield particular moral rules and are subject to interpretation. Each profession or each domain of activity has practices, understandings, and dilemmas that call for a specific fashioning of the various moral rules to deal with the particularities of its activities.

For example, in medicine the need for the physician to obtain intimate information from the patient, in addition to the fact that people generally do not want intimate information about themselves to be revealed, in conjunction with the general moral rule not to cause pain, generates the medical ethical rule "Do not breach confidentiality." Traditionally it has been understood and expected that confidences would not be violated, and formulating the rule of confidentiality simply makes it more explicit.

Another example of medicine's particularizing of general morality is in the matter of truth-telling. The general moral rule "Do not deceive," in medicine usually takes the form of "Tell the truth."[3] However, in the context of medical practice this broader interpretation makes it more useful as an action guide. Whereas in ordinary circumstances, although one is morally required not to deceive, one is not morally required to "tell the truth." (It might be none of the other person's business; if I do not tell my neighbor that my wife and I are going to be divorced, I have not deceived him.) But in medicine it is the physician's duty to disclose to the patient the relevant facts about the patient's condition, so that not telling this information is interpreted as deceiving. (There can be exceptions, but they must be justified, like all violations of moral rules.) This duty has come about by the needs and the expectations within the doctor-patient relationship. Hence in the particular circumstances of the practice of medicine, interpretation of the general moral rule is appropriate.

Similarly in the medical moral admonition to obtain informed consent before proceeding with therapy, the general moral rule "Do not deprive of freedom" is expressed in the context of the characteristic interactions and procedures of medicine. The very nature of the practice of medicine makes causing pain so everpresent (just in order to do its job) that protections against that happening without the patient's permission must be institutionalized in medicine's moral code. Thus the general moral rule prohibiting the deprivation of freedom is particularized for the special circumstances of medicine; it is expressed in the medical moral obligation to obtain informed consent, which, among other things, guards against depriving anyone of the opportunity to choose whether or not to undergo a medical or surgical procedure, especially a painful one. The American Council of Physicians, in their recent code of ethics, makes obtaining valid consent an explicit duty of physicians.

"Do Your Duty" and Professional Ethics

We have suggested that many of the particular moral rules of a profession are specifications or interpretations of the general moral rules (which are valid for all persons in all times and places) in the context of the special circumstances, practices, relationships, and purposes of the profession. Thus the particular moral rules are far more specific with respect to the special circumstances characterizing a particular domain or profession. The goal of morality remains the same, namely, to lessen the overall evil or harm in the world, but now the rules are much more precise with respect to and sensitive to a special realm of activity. This point might be more intuitively seen by considering the general moral rule "Obey the law." Obviously laws vary from place to place, depending on such matters as history, culture, and beliefs. Thus the general moral rule requiring obeying the law gets specified within particular contexts.

One of the general moral rules that is frequently expressed in particular moral rules throughout countless realms of activity is the rule "Do your duty" (or, to state it as a prohibition, "Do not neglect your duty"). Recall (from Chapter 2) the justification of this rule as a moral rule. If not followed in general, there would be a considerable increase in the amount of harm suffered. That is because everyone becomes dependent on others doing their duty; everyone comes to rely on these others and to make plans around them, expecting that they will do their duty. This is true of lifeguards, babysitters, firefighters, insurance agents, police officers, taxi drivers, and countless others. It is to the interest and well-being of everyone that no one neglects her duty.

Where do these duties come from? Who decides what they are? It should be clear that duties are normally associated with roles, occupations, relationships, and the professions. The duties constitute the expectations that everyone can legitimately have of the role, occupation, relationship, or profession. Society has certain expectations of firefighters, doctors, lifeguards, parents, and airplane pilots. How do these expectations get established?

There are many sources for role-related duties. Tradition is a major one. A group comes to provide a particular service, in a particular way, and eventually others come to count on these provisions. Thus a tradition is born. It may be a role (like that of firefighters) that develops over decades, even centuries. Sometimes the providers can develop expectations in the public by practice and by projection of image through advertising or group-promotion. Very often the groups have a code that specifies what can be expected of them by others. Certain standards evolve so that now these become "duties," because others have come to count on these actions. Thus there are "standards of practice" in medicine that become duties of the profession.

Many moral disputes pivot on the vagueness of duties: everyone may agree that one is morally required not to neglect his duty, but not everyone agrees on precisely what those duties are. The details of duties can be vague because of a variety of factors: the tradition is not clearly established; there are various interpretations of the code; and different practices and standards of practice are followed in different parts of the country. The duties of parents and of babysitters are seldom stated in codes or contracts; it is debatable whether a sports hero has a duty to live an exemplary life (inasmuch as his or her behavior influences the young.) Not infrequently these issues are settled in court (for example, whether opthamologists have a duty to screen every patient over 40 for glaucoma by measuring intraocular pressure), and the resultant court ruling then becomes another tradition relevant for interpreting duty, namely, the legal tradition. The precedents set in such cases become the standard of duty in those particular roles or occupations.

The nature of duties is a rich topic, especially important to an understanding of bioethics. Our point in Chapter 2 was to show the justification for the moral rule "Do your duty." Our point here is to show that duties grow out of various roles and relationships. The importance of duties is that they show how a general moral rule can be significantly culture-sensitive. We do not think it appropriate to talk about universal duties; we regard duties as developing around a role or relationship in any "culture," whether familial, professional, occupational, or social. If there are valid expectations that others have come to count on, then it is likely that a duty exists. The duty "grew up" in, and is indigenous to, that particular setting and culture.

Though books and articles on medical ethics frequently appeal to the "duties" and obligations of health professionals, these appeals generally are simply ad hoc declarations. There is no theory to which these duties are related and by which they are explained. Consequently, there is no way to distinguish between professional duties and moral requirements in general. In moral disputes it is important to know the difference, since it is relevant to how the points should be argued. It may well be that the so-called Principles of Biomedical Ethics should be understood as simply a rough classification of duties of health care professionals at a certain level of generality. As such, the principles are a kind of generalized grouping of duties (divided into four or five categories) that have accrued to the health care professions. There is no underlying account or explanation, but only some organizational principle at work. The context for these observations about the "principles" is provided in Chapter 4, in which we present a general critique of "principlism." We will now and again refer to the concept of duty throughout the following chapters, and it is always a role-specific obligation that we have in mind. Our goal to this point has been to show how public morality bears on professional morality, and, along the way, to show how both are sensitive to context.

Other Sources of Duties

We have discussed the integral relationship of professional ethics to common morality. We have shown how the moral rules are expressed or interpreted in the context of a profession, thus articulating moral requirements which are much more specific and appropriate to the particulars of the practice of that profession. Deceiving, cheating, breaking promises, depriving of freedom, causing pain, and the rest have their own fairly unique interpretations in various professions, so that the moral admonitions within that profession must specifically speak to those typical moral hazards.

With that as background the next step toward viewing professional ethics will be easier to understand. Our basic distinction between moral rules and moral ideals (Chapter 2) enables us to explain how the ideals play a role in professional ethics. Moral ideals express the aspirations of the profession: its pledges to go above and beyond what is required by the general moral rules. That means the profession is not content with simply not causing harm, but it commits itself to going out of its way to prevent and to relieve harm. The ideals, like the rules, are context-sensitive, that is, they are relevant to each profession's capabilities and interests; they express the ways that those in that profession can prevent and relieve harm. Doctors presumably do not turn away anyone in need of medical care; they treat regardless of ability to pay. Doctors always act primarily in the best interest of the patient rather than in their own interest. Doctors are dedicated to the prevention and cure of sickness and suffering. These are ideals set by the medical profession, though perhaps clarified and modified by law and society.

There is always some vagueness concerning the ideals. When do they cease to be accepted simply as ideals and become instead duties of the profession? In ordinary morality the ideals are characterized by being impossible to practice toward everyone, impartially, all the time. Similarly a profession treats its accepted ideals as goals, as something to be worked toward, as aspirations. It can hardly fulfill these ideals toward everyone, impartially, all the time. Nevertheless, some ideals do become duties, but others do not, and it is important to be aware of the difference. Those that doctors are expected to follow toward each of their patients might be considered duties. Necessarily those ideals that become duties need to have significant limitations, since it is humanly impossible to follow unlimited moral ideals toward all one's patients, all the time. These duties are generally limited to those that can be accomplished while in the presence of the patient: eliciting relevant information or explaining information relevant to obtaining consent for therapy. Of course there can be some dispute about how much time and effort is required of a doctor to do his or her duty and how much constitutes going above and beyond duty, and so acting on an ideal. (See Chapter 7, where *valid* or informed consent is distinguished from *ideal* consent.) Many ideals or aspirations never become duties. Medicine might pledge itself to achieving health defined as total mental, physical, and social well-being, but surely no one holds the profession or an individual physician responsible for failing to accomplish that goal.

The admonition to physicians "Always act in the best interest of one's patients" is vague and can be interpreted so as to make it impossible to satisfy completely. If a physician goes out of town for a vacation, she is hardly acting in the best interests of her patients. There is probably always someone who is in need of the physician's help, or who at least would do better or feel better if the physician were never away. The same holds true of the normal work day.

Should a physician be on call 24 hours a day, forever, in order to satisfy maximally "the best interest of her patients?" Should she spend many hours with each patient? These actions cannot literally become the duty of any individual physician, though in achieving ideals, groups of physicians might make certain rational arrangements among themselves in order to fulfill the ideal of twenty-four hour coverage for their patients, or, for that matter, for the whole town. But notice, once this achievable goal is stated and practiced, it might become a duty, because people reasonably come to count on it and may be harmed if that duty is neglected. But when it holds and when it does not, when it is clearly a duty and when it is not, becomes the focus of many law suits. However, the unclear or disputed cases do not discount the value of the distinction between duty and ideal, indeed, they make it important to become as clear as possible about the distinction in different circumstances. Most cases are clear-cut, but there are always some instances that remain vague and can only be settled by adjudication or stipulation.

Professional Rules of Conduct

Many rules that apply to individuals by virtue of their occupation or role are not the expression of general moral rules or ideals in that particular context. The "rules of conduct" for professional conduct contain a diverse collection of rule types, only some of which are directly related to the general moral rules or ideals. This fact can be confusing, since the different types of rules have different purposes; some serve general moral goals and some serve the special goals of the members of the profession. It is important to sort out these rule types so they can be understood and evaluated in terms of their purposes, their validity, and their relationship to common morality. We have already described those that are directly based on common morality (both moral rules and moral ideals), which are expressed as particular rules and ideals within the context of a particular profession. But mixed in with these clear moral rules and ideals are at least two other types of rules: preventive and group-protective.

Preventive Rules

The preventive rules are those rules that effectively rule against behavior which, though not immoral in itself, is thought to make immoral acts more tempting and thus more likely. They serve to diminish enticement to break a moral rule. Examples of this kind of preventive moral rule are the rule among baseball players that they not bet on games, and the rule among lawyers that they not be mentioned as inheritors in the wills of their clients. Usually these rules are written and agreed upon by the profession itself as part of its code of ethics. However, a rule might be imposed by law if it is thought to affect the public (for instance, the law might state that physicians may not refer their patients to facilities and services in which the physicians themselves have a financial interest.) Notice that none of these forbidden actions are immoral in and of themselves. Rather the existence of the forbidden practice is considered a "moral hazard," in that it could easily lead to immorality or at least the appearance of immorality.

The baseball player might be tempted to play poorly for his team in order to win the bet he had placed; the lawyer might be tempted to manipulate her way into receiving a portion of the inheritance from one of her clients; the physician might send his patient for unnecessary diagnostic services from which the physician gains financially. All these latter actions are, of course, immoral simply by virtue of the general moral rules (the rules, for example, proscribing cheating, deceiving, causing pain, and depriving of freedom). However, the preventive moral rules are prospective in nature, designed to help avoid infringements of moral rules. The preventive moral rules themselves then become part of the ethical code so that, now, though doing the action they proscribe does no harm in itself, breaking that rule must be considered immoral for those members within the group, because within that group, following that rule has become their duty.

Group-Protective Rules

The group-protective rules mixed in with the particular moral rules and the preventive moral rules in the various codes of conduct serve more to enhance or preserve the public image of the group, or to prevent some harm from being done to the group or to other members of the group. These rules are more like guild rules: rules to enhance and nurture the profession or occupation itself. Examples are those exhortations to engage in some activity (group aspirations) that enhances the public image of the profession, or admonitions not to lure away each other's clients, or not to do anything that has even the appearance of wrongdoing. As with the particular moral rules and ideals and the preventive rules, these group-protective rules become duties for the members of that occupation or profession.

What is the relationship of these various rules to morality? Obviously, the particular moral rules and ideals are integral parts of morality because they are contextual expressions of the general moral rules and ideals. And the preventive rules might be seen as based on moral ideals, because they are exhortations to prevent harms by urging the members not to put themselves in the position where causing harms would be easy and tempting.

The group-protective rules, however, are not really moral rules, although all members of the profession are required to obey them. As with all the rules in the codes, they are duties of the members of that group. Each member of the group benefits from obedience to these mutually agreed-upon rules, and members are required to fulfill them. The fact that "Do your duty" is a general moral rule is, no doubt, partially responsible for thinking of codes of conduct as moral codes. But the most that can be said about the group-protective rules is that they must be morally acceptable. They must not involve unjustified exceptions to any of the general moral rules. No matter how one thinks about this mixed bag of rules called "professional codes," "codes of ethics," or "codes of conduct," the important moral point is this: they are morally acceptable as long as they do not require unjustifiable violations of any general moral rules. *No one can have a duty to do something immoral.* So there cannot be a duty to protect a colleague in the group if that involves deceiving, or cheating, or causing pain, or suffering to someone outside the group.

A group or profession cannot simply construct any rules of behavior they want and make them "duties." To be considered duties, they must not only not involve unjustifiable violations of any general moral rules, they must be supportive of the goal of morality, that is, to reduce the amount of evil in the world. Notice how the preventive rules, though not proscribing immoral actions themselves, do proscribe actions that can all too easily lead to breaking a moral rule. As such they are integrally related to the moral rules, but they apply only to those who are members of the group in question. In a sense these preventive rules could be seen as turning moral ideals into duties, inasmuch as they call for some sacrifice by the member, of freedom, say, in order to achieve a prevention of harm. A group can always take on itself a more stringent morality, that is, one that not only does not violate any of the general moral rules but which demands more of its members than is required by the general moral rules. Even the group-protective rules protect other members of the profession from suffering unwanted harms, without thereby causing harm to those not in the profession, thus even they are supportive of the general goal of morality of lessening the amount of harm in the world.

Moral Expertise

An important goal of our first three chapters is to give confidence to general readers to engage in moral deliberations. They should realize that morality is basically one. Their moral intuitions, as trained and honed in everyday life, should stand them in good stead in professional ethics. All rational persons can and must participate in moral decision making. Everyone understands morality without the need for "expertise." Everyone can and does discuss moral issues in a meaningful way without having had courses in either ethical theory or professional ethics.

The technical language of professional ethics can sometimes obscure the real moral issues. Though technical language can make valuable distinctions and facilitate precision, it can also incline people to force their reflections into fixed categories and consequently to miss the obviously immoral. Technical language also tends to produce "moral experts" (distinguished by being facile in the use of the technical language), which conflicts with the nature of morality as an informal public system that applies to all rational persons. This means that moral experts should not be allowed to overrule one's own moral intuitions or to inhibit one from participating in moral deliberations. Ordinary understanding of ethics is usually sufficient, as long as one knows and appreciates the facts, purposes, understandings, and relationships of the field whose ethics he is dealing with. Common morality itself is fairly straightforward; everyone understands what it is to harm someone, to deceive, to cheat, to neglect one's duty, and so on, and even has a good sense of when and why it would be justified to violate one of these moral rules.

Notes

1. This line of reasoning is often expressed in the language of rights: "I have a right to wear my hair as long as I want, no matter what anyone thinks." See *Morality,* pp. 113–116

2. See Joel Feinberg, *Offense to Others: The Moral Limits of the Criminal Law* (New York: Oxford University Press, 1985) for a detailed discussion of these matters.

3. This formulation has drawbacks as a general injunction, for it requires far more than simply not deceiving. For a fuller discussion of this point, see *Morality,* pp. 127–128.

4

Principlism

Having presented our own account of morality, from the foundations to the practical rules and ideals that guide actions, we devote this chapter to highlighting its distinctive differences. In order for our account of morality to be clearly and accurately perceived, we contrast it with the dominant "theory" that has pervaded biomedical ethics for almost two decades. We want to minimize the chances that aspects of this dominant theory might unwittingly and automatically be read into our own account, so we highlight the significant differences between the two accounts. Inasmuch as part of the rationale for this book is to show the relevance of theory to practice, it is appropriate to bring the matter into sharper focus by examining in detail the dominant theory in use. Readers who have neither interest in nor commitment to another theory of ethics can, without significant loss of understanding, skip this chapter.

In arguing that our theory is more adequate and more useful we follow the time-honored tradition of theory replacement. We point out how our theory (1) overcomes the inadequacies of the dominant theory, (2) accounts for what is good in the dominant theory, and (3) is more readily usable, understandable, and intuitively correct than the dominant theory. Thus, in this chapter, we focus particularly on the inadequacies of the theory in question, and show how the good aspects of it are better accounted for by our theory.

The dominant view in question we have labeled "principlism."[1] It is characterized by its citing of four principles which constitute the core of its account of biomedical ethics: beneficence, autonomy, nonmaleficence, and justice. So entrenched is this "theory," that clinical moral problems are often grouped (for conferences, papers, and books) according to which principle is deemed most relevant and necessary for solving them. It has become fashionable and customary to cite one or another of these principles as the key for resolving a particular biomedical ethical problem. Throughout much of the biomedical ethical literature, authors seem to believe that they have brought theory to bear on the problem before them insofar as they have mentioned one or more of the principles. Thus, not only do the principles presumably lead to acceptable solutions, but they are also treated by many as the ultimate grounds of appeal.

We examine principlism by looking at the undeniably leading account of principlism, namely that of Beauchamp and Childress, as manifested in the editions of their book, *Principles of Biomedical Ethics.*[2] Their account is the very best the position has to offer, and it is their account which has so pervaded the world of biomedical ethics. For many years it has provided the conceptual framework of the Georgetown Intensive Bioethics Course, a one-week summer course which has been attended by thousands from the United States as well as from around the world. Beauchamp and Childress's book is outstanding for its insights into particular problems in bioethics and for its sensitivity to important issues and relevant subtleties. Our criticism focuses only on their theoretical account of morality.

As we emphasized in previous articles on principlism, we are not criticizing Beauchamp and Childress as such. We select them as the very best spokesmen for the principle-based approach to bioethics, but we are concerned about the widespread popularization of principlism throughout the biomedical ethics world, where it is not dealt with as carefully as it is in the hands of Beauchamp and Childress. This concern is more important than ever to emphasize, because principlism is still flourishing, even though Beauchamp and Childress have changed their theoretical account considerably. Their fourth edition (1994) has accommodated so well to the criticisms of principlism that Ezekiel Emanuel entitled his review of the book "The Beginning of the End of Principlism."[3] This turn of events helps to reinforce our claim that it is not particularly Beauchamp and Childress that we are criticizing, but a paradigmatic form of principlism, which has been and still is thriving throughout the bioethical world. We do continue occasionally to cite early editions of *Principles of Biomedical Ethics,* but only because those editions are the ones that have been so influential in shaping the paradigmatic form of principlism which persists in the bioethical world at large. Meanwhile, we remind the readers that the fourth edition is very different, and according to Ezekiel Emanuel may no longer even be principlism. In this edition Beauchamp and Childress appeal, as we ourselves have long done, to a basis in common morality, the claims concerning which, Emanuel says, "constitute a radical change and herald the end of 'principlism.'"[4]

To understand the historical background of principlism's pervasive influence, it is helpful to review the "Belmont Report," which seems to be the progenitor of the principles.

The Principles in Historical Context

The principles emerged from the work of the National Commission for the Protection of Human Subjects of Biomedical and Behavioral Research, which was created by Congress in 1974. One of the charges to the commission was to identify the basic ethical principles that should underlie the conduct of biomedical and behavioral research involving human subjects, and to develop guidelines which should be followed to ensure that such research is conducted in accordance with those principles.[5]

At that time there was frustration over the many and various rules for research that were spelled out in the extant codes covering research using human subjects. These codes included the Nuremberg Code of 1947, the Helsinki Declaration of 1964 (revised in 1975), and the 1971 Guidelines issued by the (then) United States Department of Health, Education, and Welfare. (The "Guidelines" were codified into U.S. federal regulations in 1974.) The assortment of rules seemed at times inadequate, conflicting, and difficult to apply. It therefore became part of the commission's charge to formulate "broader ethical principles [to] provide a basis on which specific rules may be formulated, criticized and interpreted."[6]

The higher level of generality was achieved by the commission and articulated as three ethical principles: the principle of respect for persons, the principle of beneficence, and the principle of justice. These principles comprised the "Belmont Report," so-named because their articulation was the culmination of intense discussions that took place at the Smithsonian Institution's Belmont Conference Center. In effect, these principles sought to frame in a more general and useful way the moral concerns that underlay the diverse, ambiguous, and (sometimes) conflicting rules comprising the various ethical codes related to research on human subjects.

The work of the commission was significant. It was insightful and helpful; it elegantly captured in a more general way the basic moral concerns haltingly expressed in the miscellaneous codes. The commission also went on to delineate some of the more practical consequences of the principles. From the principle of respect for persons came attention to autonomy (which from their discussion seems more like what is now regarded as "competence") and to informed consent. From the principle of beneficence came the obligation to maximize benefits over risks and not to harm. From the principle of justice came attention to fairness in the distribution of the benefits and burdens of research.

These principles were clearly intended to be generalized guides for protecting humans as subjects in biomedical and behavioral research. Also, they seem less to have been derived from a theory of any sort and more to have been abstractions from ethical rules expressing particular moral concerns. In a summary fashion the principles generalize and encapsulate a variety of moral considerations especially applicable to research using human subjects. Very likely these formulations additionally accomplished a crucial maneuver for the commission. They made possible a consensus in a setting where a more detailed account of morality would probably never have been agreed upon.

From these beginnings the application of the principles has grown and now encompasses biomedical ethics in general. Each principle has changed somewhat as its meaning is elaborated, as subdivision takes place, and as another principle or two is added (varying with each author). For example, for Beauchamp and Childress, the principle of beneficence spawns the principle of nonmaleficence. Nevertheless, in one form or another, these principles have come to dominate the field of bioethics, which is why we are investigating several of them in detail.

Our overall impression of the principles is that they express something very important, something very basic to common moral intuitions. However, for reasons to be seen, they are inadequate and misleading. Our plan is to show how our more comprehensive theoretical framework can encompass and preserve what is good about the principles, while eliminating their unfortunate features. We see them as historically providing a conceptual ladder that allowed the field to achieve certain insights and goals. But having enabled that achievement, the ladder is best set aside because it has become cumbersome and possibly dangerous.

Critique of Principlism: Our General Approach

Although we have been referring to principlism as a theory, it is not in fact a theory, but rather a collection of "principles," which together are popularly but mistakenly thought to function as a theory in guiding action. Principlism puts forward certain principles which it considers to be the high-level "action guides" most relevant for dealing with issues of biomedical ethics. A variety of principles are claimed by different authors to be "the principles of biomedical ethics," but the best known and most frequently cited principles are those labeled "the principle of autonomy," "the principle of nonmaleficence," "the principle of beneficence," and "the principle of justice." Because these four occur by far most frequently together (and thus are more apt to pose as a theory of biomedical ethics), and because these are the ones espoused by the prime expositors of principlism (Beauchamp and Childress), they are the ones we analyze in order to contrast and compare them with our own theory.

In this chapter we show that principlism is mistaken about the nature of morality and is misleading about the foundations of ethics. We argue that its "principles" are really misnomers, since, when examined carefully, they are not action guides at all. Traditionally, principles really are action guides that summarize and encapsulate a whole theory and thus, in a shorthand manner, assist a moral agent in making a moral decision. Those kinds of principles are to be clearly distinguished from those of principlism. We argue that the principles of principlism primarily function as checklists, naming issues worth remembering when one is considering a biomedical moral issue. "Consider this. . . consider that. . . remember to look for. . ." is what they tell the agent; they do not embody an articulated, established, and unified moral system capable of providing useful guidance.

These principles presumably follow from several different moral theories, though that connection is neither explicitly focused on nor clearly stated by the proponents of principlism. This is a matter of significant concern since there seem to be no underlying connections among the principles. They do not grow out of a common foundation and they have no systematic relationship among themselves. Though each may be an expression of one or another important and traditional concern of morality, there is no priority ranking among them nor even any specified procedure for resolving the conflicts that inevitably arise between principles. This serves to perpetuate what we have called the "anthology syndrome." This, as described in Chapter 1, is a kind of relativism espoused (perhaps unwittingly) by many books (usually anthologies) of bioethics. They parade before the reader a variety of "theories" of ethics (Kantianism, deontology, utilitarianism, other forms of consequentialism) and say, in effect, choose the theory, maxim, principle, or rule that best suits you or the situation. Similarly, though each of the principles of principlism embodies a key concern from one or another theory of morality, no account is given of whether (or how) they are related to each other. We conclude that principlism obscures and confuses moral reasoning by its failure to provide genuine action guides and by its eclectic and unsystematic account of morality.

We begin our analysis with a brief discussion of the principles of nonmaleficence and justice in order to set the context for our argument. Then we discuss in more detail the principles of autonomy and beneficence in order to demonstrate the force of our arguments against principlism. These latter two were chosen not only because they are the principles most often employed in discussion of biomedical ethics, but also because they best illustrate the most problematic aspects of principlism. In particular, we show that principlism manifests the inadequacies of most previous accounts of morality by failing to appreciate the significance of the distinction between moral rules and moral ideals, by misrepresenting the ordinary concept of duty, and by failing to realize that morality is a public system that applies to everyone.

The Principle of Nonmaleficence

This is the one principle for which we have a strong affinity because, as Chapter 2 makes clear, the key insight expressed by the principle of nonmaleficence is also a major orientation of our account of morality. It is the only one of the four principles that does not blur the distinction between moral rules and moral ideals. Indeed, this principle is most reasonably interpreted as merely summarizing some of the moral rules. The moral rules "Don't kill," "Don't cause pain," and "Don't disable" are clearly included in this principle, and probably the rule "Don't deprive of pleasure" is as well. Even the rule "Don't deprive of freedom" can be included in the principle of nonmaleficence, but principlism seems to prefer to include it under the principle of autonomy. However, we see no reason for distinguishing "Do not deprive of freedom" from the other four rules, for all five of these rules proscribe causing what are universally recognized as evils (or harms)—death, pain, disability, loss of freedom, and loss of pleasure.

The principle of nonmaleficence does no more than simply collapse four or five moral rules into one more general rule, "Do not cause harm." That general rule, in the form "Primum non nocere," is often taken as the first principle of medicine. It is primarily a matter of purpose and style whether one prefers to list five distinct moral rules or to have one general principle that includes them all. We prefer the former because it makes more salient the fact that there are different kinds of harms (or evils) and that rational persons can and do rank them differently. (Neglecting the fact that there are different rational rankings is one of the primary causes of unjustified paternalism—see Chapter 10.) Thus, insofar as specifying the different harms that one must avoid causing must be explicitly and carefully done sooner or later, the gain in simplicity of having just one general principle is minimal and transitory at best. Nonetheless, this principle, even as it stands, has no major problems. That fact is not surprising, since it is the only one of the principles that is not an invention of philosophers, but is a longstanding principle of medicine.

The Principle of Justice

Our discussion of justice is equally brief, but not for the same reasons. Not only is this principle not similar to any specific moral rules, it does not even pretend to provide a guide to action. It is doubtful that even the proponents of principlism put much stock in it as an action guide. The "principle of justice" is the prime example of a principle functioning simply as a checklist of moral concerns. It amounts to no more than saying that one should be concerned with matters of distribution; it recommends just or fair distribution without endorsing any particular account of justice or fairness. Thus, as used by principlism, the principle of justice, in effect, is merely a chapter heading under which one might find sophisticated discussions of various theories of justice. After reading such a chapter one might be better informed and more sensitive to the differing theories of justice, but when dealing with an actual problem of distribution, one would be baffled by the injunction to "apply the principle of justice."

The principle of justice shares an additional problem with the two remaining principles: it blurs the distinction between what is morally required (obeying the moral rules) and what is morally encouraged (following the moral ideals). Since the principle of justice cannot be taken seriously as an action guide, this blurring is not as obvious as in the two remaining principles. In this, as in other matters, principlism simply takes over errors of those theories which suggested the four principles in the first place. For example: The most prominent contemporary discussion of justice is by John Rawls. In *A Theory of Justice*, Rawls describes what he calls the duty of justice as follows:

This duty requires us to support and to comply with just institutions that exist and apply to us. It also constrains us to further just arrangements not yet established, at least when this can be done without too much cost to ourselves.[7]

Rawls includes in what he regards as a single duty (1) the moral rule requiring one to obey (just) laws and (2) the moral ideal encouraging one to help make just laws, without even realizing the significant difference between these two guides to action.[8] As we show later, this failure to distinguish between what is morally required (the moral rules) and what is morally encouraged (the moral ideals) also creates significant confusion in both the principle of autonomy and the principle of beneficence.

The Principle of Autonomy

This principle seems to be the centerpiece of principlism. It is cited more frequently than any of the others and has taken on a life of its own. The concept of autonomy has come to dominate discussions of medical ethics to the point that there is a growing and focused opposition to its predominance. Attention is being drawn to concerns that outweigh autonomy; its primacy over all of the other principles is being questioned. (It is to the credit of Beauchamp and Childress that they make it clear that other considerations sometimes outweigh autonomy.)[9] But these developments are only symptomatic of deeper theoretical problems with autonomy as a principle. As close as Beauchamp and Childress get to stating the principle of autonomy is this:

Hence, we shall here understand the principle of autonomy as follows: *Autonomous actions and choices should not be constrained by others.* . . . . It asserts a right of noninterference and correlatively an obligation not to constrain autonomous actions—nothing more but also nothing less." (2d ed., p. 62, their emphasis)

And in the third edition (p. 72, their emphasis):

> This principle can be stated in its negative form as follows: *Autonomous actions are not to be subjected to controlling constraints by others.* This principle provides the justificatory basis for the right to make autonomous decisions. The principle should be treated as a broad, abstract principle independent of restrictive or exceptive clauses such as "We must respect individuals' views and rights so long as their thoughts and actions do not seriously harm other persons." Like all moral principles, this principle has only prima facie standing. It asserts a right of noninterference and correlatively an obligation not to constrain autonomous actions.

As stated here it is surprisingly akin to the principle of nonmaleficence and, as such, we of course have little disagreement with it. In fact, it seems to pick out just one evil, the loss of freedom, and gives it a principle all to itself. Interpreted simply as an alternative formulation of the moral rule "Do not deprive of freedom," we have no objection to this principle, for it is a genuine action guide in that it prohibits constraining others' actions. However, the principle does not say simply that one should not constrain another's actions and choices, but rather it says that one should not constrain another's *autonomous* actions and choices. The principle does not prohibit constraining nonautonomous choices and actions. Consequently, the distinction between autonomous and nonautonomous actions takes on great moral significance. What counts as an autonomous choice or action becomes a matter of fundamental moral concern; thus the addition of "autonomous" causes many problems in applying the principle of autonomy.

Autonomous actions and choices. In practice the basic difficulty with autonomy, dogging it throughout all its uses, is knowing whether the actions and choices one is concerned with are autonomous. Is the choice to give up drinking the autonomous choice or is the autonomous choice to continue drinking? Is the choice to withdraw from expensive life-prolonging treatment to save one's family money and anguish the autonomous choice, or is the autonomous choice the decision to go on living a while longer? Which choice is it that one is being admonished not to constrain? If there is a conflict between people who differ on which choice of the patient is the autonomous one, each side will appeal to the principle of autonomy for support. One side may favor overruling a patient's refusal because the fact that it is irrational shows that the choice is not autonomous; whereas the other side may favor going along with the patient's explicitly stated refusal on the ground that although it is irrational, the patient is competent and therefore the refusal is an autonomous choice. Both sides can sincerely claim that they are acting on the principle of autonomy by respecting the autonomous choice. This is not merely a normal problem of interpretation, for, as discussed in the previous chapter, we realize that all of the moral rules are subject to some interpretation. However autonomy is such a fundamentally ambiguous and disputed concept that "the principle of autonomy" can be used to support two completely opposing ways of acting, even when there is no disagreement on the observable facts of the case and there are no cultural differences. Such a principle is obviously not a useful guide to action.

There may seem to be times when it is appropriate to question whether a patient has made an autonomous choice, such as when he is delirious, or intoxicated, or under the influence of drugs, and the views he expresses significantly differ from those he expresses when he is in a normal state. However, when the significant departure from previously expressed views is not temporary and not explained by medical reasons, then it is misleading and unhelpful to focus on the question of whether a patient's choices are autonomous. The correct application of the label of "autonomous" to a patient's choices is a matter of longstanding philosophical dispute, and there is no clear ordinary use of the term which is helpful in resolving any of the difficult cases. Thus, following the principle of autonomy may encourage one to act with unjustified paternalism, that is, to overrule the patient's explicit refusal, simply because one views that choice as not being autonomous. Thus the principle of autonomy may lead one to deprive a person of freedom without an adequate justification for doing so.

A much more adequate method for dealing with such problems is by using the concepts of "rational" and "irrational" as we have presented them in Chapter 2. Only if a person's decision concerning his own health care is seriously irrational is overruling it justified (see Chapter 10). If the decision is rational, overruling it is not justified. Suppose, for example, that a patient has thoughtfully and persistently throughout his life insisted that if he contracts terminal cancer, he wants no treatment at all. But now that he has cancer that is regarded as terminal (and is anxious, stressed, and drugged), he says he wants life-prolonging treatment. Health care professionals would be hard pressed to decide what to do on the basis of whether or not this was an autonomous decision (after all, it was a sudden change of mind, under the influence of drugs and stress). However, the patient's current decision in favor of treatment is clearly not irrational, and hence, on our account, should not be overridden. (We discuss this matter in considerable detail in Chapters 6 and 10.)

Moral rules and moral ideals: A fundamental distinction. At the core of many problems with the principle of autonomy, as with other principles, is its general failure to recognize the significance of the distinction between what is morally encouraged (following the moral ideals) and what is morally required (obeying the moral rules). Many philosophers, including Kant and Mill, have made this distinction, or rather one that seems closely related to it, by distinguishing between duties of perfect obligation and duties of imperfect obligation ("perfect" and "imperfect" duties). However, this indiscriminate use of the term "duty" (a matter we discuss later in connection with beneficence) has resulted in this crucial distinction not being made in the correct way. The first five moral rules, discussed in Chapter 2, are examples of perfect duties. So also are the second five moral rules requiring one not to deceive, not to cheat, not to break promises, not to disobey the law, and not to neglect one's duty (in the normal sense of "duty"). Perfect duties must be impartially obeyed all of the time. One is allowed to violate a perfect duty only when one has an adequate justification for doing so.

On the other hand, the moral ideals are imperfect duties, that is, those duties that are impossible to obey either impartially or all of the time. Working to help the downtrodden is an example. One must pick and choose not only which of the downtrodden to help, but also when and where one will provide this help. Furthermore, one may even choose not to act on that imperfect duty at all, but rather to act on some other imperfect duty such as preventing the deprivation of freedom of someone, somewhere. It seems as if an imperfect duty is a duty that one is not required to act on at all; morality certainly does not require one to work for either Oxfam or for Amnesty International, let alone both. It is not morally required to give to or work for any charity, although morality certainly encourages such behavior. Doing so is following an imperfect duty (moral ideal), not a perfect duty (moral rule).

Because this traditional distinction between perfect and imperfect duties embodies a confusion about the notion of duty, we make the distinction in a different and less misleading fashion. Moral rules prohibit acting in ways that cause, or increase the risk of, others suffering some harm. That is precisely what morality requires. Moral ideals, on the other hand, encourage the prevention and relief of harm, but morality does not require following those ideals (unless a moral rule, such as "Do your duty," requires such prevention or relief, but then the circumstances are specified and limited, as discussed in Chapter 3). The moral rules must be followed all the time, toward everyone, impartially, but that is impossible in the case of the moral ideals. Doing what morality requires (obeying the moral rules) is usually not praiseworthy; rather it is expected, and failing to do it makes one liable to punishment. Doing what morality encourages (following the moral ideals) is usually praiseworthy and failing to do it is not punishable. The distinction between moral rules and moral ideals is crucial for a proper understanding of the moral system.

The phrases "perfect duties" and "imperfect duties" obscure this crucial distinction between moral rules and moral ideals. The ordinary use of "duty" suggests that punishment is deserved when one fails to do one's duty. After all, it is morally required to obey the moral rules impartially all of the time. For example, whenever one deprives persons of freedom (principlism might call this violating their autonomy), one needs an adequate justification for doing so. But one does not need a justification for failing to help them to increase their freedom (principlism might call this promoting their autonomy), unless one has a duty to do so, for example, because of one's profession. In the absence of such a duty, helping someone to increase her freedom is following a moral ideal. Morality certainly encourages doing that, but morality does not require doing it.

Autonomy as rule and ideal. The principle of autonomy requires respect for autonomy, but it fails to distinguish clearly between "respecting (not violating) autonomy" and "promoting autonomy." Not distinguishing clearly between "respecting autonomy" and "promoting autonomy" inevitably leads to confusion. Compounded by the search for the "genuinely" autonomous actions and choices, the principle of autonomy invites a kind of activism in which an agent promotes those choices and actions of another that the agent regards as the other's autonomous choices and actions, even though that involves depriving that person of freedom. For example, suppose a woman is pregnant with a fetus that tests have shown to be severely defective. The woman, wanting an abortion, consults a counselor, informing the counselor that she has "always been a good Catholic." The counselor, seeking to abide by the principle of autonomy, faces a dilemma. The principle commits him not only to never overriding a client's autonomous decision, but to actively promoting the client's autonomy. But what is the pregnant woman's autonomous self in this case? Her "real self" may be her firm and life-long commitment to Catholicism, in which case the counselor should, in the interests of promoting autonomy, lead her back to those foundations. On the other hand, moving her back to her religious commitments could be seen as an intrusion on her apparently autonomous decision to have the abortion. Thus the dual demands of the principle of autonomy not only lead to confusion, but could be seen as leading to immoral manipulation of a vulnerable patient in order to promote what one decides is (or should be) the patient's autonomous choice.[10]

Thus, principlism's centerpiece "principle of autonomy" embodies a dangerous level of confusion. That confusion is created by unclarity as to what counts as autonomous actions and choices and the additional blurring of a basic moral distinction between moral rules and moral ideals. This unnecessary introduction of the confused and disputed concept of autonomy inevitably results in making it more difficult to think clearly about moral problems. The goal of moral philosophy is to clarify moral thinking, not to introduce new and unnecessary complications.

As an aside, it is worth observing that the principle of autonomy probably caught on so tenaciously in the last three decades for many reasons. One is that Kantian ethics was experiencing a renaissance and that Kant's notion of autonomy was central to his account of morality. A second is that the society became increasingly aware that the medical profession was so markedly paternalistic that patient self-determination was almost nonexistent. A third was that the increase in medical technology resulted in alternative treatments for most maladies. A fourth was the aging of the population and the resulting increase in chronic diseases that could not be cured, only managed, and patients often knew almost as much about managing them as their physicians. A fifth, the combination of the increase in medical technology that could keep extremely sick people alive for a long time, together with an aging population that often had a rational desire not to be kept alive, even made it rational to refuse life-prolonging treatment. So the emphasis on autonomy became the banner under which forces rallied to gain for patients more control over their own health care. Allowing the patient to decide what, if any, treatment he would receive became the main issue, and thus momentum and conviction, rather than conceptual clarity or theoretical soundness, perpetuated the emphasis on autonomy. Even the fact that the principle of autonomy did not really embody Kant's notion of autonomy did not detract from the overwhelming political appeal of invoking the principle.

An example of how confused the general understanding of autonomy is can be seen by examining Kant's view of autonomy. On Kant's view a person is not acting autonomously if he kills himself or allows himself to die because of intractable pain. To do so is to allow pleasure and pain (which, according to Kant, are not part of the rational self) to determine one's actions. Thus, such suicide or allowing oneself to die is not an autonomous action of the rational self. To act autonomously one must always act in accord with the Categorical Imperative. In *The Grounding of the Metaphysics of Morals,* Kant explicitly states that the Categorical Imperative requires one not to commit suicide because of pain. By way of contrast, note that one of the major arguments in favor of allowing people to die when they are suffering from intractable pain is the principle of autonomy. The seeds of confusion were present in the initial planting of the concept of autonomy. This explains, in part, why we prefer the simple rule "Don't deprive of freedom" to the principle of autonomy for protecting patient self-determination.

The Principle of Beneficence

As used by principlism, this principle suffers shortcomings similar to those of autonomy. As popularly used in the biomedical ethics literature this principle is cited simply to give "validation" both to preventing or relieving harm and to doing good or conferring benefits. Beauchamp and Childress, though much more cautious in their discussion of the principle of beneficence than many, do not avoid the errors. For them the principle of beneficence "asserts the duty to help others further their important and legitimate interests."[11] As such it is morally required. In the biomedical context, the principle becomes the duty to confer benefits and to actively prevent and remove harms, in addition to balancing the possible goods against the possible harms of an action. Even though Beauchamp and Childress are well aware that many philosophers treat beneficent acts as "morally ideal," they still regard beneficence as morally required. But how can benefiting others always be morally required of everyone? As we have shown, impartiality is an essential feature of moral requirements, but the requirement of beneficence cannot be impartially followed toward everyone all the time.

Thus the principle of beneficence not only succumbs to the same criticisms that we earlier leveled at the principle of autonomy, by ignoring the distinction between moral ideals (preventing harms) and moral rules (avoiding causing harms), but it adds a new one, namely, failing to distinguish between the preventing or relieving of harms and the conferring of benefits (promoting goods). This distinction is especially important for medicine, inasmuch as preventing or relieving harm often justifies violating a moral rule without consent, whereas conferring benefits (or promoting goods) rarely, if ever, does.

Beneficence and the concept of duty. Another major confusion perpetuated by the principle of beneficence concerns the concept of duty. Although it arises from the mistake of turning moral ideals into duties, the problem itself has nothing to do with the rules/ideals distinction. Principlism considers it a duty to follow the principles. This becomes especially clear in the frequent references to "the duty of beneficence." That beneficence is a moral ideal is not the only reason it is incorrect to call it a duty; it is equally incorrect to call "not killing" a duty, even though it is a moral rule. Rather it is incorrect because such usage distorts and obscures the primary meaning of "duty," which specifically refers to the particular duties that come with one's role, occupation, or profession. Though it is correct to say "one ought not to kill" or "one ought to help the downtrodden," it creates significant confusion to regard these "oughts" as duties. For some philosophers "Do your duty" has come to mean no more than "Do what you morally ought to do." But using the term "duty" in this way makes it very difficult to talk about real duties, such as those associated with people's occupations and whose content is determined by the members of those occupations or professions and the society in which they live. For reasons of conceptual soundness and clarity, we use the term "duty" only in its ordinary sense, that is, to refer to what is required by one's role in society, particularly by one's occupation, profession, or relationship as family member. It is not only misleading to talk of the moral ideals as imperfect duties, it is also misleading to talk of the moral rules as perfect duties.

Thus "Do your duty" is a distinct moral rule and on a par with the other moral rules; it is not a metarule telling one to obey the other moral rules. However, morality does put a limit on what counts as a duty: there can be no duty to violate unjustifiably any of the other moral rules. "Do your duty" is justified as a moral rule because of the harm, or significantly increased risk of harm, that is caused by one's failure to do that which others are justifiably counting on being done. One is morally required to do his duty, but it generates confusion to say that one has a duty to do his duty.

In medicine it is especially misleading to use the principle of beneficence as if it creates a general duty for all health care workers. Again, this obscures the role of real duties, that is, the specific duties that come with one's role or profession. Beauchamp and Childress seem to recognize the significant difference between what they call the general duty of beneficence and the specific duties of beneficence. They state: "Even if our general duty of beneficence derives in part from reciprocity and fair play, our specific duties of beneficence often derive from special moral relationships with persons, frequently through institutional roles."[12] A later version (third edition) is even clearer: "Even if the general obligation of beneficence derives largely from reciprocity, specific obligations of beneficence often derive from special moral relationships with persons, frequently through institutional roles and contractual arrangements. . ."[13] They are clear that doctors, nurses, and others in the health care field have specific duties to their patients that are determined by their profession and by the practices of their specific institution. However, to lump these varied and detailed professional duties together with the misconceived "general duty of beneficence" and place it all under one principle of beneficence is to substitute a slogan for substance.

Beneficence and "morality as a public system." Principlism fails to appreciate that morality is a "public system," that is, it must be known and understood by all moral agents, and it cannot be irrational for them to follow it. This failure to recognize that all justified violations of a moral rule must be part of a public system that applies to everyone, that is, that everyone must know that this kind of violation is allowed, is a serious flaw. This failure to appreciate that morality is a public system is most clearly seen in act utilitarianism (see Chapter 2). If act utilitarianism is thought of as a code of conduct requiring everyone always to act so as to produce the best overall consequences, regardless of the consequences of everyone knowing that they are allowed to act in that way, then it is appropriately criticized for not recognizing the public nature of morality, that is, that morality must be a public system that applies to all moral agents.

Rule utilitarianism is, properly speaking, not a consequentialist moral system, for rules as well as consequences seem to be involved in making a moral judgment on a particular act. Nonetheless, even rule utilitarianism does not appreciate the fact that morality is a public system. It claims that those rules which would have the best consequences if generally obeyed, are the moral rules. It does not require that those rules be known by all those who are subject to them. More important, a rule utilitarian has significant problems in dealing with exceptions to the rules. If a rule utilitarian tries to avoid the problem of justified exceptions by incorporating the exceptions into the rule itself, the rule becomes indefinitely long; as such, it cannot be part of a public system, because it cannot be understood by all rational persons. Common morality has rules that are simple and general.

If a rule utilitarian adopts simple and general rules, she must determine how particular violations of a rule are justified. She must decide whether to (1) consider only the consequences of her doing this particular act at this particular time or (2) consider the consequences of everyone knowing that they are allowed to do that act in the same morally relevant circumstances. If a rule utilitarian is contemplating cheating on an exam or deceiving someone and chooses (1), then her decision is often at odds with what morality requires. If she chooses (2) she is no longer a rule utilitarian. Rule utilitarianism must determine justified exceptions by appealing to actual or foreseeable consequences of the particular act. Common morality determines justified exceptions by appealing to the purely hypothetical consequences of *everyone knowing* that they are allowed to break the rule in the same morally relevant circumstances. If they are better than the consequences of *everyone knowing* that they are not allowed to break the rule, the violation is justified. Common morality requires consideration of these hypothetical consequences because such consideration is essential for impartially obeying the moral rules.

Neither act nor rule utilitarianism appreciates that for an act to be morally acceptable it must be one that can be publicly allowed. Thus, no principle derived from utilitarianism, such as the principle of beneficence, can be relied on to produce valid moral conclusions. Not surprisingly, the principle of beneficence, more than the other principles, is most affected by this failure to appreciate that morality is a public system. When the consequences of a particular rule violation, such as cheating, are good, but the consequences of that kind of violation being publicly allowed are bad, principlism has serious problems. Since the principle of beneficence considers only the consequences, direct and indirect, of a particular violation of a moral rule, it often encourages acting in a kind of way which if publicly allowed, would lead to bad consequences. Indeed we suspect that it is because of this tendency of the principle of beneficence to lead to what everyone regards as morally unacceptable conclusions, that the principle of autonomy has attained such prominence in principlism. That is, the principle of autonomy serves to overrule beneficence in all those cases where no rational person would publicly allow the kind of behavior that the principle of beneficence seems to require.

Consider a case in which a physician's breach of confidentiality results in some very good consequences for her patient. Yet, if intuitively it seems clearly wrong to commit the breach, the principle of autonomy can then be brought in as the reason for not following the principle of beneficence. The problem, of course, is that sometimes beneficence should outweigh autonomy, but principlism provides no systematic way of determining which should prevail in any particular conflict. Principlism simply says to weigh or balance the principles against each other without providing any instructions on how to do that weighing or balancing.[14] Common morality has a clear procedure for handing such conflicts: compare the consequences of any proposed violation being publicly allowed with the consequences of its not being publicly allowed. Since the only cases in which an account of morality needs to be invoked explicitly are those in which the principles (or rules and ideals) conflict, it is pointless to have an account of morality which provides no guidance on how to deal with such conflicts.

Summary

The traditional concept of an ethical principle has been one that embodies the moral theory that spawns it. As shorthand for the theory, it is used by itself to enunciate a meaningful directive for action because it has an established, unified theory standing behind it. "Act so as to bring about the greatest good for the greatest number," "Maximize the amount of liberty compatible with a like liberty for all." The thrust of the directive is clear; its goal and intent are unambiguous. Of course there are often ambiguities and differing interpretations with respect to how the principle applies to a particular situation, but the principle itself is never used with other principles that are in conflict with it. Furthermore, if a genuine theory has more than one general principle, the relationship between the principles is clearly stated, as in the case of Rawls's two principles of justice. Unlike principlism, one is not given a number of conflicting principles without being told how to rank them or how to resolve the conflicts between them.

The principles of principlism are quite different. In general, they seem to function more as reminders of topics or concerns which the moral decision maker should review prior to decision. Except for the principle of nonmaleficence, they are not true action guides. The principle of justice is the clearest example of that. The principle of nonmaleficence is acceptable since it simply prohibits the causing of harm, and as such merely summarizes the first four or five moral rules. But since it does not specify what counts as the harms one is prohibited from causing, it is less useful than it might be. Furthermore, since it does not make clear that there are different harms which different people rank differently, it is more misleading than it might be. Nonetheless, insofar as the principle of nonmaleficence is interpreted as "Don't cause harm," it at least meets the criterion of being morally required.

The principles of autonomy and of beneficence are more complicated. They actually sound like action guides; they seem to tell one how to act. But closer inspection shows that they generate confusion. If the principle of autonomy were an action guide, like nonmaleficence, simply telling one not to deprive of freedom, then of course we have no objection to it because it is now synonymous with that moral rule. But unhappily the principle of autonomy goes beyond that clear and defensible rule. It injects confusion because there is confusion and disagreement over the proper meaning of "autonomous action." Another troubling feature, as shown earlier, is that the principle also requires that moral agents promote each other's autonomy. That move, which fails to recognize the crucial moral distinction between moral rules and moral ideals means that the principle cannot be taken seriously as a moral requirement. If the principle is interpreted loosely to mean simply "Respect persons" (the original principle from which the principle of autonomy seems to have been derived), it is still not clear what that entails. At best it might mean, "Morality forbids you from treating others simply as you please. Some ways are acceptable and some are not. Think about it." So then one is back to interpreting the principles as a list of concerns.

The principle of beneficence also has an action-guide appearance. It seems to be saying one has a duty to prevent harm as well as to help others "further their important and legitimate interests." Besides the conceptual confusion over the notion of duty, this principle seems to be concerned primarily with what we call utilitarian ideals. It is certainly not a moral rule, for a person cannot possibly follow this principle impartially, all the time. It is not even a clear moral ideal, for the charge to confer benefits (unlike prevention of harms) usually cannot be used to justify the violation of a moral rule. As in the case with utilitarianism, from which this principle is derived, following it might lead to unjustified transgressions of moral rules toward the few in order to confer benefits on the many, thus triggering deployment of the principle of autonomy.

Lastly, we highlighted the more general difficulties with principlism. We noted that even if the individual principles are interpreted as action guides, they often conflict with each other. Since they are not part of a public system, there is no agreed-upon method for resolving these conflicts, or even understanding why a particular conflict cannot be resolved. Since they do not share a common ground, there is no underlying theory to appeal to for help in understanding or resolving conflicts. Indeed, each of the principles in effect seems to be a surrogate for the theory from which it is derived. The use of the principles seems to be an unwitting effort to allow the use of whatever ethical theory seems best suited to the particular problem one is considering. It is simply a sophisticated technique for dealing with problems ad hoc.

The appeal of principlism is that it makes use of some features of standard ethical theories that seem to have popular support. But there is no attempt to see how these different features can be blended together as integrated parts of a single adequate theory, rather than disparate features derived from several competing theories. So in effect principlism tells agents to pick and choose as they see fit, as if one can sometimes be a Kantian and sometimes a Utilitarian and sometimes something else, without worrying about consistency or whether the theory one is using is adequate or not. Principlism does not recognize that for a moral decision to be correct it must be one that can be publicly allowed. It not only does not recognize the unified and systematic nature of morality, it does not recognize that the moral system, or morality, must be public.

The upshot of having principles with an unclear content which are not part of any unified public system is that an agent is not aware of the real grounds for his moral decision. Because the principles are not clear and direct imperatives at all, but simply a collection of suggestions and observations, occasionally conflicting, the agent cannot know what is really guiding his action. Nor do these principles tell him what facts are morally relevant, such that a change in them may change what he should do; thus he is not able to propose better alternatives. Though the language of principlism suggests that the agent has applied a principle which is morally well established, a closer look shows that in fact he has looked at and weighed many diverse moral considerations, which may be only superficially interrelated, having no unified, systematic underlying foundation. Principles seem to be involved in complex decisions only in a purely verbal way; the real guiding influences on the moral decision are not the ones the agent believes them to be. Rather, the agent is, in fact, guided by his basic understanding of common morality, and only later cites principles when stating his conclusions, giving the illusion of theoretical support.

Concerning Specification

Our critiques of principlism have led those espousing it to search for a method of transforming the principles into actual action guides instead of a checklist of concerns.[15] The most prominent of these methods is known as "specification." Several articles put this method forth as the solution to some problems of principlism that we have pointed out.[16] Beauchamp and Childress incorporate the notion in their most recent revision of *The Principles of Biomedical Ethics.*[17] Indeed that may be part of the reason that the reviewer of this edition proclaimed it the death of principlism.[18]

Although the addition of "specification" to principlism might be indicative of its demise (no longer being the atheoretical principlism we have known and criticized), there is no doubt that specification is a move in the right direction. The notion of specification and its refinement seems to have originated with the work of Henry S. Richardson in his article, "Specifying Norms as a Way to Resolve Concrete Ethical Problems."[19] Richardson's attempt to make principlism more systematic is certainly a move in the right direction, but it is just a beginning. Richardson states that specification qualifies the norm "by substantive means . . . by adding clauses indicating what, where, when, why, how, by what means, by whom or to whom the action is to be, is not to be, or may be done. . ."[20] These clauses certainly encompass some of the morally relevant features of a situation or problem, but his questions (what, where, when, why, and so forth) do not help to determine what features are morally relevant, or why they are relevant. Nor does he provide any kind of theory which identifies which "substantive means" should be used to determine that any particular feature is morally relevant.

We applaud the embracing of specification by principlism, for it shows that those supporting principlism recognize the need for a theory to explain and support it. However, as far as we know, neither Richardson nor those who embrace his modification of principlism provide any theory. There is no explanation of where the appropriate specifications come from or how the narrowing of the application of the norms takes place. The theory that we describe in Chapter 2 can explain and support how norms are specified, and also provides a list of the features that are morally relevant. Our theory does not, however, as Richardson assumes that specification of norms does, eliminate all disagreement. We not only acknowledge but indeed emphasize that equally informed, impartial, rational persons can differ, not only in how they specify a norm, but also in how they apply the same specified norm. Richardson recognizes that in applying a norm to a situation, one must identify its morally relevant features, but, having no theory, he provides no clue about how one determines what those morally relevant features are.

One of Richardson's problems is his identification of "universal" with "absolute."[21] However, a norm can be universal without being absolute. The rejection of absolute norms, that is, the recognition that all moral rules have exceptions, is completely compatible with the claim that moral rules are universal, that is, that they apply to all rational persons. Richardson does not recognize that in order to make norms culturally sensitive, it is necessary to allow for some degree of interpretation of the norms. Perhaps most important, Richardson, like all principlists, does not appreciate a central feature of morality, that it is a public system. This explains why he cannot formulate criteria for, or develop a list of, morally relevant features.[22] Finally, his failure to realize that some moral disagreements are not resolvable, makes understandable his failure to formulate any procedure for dealing with conflicts between specified norms.

We conclude that specification helps principlism move in the right direction, namely, toward our account of morality. But if it moves far enough in that direction, it will no longer be appropriate to call it "principlism." So far, however, specification has not moved principlism very far; it has simply pointed it in the right direction and made it clear that it has a lot farther to go. Specification still fails to make critically important moves: listing and defending the morally relevant features of situations, relating those features to a moral theory, and incorporating the requirement that morality be a public system. Specification shows the need for these accomplishments, but does not achieve them.

One article, describing several approaches to bioethical theory, criticizes our account of morality, describing it as "deductivism," and concludes that "specified principlism" is "the most promising model—though it requires development."[23] What the author of that article does not realize is that if specified principlism develops properly, it will become our account. In most cases, our theory is deductivist in that the immorality of an action can be deduced from its description. For example, a clear case of harmful, self-serving deception is seen to be immoral by "deduction" from the moral rule prohibiting deception. However, although that is the most common and frequent kind of application of a moral rule to a situation, it is almost never discussed because there is no practical or theoretical reason to discuss it. No one doubts that the action is immoral, and because of this there is no point in discussing it. But an adequate moral theory must account for the common and uninteresting cases as well as the uncommon and interesting ones.

For these uncommon and interesting cases, the ones that are described in the medical ethics case books and discussed in all of the medical ethics anthologies and textbooks, our account of morality is not deductivist. What our critics do not appreciate is that we recognize that morality is an informal public system. Like sandlot baseball, there is unspoken agreement on the point of the game and all of the fundamental rules. What causes problems is how one interprets the rules in the nonobvious cases. But without overwhelming agreement on most matters, the game would never even get started. Similarly, there is overwhelming agreement on the point of morality, the lessening of the suffering of evil or harm, and on all of the fundamental rules. But equally informed, rational, impartial persons can disagree on almost all interesting, nonobvious cases.

Our account of the moral system explains how this can happen; for example, people can disagree on the ranking of harms to be avoided, they can disagree on the consequences of publicly allowing a kind of violation, or they can disagree on the interpretation of the particular moral rule. We do not believe, and the moral system does not require, that one and only one solution exists for each moral problem. We do not criticize principlism because it does not provide a unique answer to every moral problem, but rather because it does not explain in any useful way what is responsible for the disagreement and, hence, provides no help in resolving the disagreement.

Like principlism, we borrow from all of the classical theories. Unlike principlism, we do not merely formulate principles which call attention to the insights from these theories. We integrate the best features of each of these theories into a new theory, one that eliminates those features of the previous theories that result in so many devastating counterexamples. Our theory, like all theories, still has problems, but for the most part these are the result of a poor statement of the theory. We look forward to legitimate criticisms of the theory and its applications that we put forward in this book, so that we may continue to revise and improve our statement of it.

Notes

1. K. Danner Clouser and Bernard Gert, "A Critique of Principlism," *The Journal of Medicine and Philosophy* 15 (1990), pp. 219–236, and "Morality vs. Principlism," in *Principles of Health Care Ethics,* ed. Raaman Gillon (New York: John Wiley and Sons, Inc., 1994), pp. 251–266. See also K. Danner Clouser, "Common Morality as an Alternative to Principlism," *Kennedy Institute of Ethics Journal,* 5 (1995), pp. 219–236.

2. Tom L. Beauchamp and James F. Childress, *Principles of Biomedical Ethics* (New York: Oxford University Press, 1979; 2d ed., 1983; 3d ed., 1989, 4th ed., 1994).

3. Ezekiel J. Emanuel, "The Beginning of the End of Principlism," *Hastings Center Report,* 25 (1995), pp. 37–38.

4. Ibid., p. 38.

5. This section is based on the *Federal Register,* Vol. 44, No. 76 (Wednesday, April 18, 1979), pp. 23192–23197.

6. Ibid., p. 23193.

7. John Rawls, *A Theory of Justice* (Cambridge, Mass.: Harvard University Press, 1971), p. 115, see also p. 334.

8. For further discussion of Rawls on this point, see Bernard Gert, *Morality* (New York: Oxford University Press, 1988), ch. 13.

9. Beauchamp and Childress, *Principles,* 3d ed., pp. 122–125.

10. For a more detailed account of the problems caused by autonomy in genetic counseling, and of the way in which using the common moral system can help deal with these problems, see Chapter 6 of Bernard Gert, Edward M. Berger, George F. Cahill Jr., K. Danner Clouser, Charles M. Culver, John B. Moeschler, and George H. S. Singer, *Morality and the New Genetics: A Guide for Students and Health Care Providers* (Sudbury, Mass.: Jones and Bartlett Publishers, 1996).

11. Beauchamp and Childress, *Principles,* 2d ed., pp. 148–149.

12. Ibid., p. 156.

13. Ibid., 3d ed., p. 204.

14. Specified principlism attempts to resolve this problem, but it is not well worked out. Indeed it seems to be merely a way station on the path of principlism to our more complex and systematic account of morality, which does have a procedure for resolving conflicts. See the last section of this chapter for a fuller discussion.

15. See K. Danner Clouser and Bernard Gert, "A Critique of Principlism," *The Journal of Medicine and Philosophy,* 15 (1990), pp. 219–236, and "Morality versus Principlism," *Principles of Health Care Ethics,* ed. Raanan Gillon (New York: John Wiley and Sons, 1994), pp. 251–266.

16. For example, David DeGrazia, "Moving Forward in Bioethical Theory: Theories, Cases, and Specified Principlism," *The Journal of Medicine and Philosophy* 17 (1992): 511–539.

17. Beauchamp and Childress, *Principles,* 4th ed., 1994.

18. See note 3.

19. Henry S. Richardson, "Specifying Norms as a Way to Resolve Concrete Ethical Problems," *Philosophy and Public Affairs* 19 (1990), pp. 279–310.

20. Ibid., pp. 295–296.

21. See ibid., pp. 292 ff.

22. For the connection between morality being a public system that applies to all rational persons and morally relevant features, see Chapter 2.

23. DeGrazia, op. cit., p. 512.

5

Malady

The proper definition of "disease" (we subsume "disease" under our concept of "malady") is an issue that has been weaving in and out of bioethics for a long time.[1] There are some areas of bioethics in which the concept of disease has seemed pivotal, and others in which it has seemed to play little or no role at all. Furthermore, not everyone agrees about when the concept applies and when it does not. But in any case, the concept of disease deserves an in-depth explication since it is so central to medicine and can and does so easily surface in discussions of and within the health professions.

The concept of disease is interesting in and of itself, apart from any moral implications. It is the central concept of medicine and yet, at its core, it involves values, though what values and to what extent they play a role in defining the concept constitute much of the debate in the literature. Compare medicine's basic concept of disease with the basic concepts of other sciences—cell, molecule, gene, neuron, electron, proton, positron—all of which are empirically, operationally, or contextually defined, without any element of values. Admittedly, medicine may not be a science, but it is certainly very closely related to science, so the possibility of a value element at its core is noteworthy.

Our plan is to explicate the concept of disease (as malady) because it is so basic and because we believe it does enter into important bioethical issues. A direct and significant consequence of our analysis is the clear conclusion that abnormality alone does not constitute a malady, and thus deviancy (for example, in sexual behavior) is not in and of itself sufficient for a condition to be a malady.

An Overview of Malady

Such terms as "disease," "illness," "sickness," "lesion," and "disorder," are often used interchangeably, but each has a unique connotation. The phrase "the concept of disease" is sometimes used to include all of them. Such all-inclusiveness can be awkward in certain contexts, especially in light of all the other conditions that "the concept of disease" must refer to—injury, wound, defect, syndrome, trauma, disfigurement—if it is to be sufficiently inclusive. All these terms have specific connotations, so that in certain situations one term may seem the most accurate label: for example, "wound," if one has been stabbed with a knife. It is odd to refer to a knife wound or a leg broken in an accident as a "disease," and it is equally odd to refer to chicken pox as an injury. Nausea or a headache is probably better called an illness than a disease, since "illness" connotes the presence of symptoms; the afflicted individual is aware of pain or discomfort. On the other hand, "disease" suggests an identifiable underlying physiological process with an etiology and with distinct stages of development, all the signs of which can be present without the victim being aware of them. In fact, many people have diseases but do not yet feel ill.

Additional confusion exists because the conditions to which these terms refer overlap to some extent and the terms do not have consistent connotations. Ordinarily syndromes advance to being diseases as the causes and stages become more clearly understood, yet often the syndrome label persists simply because of tradition; for example, Down syndrome. An occasional pathology textbook uses the term "traumatic diseases," presumably to avoid the limiting connotations of the separate terms "trauma" and "disease." Another example of the arbitrary nature of disease-concept labeling is the condition experienced by deep-sea divers who return from the depths too quickly. It is called either "caisson disease" or "decompression illness," yet essentially all the ill effects are due to the cellular *injury* caused by nitrogen bubbles forming in various bodily tissues. Other conditions do not fit comfortably with any of the standard disease terms, for example, hernias and allergies.

Because of the plethora of terms with overlapping meanings and special connotations, we propose to give a new sense to the infrequently used general term "malady," so that it includes the referents of all of the other terms. As we use the term, "malady" refers to that which all the other disease words have in common: injury, illness, sickness, disease, trauma, wound, disorder, lesion, allergy, headache, syndrome, and so on. We call all of them maladies. What do they all have in common? Answering that question constitutes much of the work of this chapter. Our analysis of malady can be taken as an analysis of the expanded sense of "disease" as it is often used in medical textbooks, namely to include the referents of all these other terms. We choose to use the term "malady" because such an expanded sense for the word "disease" is a significant distortion of the ordinary use of that term among both health professionals and lay individuals.

We approach the analysis of malady much as we approached the analysis of common morality in Chapter 2. We want to capture what is common in the meaning of all the disease terms. We are not inventing a new concept, but we are making explicit and thereby calling attention to what is common in the meaning of all these terms. We are giving that commonality the name "malady," which is an old but very useful term that carries its meaning on its sleeve. There seems to be no word in the English language that serves this overarching purpose.[2] However, there is a need for such a word in order to refer to all of these conditions without being locked into one or another of their special connotations. The all-encompassing word "malady" also helps to maintain focus on the search for what the individual terms all have in common.

During the last twenty-five years analyses of "the concept of disease" have dwelt on the term's purported subjectivity and value-ladenness, as if those two terms necessarily went together. We argue strongly for the term's being value-laden but nevertheless objective. Our goal is to put the concept on a more stable footing, less subject to whimsy and manipulation. In the past the disease label has been used to try to accomplish a variety of personal and political agendas; it has been treated as a very malleable concept. It has been manipulated to force "treatment," to block entry into a country, to deny reimbursement, to forbid marriage, to restrict freedom, to enforce morals, and to "medicalize" a variety of human conditions.

An ordinary example of this malleability is alcoholism. When it is important to impress upon the alcoholic that he must share some of the responsibility for his condition, and that he must exercise some willpower, he may be told that alcoholism is not a disease, but more of a bad habit. On the other hand, when it is important for the alcoholic to be freed from a burden of guilt and blame, it may be emphasized that alcoholism is a disease, the connotation of which is that it is an unfortunate condition that has befallen the alcoholic, victimizing him, and requiring expert medical treatment. Our concept of malady makes it clear that alcoholism is a malady, even though the alcoholic must bear some responsibility for controlling the symptoms of that malady.

Our account eliminates as much of the subjectivity as possible, allowing much less room for manipulation. We provide a precise and systematic account of maladies, thus enabling a more fruitful discussion of controversial cases. Nevertheless, there are places where some vagueness remains. We give an account of these, showing what causes the vagueness and why it is unavoidable. Inevitably there will be borderline cases. Our explication shows what aspects of these conditions make them borderline and what about these conditions would have to change for them to be clear cases of maladies or clearly not maladies.

Our account of malady has some important conceptual connections to our account of morality. The harms that rational individuals want to avoid are the very harms or risks of harms that, when caused in a certain way, constitute maladies. So, like morality, the concept of malady is grounded in universal and universally agreed-upon features of human nature. Though this means that values remain at the core of the concept of malady, the values are not only specified, but they are objective and universal. Our account of malady also includes mental as well as physical maladies. Finally, our definition of malady not only includes all the harms that are collectively included in the disease-illness-injury terminology, but it also includes all of the other essential features that these terms share.

Thus, to summarize, (1) we believe that all "disease-terms" have something in common, (2) we use the term "malady" to capture that commonality, and (3) our account of "malady" is grounded in the same universal values that ground our account of morality.

We provide an objective analysis of the concept of "malady." We believe that the objective criteria we specify describe the necessary and sufficient conditions under which disease-terms are actually used in ordinary language. We do not intend to introduce a new concept, only a new word to refer to it. However, although analyses of concepts do not intend to change the concept, they often intend to sharpen it. A good analysis can make people more aware of the criteria for the use of a concept than they were previously and they may then be less apt to make loose or hasty errors. Good analyses of concepts also usually help in classifying some previously borderline situations, where it has not been clear whether the concept applies. Even if the application of a concept in a particular situation does remain borderline, the analysis usually makes it clear why the concept is in fact borderline in that situation. We consider several borderline situations later in the chapter.

Some Background

There have been many attempts to set out a formal definition of "disease," but among medical professionals "disease" has often been used in a technical sense, not in its ordinary-language sense in which there is a distinction between a disease, an illness, and an injury. Consequently, "disease" is often used interchangeably with "illness," and injuries are regarded merely as a subclass of diseases. What most formal definitions of disease have been intending to define is what we call a malady, that is, they have taken "disease" to refer to injuries, illnesses, headaches, lesions, disorders, and so on.

A characteristic definition is the following one, from a pathology textbook:

Disease is any disturbance of the structure or function of the body or any of its parts; an imbalance between the individual and his environment; a lack of perfect health.[3]

This offers three separate but presumably equivalent definitions. According to the first definition, recently clipped nails and puberty are diseases, as is asymptomatic situs inversus (right-left reversal of the position of some internal bodily organs). The second definition is too vague to be of any use, and the third is circular. Although the "disturbance of structure or function of the body" is inadequate when considered as a complete definition, it can be incorporated as a feature of a more complex and adequate definition.

Another medical textbook definition states that

disease may be defined as deprivation or lack of ease, a discomfort or an annoyance, or a morbid condition of the body or of some organ or part thereof.[4]

Here two separate definitions are offered. The second one is obviously circular and hence of no help. The first may characterize many illnesses but certainly includes far too much. It rightly includes heartburn, an earache, and an infected toe, but it also includes an overheated room, tight-fitting shoes, and irritating neighbors. Our definition of malady avoids this problem by requiring as a necessary condition that the malady be a "condition of the individual."

An early definition of disease expresses what many subsequent definitions have emphasized, portraying the disease as a result of an unfortunate interaction between the individual and his environment:

Disease can only be that state of the organism that for the time being, at least, is fighting a losing game whether the battle be with temperature, water, microorganisms, disappointment or what not. In any instance, it may be visualized as the reaction of the organism to some sort of energy impact, addition or deprivation.[5]

On this definition, one wrestler held down by another or an individual getting increasingly annoyed by loud music is suffering from a disease. We avoid the flaw in such definitions by requiring that the harm being suffered have no "distinct sustaining cause."

Several authors have correctly identified various aspects of the concept of disease. Spitzer and Endicott include in their definition of "a medical disorder" that it is intrinsically associated with distress, disability, or certain types of disadvantage.[6] We think this definition is on the right track. It begins to sort out specific harms that are at the core of disease, though it fails to capture all of them.

Goodwin and Guze significantly improve on Spitzer and Endicott's list of harms in their 1979 definition and add a condition that most others fail to consider in their definitions. Goodwin and Guze define disease as

any condition associated with discomfort, pain, disability, death, or an increased liability to these states.[7]

The important added feature that we discuss and clarify in our definition of malady is the "increased liability." It is a necessary amendment if asymptomatic conditions such as high blood pressure are to count as diseases or, to use the new term, as maladies.

The foregoing examples of definitions are typical of those found in medical and pathology textbooks. Our primary interest is not in criticizing them, but in using them to introduce our concept of malady. They show there is a need for a more adequate definition, and they suggest and exemplify some of the flaws that need to be addressed.

One kind of definition in particular directly raises moral issues: that kind of definition that makes abnormality a central feature of disease. We have not yet cited an example of this kind of definition, but many formal definitions in the literature make this feature central. For example, in the 1992 (third) edition of *Medicine for the Practicing Physician,* editor-in-chief J. Willis Hurst, in his own chapter "Practicing Medicine," says, "A disease is defined as an abnormal process." and he defines abnormality as "a deviation from the normal range."[8]

Although the concept of disease that one adopts has wide-ranging repercussions for everything from establishing the goals of medicine to the distribution of health care in society, for us the "abnormality" definition of disease has the most immediate moral implications. As we show in our explication of malady in general and mental maladies in particular, abnormality is neither a necessary nor a sufficient feature of disease or malady. However, abnormality does play an important, though limited, role in defining some of the terms that are used in our definition of malady. Consequently, it plays a role in the determination of some maladies, and it is that role that needs careful discussion and specification.

Constructing a Definition of Malady

Our plan for this section is to lead the reader through a series of thought processes in order to produce a definition of malady. This is in contrast to simply stating the definition and defending it against possible objections. We believe this "method of discovery" helps with comprehension of the problem, its subproblems, and their solutions. A step-by-step process should make the nuances and maneuvers more accessible to the reader.

Something Is Wrong

In the very broadest sense, when one of the disease terms correctly applies to an individual or, as we say from now on, when an individual has a malady, there is something wrong with that individual. As was shown in our earlier discussion of textbook definitions, however, to note that "something is wrong" is much too inclusive. Many things can be wrong in an individual's life without her having a malady: for example, being in poverty, being neglected, or being in a runaway truck. But before we specify when having "something wrong" with oneself does constitute having a malady, we must make clear what it is to have "something wrong" with oneself.

What is wrong with someone who has a malady? A typical and frequent answer is: he is in pain, he is disabled, he is dying. But do these states or conditions have anything in common? What is the genus of which pain, disability, and death are species?

The answer is: they are all harms (or evils).[9] Harm is the genus of which pain, disability, and death are species. What characterizes these harms is the fact that no one wants them. In fact, everyone wants to avoid them. At least all individuals acting rationally want to avoid them unless they have an adequate reason not to, as elaborated in Chapter 2. The very definition of an irrational action is an action of an individual who chooses not to avoid harm for himself even though he has no adequate reason for not avoiding that harm. However, people who choose to die rather than suffer unrelenting pain, or who choose to endure great pain to avoid a certain disability, are not acting irrationally because they have adequate reasons for choosing the particular harm in question.

"Pain," as we use the term, includes unpleasant feelings of anxiety, sadness, and displeasure, and all the other kinds of mental suffering. Similarly, disabilities are not limited to physical disabilities, but include mental disabilities and volitional disabilities as well. Examples of mental disabilities are aphasia and dementia; volitional disabilities include addictions, compulsions, and phobias.

Furthermore, death, pain, and disability are not the only basic harms. Two other significant harms are loss of freedom and loss of pleasure. So we anticipate that these also play a role in maladies, even though they do not immediately suggest themselves when one considers maladies. However, there are instances where one or the other of these harms underlie conditions that are intuitively considered maladies. For example, if an individual has an allergy, he may be able to avoid the circumstances and the places that trigger the allergic reaction, so that in effect he appears not to be suffering any harm. However, his freedom with respect to those circumstances and places has been limited, so in fact he is suffering a harm, namely, the loss of freedom. The loss of pleasure, independent of the other harms, is fairly limited in scope, but one example is anhedonia, which is the failure to feel pleasure. It is sometimes associated with schizophrenia, although its presence is neither necessary nor sufficient to establish that diagnosis. However, any condition of an individual that was characterized solely by a significant loss of pleasure, even without such negative feelings as sadness or anxiety, would qualify as a malady. Possible examples are a condition that leads to failure to experience sexual pleasure or a stroke that affects the limbic system, blocking out the experience of pleasure. Some forms of mutilative operations on a young woman's genitalia result in her later failure to experience sexual pleasure, so that condition counts as a malady as well.

Maladies vary in the intensity of the harms being suffered, from relatively minor to very great. However, a threshold exists in applying the concept such that trivial harms are not usually regarded as maladies. Thus an individual might experience, the day following a mild degree of exercise, a slight twinge of muscle stiffness in one of his legs. This twinge qualifies as a physical pain, but it is quite trivial, and without the addition of the phrase "nontrivial" the condition would satisfy all the criteria for applying the concept of malady (see below, page 104), even though the condition is not ordinarily regarded as a malady. We use the phrase "nontrivial" to modify "harms" because it makes clear both that trivial harms are not sufficient to make a condition a malady, and because it explains one source of some disagreement in labeling a condition a malady. We prefer to make the locus of those disagreements as obvious as possible, so it is helpful to realize that people do not always agree on when a harm is "trivial."

Thus far, then, we can say that a malady is a condition that involves the suffering of nontrivial harms. All the harms involved are instances of the basic harms: death, pain, disability, loss of freedom, and loss of pleasure. These are harms that every individual acting rationally wants to avoid. This explains why and in what way malady (or disease) is a normative term. The concept involves values, certainly, but they are objective and universal values. Like colors, these values are universal and objective because there is general agreement about them. Most people make a distinction between different colors, such as red and green, in the same way; those who cannot are regarded as color-blind. There is a similar universal agreement among people about the nature of the basic harms and about the undesirability, absent an adequate reason, of experiencing any of them. For a term to involve values in no way entails that the application of that term is subjective, whimsical, or "culturally relative."

Significantly Increased Risk of Suffering Nontrivial Harms

The notion of malady (or disease) involves more than an individual currently experiencing a nontrivial harm such as pain or disability. Many maladies do not initially involve suffering a harm; they can be at first asymptomatic. Such a condition may be regarded as a malady, even though it is not yet causing any suffering of harms, if it is a condition that will definitely lead to the suffering of nontrivial harms, like a positive HIV status, or that has a significantly increased risk of leading to the suffering of nontrivial harms, like elevated blood pressure.

We use the adverb "significantly" to modify "increased risk" because it highlights not only that insignificantly increased risks are not sufficient to make a condition a malady, but also because it explains another source of some disagreement in labeling a condition a malady. We prefer to make the locus of those disagreements as obvious as possible, so we think it is important to point out that people do not always agree on when an increased risk is "significant." Other variables enter into determining whether or not to call something a malady on the basis of increased risk. A small increase in the risk of suffering a serious harm is likely to lead to labeling that condition of an individual as a malady, whereas a greater increase of a mild harm might not. For example, a condition of a 20-year-old associated with a 3–5% greater risk of dying before the age of 50 would probably be regarded as a malady, while a 3–5% greater risk of experiencing mild joint pain before the age of 50 probably would not be. Still another variable may be whether or not there is a cure. If a cure is available, there is some advantage to labeling a condition as a malady, even if the increase in risk that justifies the labeling is for a relatively mild harm in the relatively distant future. Our point in stressing the role of "significantly" in the important component of our definition "significantly increased risk of suffering nontrivial harms," is to alert the reader to a source of reasonable variation in how and what conditions are labeled maladies.

A Condition of the Individual

"A condition involving the suffering of nontrivial harms or the significantly increased risk of suffering nontrivial harms" still includes too much. There must be an identifiable condition of the individual that is associated with the predicted harm. It is not sufficient that the individual be at risk of harm simply by being in a statistical cohort of some sort. For example, if all families living within a 10-mile radius of an atomic power plant have a 2.0% greater risk of developing thyroid problems than a matched cohort living elsewhere, it does not follow that all of these individuals have a malady. Similarly, women whose mother or sisters have or have had breast cancer may be at increased risk of getting breast cancer themselves, but they do not all therefore have maladies. Being in a statistical cohort, as explained below in discussing genetic maladies, is not a condition of the individual. Unless the condition that leads to the increased risk is identified as a condition of the individual, we do not say that she has a malady.

Thus we need to add to our nascent definition of malady that it is a condition of the individual that involves suffering a harm or the significantly increased risk of suffering a harm. The condition must pertain only to what is within the integument of an individual's body: it is limited to what is contained within that zone marked by the outer surface of the skin and inward. This distinguishes the condition from the situation or circumstances the individual is in. For example, an individual could be in an elevator with a broken cable, hurtling downward. That individual is at significantly increased risk of harm, yet it is incorrect to describe him as having a malady, at least at the moment. Likewise, an individual who is in jail is suffering a harm, namely, a loss of freedom. Yet this surely is not a malady. It is a situation the individual is in, rather than a condition of the individual himself.

The condition which significantly increases the risk of suffering harm must have a locus within an individual. This requirement distinguishes it from a mere statistical probability associated with membership in a group, in which case there is no identifiable condition having a locus within the individual person that causes the increased risk of suffering a harm.

In order to make sure that the malady is within the individual and not identified with some circumstance of the individual, this aspect of malady must be more carefully described. We started our construction of the malady definition by talking about an individual with whom something was wrong. Occasionally we have used the phrase "condition of an individual." It is tempting to speak of a "bodily condition" in order to emphasize that the malady must be in the body and not a situation the body is in. That phrase, however, makes it impossible to include mental disorders within the malady label because, though at least some mental maladies are very likely to be conditions of the body, they need not be in order to qualify as maladies (see mental maladies, below). Referring to "a condition of the individual" leaves the condition's ontological status an open question but still individuates the locus of the malady.

On the other hand, "malady" not only has the same meaning in "mental maladies" as in "physical maladies," but it also has the same meaning when applied throughout the plant and animal world, at least insofar as particular plants and animals are capable of suffering any of the basic harms. Therefore we properly should refer to the locus of maladies as "a condition of an individual organism." That phrase, however, seems somewhat stilted and given that our primary concern is with human maladies, we shall continue to use the simpler phrase "a condition of an individual" or, occasionally, "a condition of the person."

Except for Rational Beliefs and Desires

So far our developing but still incomplete definition of malady is "a condition of an individual such that he is suffering or is at significantly increased risk of suffering some nontrivial harm (death, pain, disability, or loss of freedom or pleasure)." But "condition of an individual" can cover a lot of territory, so a certain narrowing and certain exclusions are necessary to trim the concept down to something more intuitively correct. Beliefs and desires are part of an individual and certain beliefs and desires can have the effect of causing harm or increasing his risk of suffering harm. A belief that one has lost all his money in the stock market or a belief that one's child is very sick causes suffering, but neither is regarded as a malady. Similarly, desires to climb mountains, ride motorcycles, and fly hang gliders are conditions of individuals such that they are at increased risk of suffering harms, yet no one regards having those desires as constituting maladies.

On the other hand, there are beliefs and desires that not only cause harms to be suffered, but are themselves symptoms of maladies, usually mental maladies: for example, irrational beliefs and desires. One might have a belief that he is being tortured by demons and thus be currently suffering. Or a man might believe that he could fly if he leaped from a high window, and thus be at increased risk of suffering harms. A desire to commit suicide to see what it would be like to be dead puts one at significantly increased risk of harm. These cases do seem like maladies, and they do involve beliefs and desires.

The way we sort this out is to make "rational beliefs and desires" an exception to the conditions of individuals that can be maladies. Our expanded definition thus reads, "a condition of an individual, other than his rational beliefs and desires, such that he is suffering or is at significantly increased risk of suffering some nontrivial harm (death, pain, disability, or loss of freedom or pleasure)." As shown in the previous paragraph, irrational beliefs and desires must not be ruled out as being involved in maladies since they may, in fact, constitute a malady. A belief is irrational only if its falsity is obvious to almost everyone with similar knowledge and intelligence.[10] A desire is irrational when it is a desire for any of the harms or a desire for something which one knows will result in her suffering a harm, and she does not have an adequate reason for that desire.

Distinct Sustaining Cause

We have focused the condition constituting the malady within the individual organism; now it must be noted that though that is a necessary condition of being a malady, it is not a sufficient condition. There are many instances of conditions of individuals such that they are suffering harms not because of a rational belief or desire, and yet no one regards that condition as a malady. A wrestler could be experiencing the pain induced by an opponent's hammerlock; a gardener could be experiencing the discomfort of the relentless sun beating down on her; an individual might be trapped in a tightly closed space and therefore be experiencing aching muscles and anxiety. Yet none of these people necessarily has a malady. We need to make some kind of conceptual move in order to distinguish these cases from those conditions which are regarded as maladies. We need to distinguish between those harms being suffered by the individual due to factors within the individual and those caused from without.

Many harms are of course caused by agents from outside the individual: for example, allergens, germs, car accidents, and bright sun rays. Nevertheless as long as the external circumstances are actively responsible for perpetuating the harm (for example the anxiety is being suffered because one is in a runaway car), then we do not regard that anxiety as constituting a malady. If someone suffers a loss of freedom due to something internal to the individual, for example because of allergies or a fear of heights or open spaces, then we say he has a malady. But if his freedom is restricted by being in jail, we do not. When a change in the external circumstances immediately, or almost immediately, removes the harm being suffered, we do not call the condition a malady. We believe that all of this is in accord with the ordinary use of malady terms like "disease" and "injury."

To accomplish this conceptual move with a bit more finesse, we introduce the notion of a sustaining cause. As long as the harms are sustained by a cause distinct from the individual, the harms do not constitute a malady even though they do involve a condition of that individual. But these causes must be clearly distinct from the individual in whom the harms are being experienced. Thus we include as a necessary condition for a malady that the condition of the individual giving rise to his suffering harms has no sustaining cause that is distinct from the individual.

A distinct sustaining cause is a cause whose effects come and go simultaneously, or nearly so, with the cause's respective presence or absence. A wrestler's hammerlock may be painful, but it is not a malady because when the hammerlock ceases, so does that individual's pain. Of course, if the pain persists a considerable length of time after the hammerlock ceases, then a malady is present because the pain, initially caused by an external source, is now being generated by the condition of the individual himself. A malady is a condition of an individual such that, whatever its original cause, it is now part of the individual and cannot be removed simply by changing his physical or social environment.

Our complete definition of malady now looks like this: *An individual has a malady if and only if he has a condition, other than his rational beliefs or desires, such that he is suffering, or is at a significantly increased risk of suffering, a nontrivial harm or evil (death, pain, disability, loss of freedom, or loss of pleasure) in the absence of a distinct sustaining cause.*

The Role of Abnormality: Disabilities, Significantly Increased Risk, and Distinct Sustaining Cause

Thus far we have been able to discuss maladies independently of any reference to normality. We have explicated malady in terms of something being wrong with an individual. We have explained that to have something wrong means to be suffering a harm or to be at significantly increased risk of suffering a harm. And we have explained under what circumstances suffering a harm counts as a malady. Now, however, we come to some aspects of the definition of malady in which reference to the notion of normality is necessary.

One reason for relegating this discussion to a separate section is to emphasize that, contrary to most definitions of disease, abnormality is, for us, neither necessary nor sufficient for applying the disease or malady label. Earlier, we provided a recent example where abnormality was cited as the essence of disease in a book on medicine for the practicing physician. As we show later in this chapter, some editors of the American Psychiatric Association's Diagnostic and Statistical Manuals have made this same error. We believe that this is both wrong and potentially dangerous. Making abnormality the essence of disease has serious moral consequences, and that is why we need a clear account of abnormality's proper role. Labeling sheer deviancy as a disease mislabels, misdirects, and eventually may even lead to mistreatment. However, normality is a necessary feature for determining what counts as a disability, what counts as a significantly increased risk, and what counts as a distinct sustaining cause.

Disabilities and Inabilities

One of the basic harms whose presence can in part define a malady is a disability. However determining what counts as a disability requires use of the concept of normality.

How do we determine when someone has a disability? Most cases are clear: if an individual cannot see, unless she is a fetus, she has a disability. If an adult cannot walk, or has a limited range of motion in his joints, then he has a disability. But problems of labeling come in the borderline cases. Does an individual have a disability if he can walk but cannot run, or if he does not have full and complete range of motion in all his joints, or if he has less than perfect vision? What if someone who is only four months old cannot walk? Or what if an individual cannot jump to the top of a two-story building at any age? What if an individual cannot walk more than a quarter mile without tiring? These are the kinds of labeling problems that need to be worked through in order to have a grasp of the variables at work in the use of malady labels.

It is obvious that the lack of some abilities is properly called an inability rather than a disability. That humans cannot fly is a clear example of an inability. No humans can fly. Further, there are some extraordinary abilities that a very few humans have, but that does not mean that everyone else is disabled. It is at this point that the concept of the norm for the species becomes relevant. The lack of an ability to run a mile in four minutes is an inability rather than a disability. Even though there are a handful of humans who can actually run that fast, it is so far from the norm that there is no question that an individual is not disabled because he cannot do it. Labeling is more difficult as less rare abilities are considered. Just how far should one be able to walk or run, and how quickly, in order not to be considered disabled? Invariably the norm for the species must be consulted, and that which takes special training, for example, pole vaulting, jumping hurdles, or playing chess, must be taken into account. Many athletes can do extraordinary things, but again that does not mean that everyone else is disabled. For one thing, the athlete's feats are outside the normal range of what people can do, and for another, they require special training that others may not have an opportunity to acquire. If an ability is present in only a small subset of the human species, the lack of that ability is not regarded as a disability; and if an ability requires special training the lack of that ability is also not regarded as a disability. In both these cases the lack of ability is more accurately described as an inability.

A baby is unable to walk when she is only four months old. Is she disabled? Many very elderly persons cannot walk even a hundred feet. Do they have a disability? The baby does not have a disability but the very elderly individual does. We believe that a clarifying conceptual move in this regard, and one that parallels the intuitive understanding of the matter, is to conceive of a stage in normal human development when abilities are at their peak. Until an individual reaches that point, she may lack the ability but is not properly said to have a disability. It would simply be said that she is unable to do such and such or that she cannot yet do such and such: for example, the baby cannot yet walk. If she still does not have the ability in question after the time when it usually appears in the human species, or if she has had it but no longer does, then the lack of the ability is regarded as a disability, and hence a malady. For common abilities, after particular points in human development, the ability in question is simply regarded as the norm. After that maturation point, whoever does not have the ability has a disability no matter how many of the population, for example, 95%, also do not have the ability at that stage. It is not inconsistent to say it is normal for the very elderly to have a significant loss of flexibility. Just because it is normal in one sense (it is statistically common) does not mean that it is not a disability, at least not after one has reached that stage of life when having the ability is the norm.

In summary, both inabilities and disabilities involve the lack of abilities. An inability is not a malady. A lack of ability is an inability if either (1) the lack is characteristic of the species or of members of the species prior to a certain level of maturation, or (2) the lack is due to the lack of some specialized training not naturally provided to all or almost all members of the species. A lack of ability is a disability if one has reached a stage of life at which that ability is the norm for the species. Furthermore, having reached that point of maturation, one has a disability even if most others in his age group also lack that same ability. Abilities which only one gender has are not abilities that are the norm for the species, thus lacking that ability is not a disability in those of a different gender (men are not disabled because they cannot bear children), but if a male or a female lack an ability which is the norm for males or females, then they do have a disability.

That disabilities exist along a continuum leads to some inevitable vagueness in using the malady label. When should a low level of an ability be called a disability? The gradations are sometimes so gradual that there is no definitive way to draw lines. Obviously one must rely considerably on the norms for the species, the norms apart from any special training to enhance abilities. For example, an individual who cannot walk even after the maturation point at which a member of the human species generally acquires that ability obviously has a malady. But how far must he be able to walk so as not to be considered as having a malady? If he is limited to a few steps, or even to 50 yards, he is considered disabled. But a mile? Two miles? One must rely on a comparison with the ability of the vast majority of humans at their prime for that ability. If that ability is distributed along a normal curve, as abilities commonly are, then those falling in that range, no matter how wide that range is, are considered normal, that is, without a disability. Those few at the very low ability end of the curve are disabled, though, of course, those few at the high end of the curve are not. They have super abilities.

Something of this sort is already done in general intelligence testing. Intellectual ability is normally distributed and an IQ of 100 denotes average intelligence. Those having somewhat lesser IQ scores, for example between 70 and 80, are not regarded as mentally disabled but merely as having lesser ability. But those scoring 69 and under are regarded as being mentally disabled to varying degrees. Everyone knows that this is somewhat arbitrary and that there is no bright line distinguishing those who have a lesser normal intelligence (for example, an IQ of 71) from those who are mentally retarded (for example, an IQ of 69).

An individual who develops an extraordinary ability, such as the ability to run a marathon in less than three hours, and then subsequently loses that ability, does not thereby have a disability, even if she loses it because of disease or injury. As long as she still falls within the normal range of ability, she is not disabled even though her own ability is significantly less than it was. Only if she reaches a point where she falls outside the normal range of ability, for example, can barely walk, is she said to have a disability. And that is true no matter how many individuals her age have the same problem. The comparison group for making these determinations is always the human species at its prime for that particular ability.

Significantly Increased Risk

We want to forestall some conceptual confusions that can arise from the notion of "being at a significantly increased risk." As has been shown, this is an important phrase in our definition. These possible confusions relate to the matter of normalcy in the species.

We noted earlier that it was necessary to use the phrase "being at significantly increased risk." Some conditions of the individual that need to be labeled maladies are not yet causing perceptible harm, but they nevertheless put one at significantly increased risk for eventually suffering harm. High blood pressure is a good example, as is presymptomatic arteriosclerosis. In these examples it is clear that the significantly increased risk is based on empirical studies showing that having the condition often leads to suffering some harm in the future. In most of these cases even the causal mechanism is well understood. So the clearest instances of "significantly increased risk" are empirically based.

One of the possible interpretations of "increased risk" that we want to avoid is the one that applies to an individual who had been in extraordinarily good health and has now slipped from that peak condition. Perhaps she had been a highly trained athlete who ate carefully and exercised vigorously. But now she has ceased training and has relaxed her nutritional regimen. She is now more at risk for a malady—arthritis, high blood pressure, obesity—than she had been before. We do not label this kind of increased risk a malady. The increased risk criterion is not a matter of comparing two states of the same individual, but a matter of comparing the state in question with conditions known to put humans at increased risk.

The key to understanding the meaning of "increased risk" is seeing it as a comparison with what is normal for the human species. Given that the human condition itself puts one at risk for all kinds of harms, the only conditions which count as maladies are those which significantly increase the risk of such harms. Maladies designate those conditions of the individual that put him or her at significant risk of harm over and above what is normal for members of the species in their prime.

Allergy, Abnormality, and Distinct Sustaining Cause

Many maladies become apparent only in certain settings. When an individual is suffering discomfort and pain during an allergy episode, there is no doubt about his having a malady. At first impression it might seem as though this is a case of a distinct sustaining cause, since if the allergen were removed, the bad effects of the malady would disappear. But usually that does not happen quickly, and the individual continues to suffer for a period of time even in a changed environment.

But what about such an individual who is in an environment free of allergens, does he still have a malady? Certainly he has a condition that puts him at risk of a malady. If he is living in a place where there are no allergens, then he is not very much at risk, but he still has the malady. He is not only at some risk of suffering a harm, he is, as explained earlier, already experiencing a harm, namely, the loss of freedom. His choices of environment are limited because of his condition. Hence he definitely has a malady, though it may not be a very disturbing one for him.

It is in this context that another need for the concept of normality becomes evident. It is necessary for determining which reactions to one's environment are normal and which ones are indicative of a malady. If all humans gasp for air in a densely smoked-filled room, then gasping for air in a densely smoked-filled room does not indicate that one has a malady. The harm is regarded as caused by the environment, not by something within the individual. If only a small number of individuals develop shortness of breath in the presence of a cat, then the problem is regarded as being within those individuals. They have a malady and the harm is regarded as being caused by their condition, not by a distinct sustaining cause. Similarly, if an individual becomes anxious in the presence of almost everyone she meets, then she has a malady. In certain circumstances almost everyone becomes anxious, but if someone gets anxious in circumstances where most others do not, she has a condition that is causing the problem. The cause is not in the environment, but in her. Thus "abnormality" is important here, too, in deciding whether someone has a malady, for it determines whether an experienced harm does or does not have a distinct sustaining cause.

Society's Reaction

The final aspect of malady that employs the concept of normality is an unusual consideration. It is best seen when stated as a problem: if a malady is a condition of the individual such that he suffers harms, then might not race be a malady? Race, after all, can lead to individuals suffering death, pain, disability, loss of freedom, and loss of pleasure. But it is certainly wrong and counterintuitive to think of race (or ethnic origin, or gender) as a malady. On the other hand, how should a grotesque deformity, or a significant disfiguration caused by accidents or surgery, or an extreme abnormality of someone's body, be regarded? A significant part of the suffering associated with these latter conditions may be based on society's reaction to the condition, and here the malady label seems more appropriate. If the latter set of conditions are maladies, how can they be distinguished from the first set, which are not regarded as maladies?

It may seem that in the case of race, society's reaction could be regarded as a sustaining cause that is clearly distinct from the individual, and therefore that race (or gender, or ethnic origin) is not a malady. But what of deformities, disfigurations, and extreme abnormalities? Do these not also depend upon society's reaction? These extreme deformities usually involve some pain and disability and that alone makes them maladies without even considering the reaction of others to the deformity. For example, there can be organ and joint involvement in extreme abnormalities of size; there can be difficulties in using one's hands and legs in deformities; there can be disabilities of seeing, blinking, breathing, and hearing in disfigurations. So, in general, the pain and disabilities connected with abnormalities and deformities are sufficient themselves to classify the conditions as maladies.

Suppose, however, that there were no disability or pain connected with a severe disfigurement. Is the disfigurement or deformity still a malady? If there is a "natural" or "universal" shock to others who first observe such individuals (for example, a person without a nose), they do have a malady according to our definition. If this is not a learned, acculturated response, but rather is a basic emotional response of all humans upon first encountering these abnormal features, then the condition is a malady. In this sense such conditions are similar to allergies. In allergies, a condition of the individual interacts with certain elements of the environment resulting in harmful effects to the individual. One can avoid that environment, but having to do so constitutes another harm the individual is suffering, namely, loss of freedom. The natural, spontaneous reaction of other humans to these physical abnormalities is like the natural environment. The abnormalities of the individual, not the natural reaction of others, are regarded as the cause of the pain and suffering to the individual. As a general rule, any deformity, abnormality, or disfigurement that is highly unusual and normally provokes an unpleasant response by all others should be regarded as a malady. That, of course, leaves a certain amount of vagueness, but at least the features essential for deliberating about each case are clearer.

Race was dismissed as a malady because society's negative reactions were considered to be a distinct sustaining cause. But this is an inadequate reason. Allergies also have a distinct sustaining cause, but the condition of the individual is regarded as a malady because the overwhelming majority of the species do not suffer harm when they encounter that environment. So are race and similar features like ethnic origin really maladies? They are not, because the cause of the harm, unlike the example of disfigurement, is not normal for the species. Indeed, in other societies, an individual being of that race or ethnic origin might provoke a positive response. When the reaction is characteristic only of a society, not of the species as a whole, we regard the reaction as a distinct sustaining cause, and do not regard the object of that reaction, for example, race, as a malady.

This suggests that if animals respond viciously to certain individuals who have a certain condition, that condition is a malady since it puts the individuals at a significantly increased risk of harm and deprives them of freedom. We accept that implication. Some individuals attract mosquitoes much more than others, and that condition should be regarded as a malady, although perhaps not a major one. All humans attract mosquitoes to some extent, so do they all have maladies? No, because attracting mosquitoes to some extent is normal, thus they do not have a condition that puts them at significantly increased risk of harm. This is an instance of our meaning of "significantly increased risk" as "significantly more than is normal for the human species." This is how it is determined if it is the individual who has the malady or if it is simply an abnormal environment. For example, submerged in water or in a smoke-filled room, all humans have difficulty breathing; such difficulty is caused, not by an abnormal condition of the individuals involved, but by an abnormal environment. That is because the standard is what is normal for the species. It is the norm for the species to be unable to breathe underwater or in dense smoke. So the problem is not in particular individuals. However, if an individual cannot breath because there is a cat in the room, then the problem is within that particular individual, because it is normal for an individual to be able to breathe in such circumstances.

Thus the norm for the species is essential for determining whether the lack of an ability counts as a disability or only as an inability. It is also essential for determining what counts as a significantly increased risk of harm. Finally, what is normal for the species sometimes even determines whether the harm has a distinct sustaining cause and, consequently, whether the individual suffering that harm has a malady.

Some Special Concerns

Cross-Cultural Issues

One sometimes hears accounts of diseases that appear to conflict with the labeling of one's own culture. For example, conditions that American society regards as maladies, other cultures regard as a sign of beauty or a gift of the gods. St. Vitus dance, a neurological disorder associated with uncontrolled movements, is claimed by some to be a visitation from the gods; dyschromia spiraccotosis, a bacterial infestation, is regarded by some as a beauty mark. Is the labeling of maladies purely a relative matter?

We believe the relativity of maladies is analogous to the relativity of morality. We regard both maladies and morality as basically universal, because both involve those harms that all rational persons everywhere avoid unless they have an adequate reason not to.

However, a different culture could have a rational belief which leads it to interpret a particular pain, disability, or loss of freedom differently from other cultures. In our definition of malady, we have excluded rational beliefs and desires as conditions of the individual that can count as maladies. Thus we do not deny that another culture may welcome a condition that most cultures regard as a malady, but this does not show that the concept of malady is society-relative. In all cultures, a malady is occasionally welcomed: for example to avoid work, to avoid being drafted, to avoid being chosen for a dangerous mission, or to receive compensation. But the condition involved is still a malady if intrinsically, it causes death, pain, disability, and/or the loss of freedom or pleasure, or a significant risk of suffering these harms. St. Vitus dance is a disability in any culture, yet it may still, on balance, be desired if it is thought to be a favor of the gods. In short, though maladies are intrinsically bad, they can be instrumentally good.

The matter is sometimes even more complex. What are regarded as good or bad ends are sometimes a function of the beliefs of that culture. For example, some cultures have ceremoniously inflicted severe wounds on members of their group because of beliefs that regard these wounds as associated with significant goods: purification, the passage to manhood, or some other spiritual benefit. Although these wounds may not be thought of as maladies by those cultures, one suspects that a closer look at behavior would reveal that those wounds were attended to in the same manner that similar wounds incurred under different circumstances are managed. It also seems likely that a similar wound on some other part of the body—not involved in the belief system—would be regarded and treated as a malady.

There is another reason that the very same condition of an individual might not be labeled as a malady by all societies. Some societies may not know that a certain condition is a malady because it is so endemic in their culture (for example, schistosomiasis, a parasitic infestation) that they believe its signs and symptoms are a normal feature of the species. However they can be mistaken about this, just as they can be mistaken about any matter of fact.

Distinct Sustaining Cause within an Individual

Another point of ambiguity concerns distinct sustaining causes. The issue at hand is whether the harmful effects experienced by the individual stop when the external cause ceases. A clear case is the wrestler's hammerlock, or being in jail, where the pain or the loss of freedom may stop immediately and coincidentally with the cause being withdrawn. But sometimes there are lingering pains or disabilities. Here, as in many of these issues, practical considerations guide the labeling process. Someone who coughs for only one or two minutes after leaving a smoke-filled room is not said to have a malady. There is little point in so labeling her momentary condition. If the coughing continues for a significant amount of time, even an hour, depending on its severity, it might be regarded as a malady. That is because what had been a distinct sustaining cause is now seen to have caused a condition within the individual which continues independently of the original cause. At that point the cause of the pain and suffering is not distinct from the individual. Similar reasoning applies to the wrestler's hammerlock if the pain continues for a significant time after the hold is released. At some point, the condition of the individual that is producing the pain is not distinct from that individual. To state it somewhat more precisely, we say that the individual has a malady if and only if the harm she is suffering does not have a sustaining cause that is distinct from the individual. That keeps us from having to locate it precisely within the individual; rather it requires only that it be shown that the harm is not in continuing dependence on the distinct sustaining cause.

Our account of a distinct sustaining cause may suggest that these causes are always externally located, that is, outside the individual's body. Most are, but an increased risk of harm may have a sustaining cause that, though "clearly distinct" from the individual, is nevertheless within that individual, for example, a cyanide capsule held in the mouth. What if the poison capsule is swallowed but is still undissolved? At what point does a "clearly distinct" sustaining cause become one not so clearly distinct from the individual? A quantity of heavily encapsulated cyanide inside an individual's mouth is a "clearly distinct" sustaining cause because it has not yet been biologically integrated into the individual's body and it can be easily and quickly removed. If it were removed the individual would instantaneously be rid of the risk of harm. If it is swallowed and in the body of the individual, so that it cannot be easily and quickly removed, it is no longer a distinct sustaining cause; if it causes a significant increase in the risk of harm, its presence constitutes a malady.

An example of a foreign substance in the body that is not a distinct sustaining cause is the defoliative poison dioxin. It may become absorbed in the body's fat tissue and not have a harmful effect until the individual loses weight and the dioxin is released into the body, becoming metabolized within the body's circulation. Thus the individual whose body is storing dioxin certainly has a malady because he has a condition that increases the risk of his suffering an evil. This case is even clearer than the encapsulated cyanide that has been swallowed, for the dioxin has been biologically integrated with his body, even though it has not yet caused any harm.

When we speak of biological integration of a substance, we mean that the substance has become a part of the individual, unlike, say, a marble that a child has swallowed. Biological integration means that body cells are invaded and interacted with, biochemical exchanges take place, and/or body defenses react. But biological integration is not necessary for something in the body to cease to be a distinct sustaining cause. We do not consider a clamp or sponge in the stomach (left after surgery) or food in the windpipe to be distinct sustaining causes. They may appear to be instances of internal distinct sustaining causes because they are not biologically integrated but, for us, anything in the body that is difficult to remove without special training, skill, and/or technology, does not count as a distinct sustaining cause.

It is universally recognized that if the cause of harm or increased risk of harm is inside the body, and has become biologically integrated or physiologically obstructive, then the cause is not a distinct sustaining cause and the individual has a malady. It has not been universally recognized that if the cause of harm or increased risk of harm is inside the body and cannot be quickly and easily removed without special training or skill or equipment, then the cause is not a distinct sustaining cause. Conditions involving these items significantly increase the risk of suffering harm and so, when discovered, require swift medical intervention. Such conditions have all the features of a malady even though there is no ordinary malady term that refers to them. In persisting to the fine points of using the malady label, we are making distinctions at a level not ordinarily recognized or considered. We regard the ability of our analysis of the concept of malady to provide guidance, not provided by ordinary disease terminology, as an indication of its utility and precision.

Genetic Maladies

We explore in this section several interesting issues concerning the application of the term "malady" to an individual's genetic status. It is likely that soon it will be possible to map an individual's entire genome and sequence her individual genes. When that happens it is also likely that a great deal will be learned about the correlation between individual genes and the occurrence of particular physical and psychological conditions, some of them maladies, some of them not. In some cases the discovered correlation will be between a single gene (either a dominant gene as in Huntington disease or a recessive as in Tay Sachs) which is only slightly modulated by other genes, and its physical or behavioral manifestations. In other cases the manifestations will be under polygenic control. Sometimes this correlation may be exact, with the environment controlling only the timing and the severity of the malady. Thus the discovery of particular genetic sequences early in life may predict unerringly the appearance of a particular malady in the future. In other cases the correlation between the genes and the malady will be lower, for some specific environmental circumstances will be necessary for its appearance, but knowledge of the genome will still allow better predictions than are now possible.

What Conditions Qualify as Genetic Maladies?

When, according to our definition, is it true that conditions which are correlated with particular DNA sequences constitute genetic maladies?

An individual clearly has a genetic malady if he is directly suffering harms because of his genetic condition (for example, he has Tay-Sachs disease) or his chromosomal structure (for example, he has Down syndrome). Such conditions qualify according to the definition because harms (for example, mental and physical disabilities) are being suffered, and these harms are caused by the individual's genetic makeup or his chromosomal structure.

By contrast, there are a great many conditions which are genetically determined, fully or partially, but which are not maladies because they do not involve the suffering of harms. Eye color and fingerprint patterns are two clear examples. Having hazel eyes is not a malady. Neither is having all ten fingers each with a fingerprint pattern of an arch (or having ten loop patterns, or ten whorls), though this is statistically extremely rare. Although eye color and fingerprint pattern are genetically determined, neither condition involves suffering, or an increased risk of suffering, harms. Therefore, neither can be considered a malady, hence they cannot be genetic maladies, either intuitively or according to our definition.

It also follows from the definition that an individual has a genetic malady if her genetic structure is primarily responsible for her having a significantly increased risk of suffering harms in the future. Huntington disease is a clear example: if a young woman in her twenties is discovered to have the Huntington disease gene, she is usually regarded as having a genetic malady even though she is not yet suffering any symptoms. The definition thus accords with ordinary intuitions. The situation is similar to someone having a significantly elevated blood pressure but not yet having any target organ symptoms, or someone being HIV + but not yet symptomatic with AIDS. The Huntington-positive and the HIV + individual will certainly or nearly certainly suffer harms in the not too distant future. The individual with the Huntington disease gene is even more likely than the hypertensive individual to suffer harms in the future, and nonsymptomatic hypertension is widely regarded as a malady.

Genetic testing may soon reveal many conditions that, if suitable prophylactic measures are taken, will not develop symptoms. PKU is a well-known example of this kind of condition: if the condition is diagnosed sufficiently early and appropriate dietary precautions are followed, serious symptoms may be prevented. Other conditions may be discovered in the future in which a suitable diet or the chronic administration of a drug may prevent symptoms from occurring. However, even in the fortunate cases where prophylaxis results in the genetic malady's symptoms being completely avoided, people would still be regarded as having a genetic malady. This is because they suffer the loss of freedom to eat certain foods, at least for some period of time. As long as one cannot eat certain foods, or must take some drugs chronically, then one continues to have the genetic malady. This situation is closely analogous to the condition of having an allergy. An allergy is a malady even if the individual can eliminate symptoms totally by taking a drug or moving to another part of the country: her freedom has been curtailed by having always to take the drug, or by having to live in one place and not another. Indeed, it is quite likely that allergies are genetic maladies.

Genetic maladies (like Huntington disease and PKU) are far more likely than nongenetic maladies to include conditions in which harms are not currently being suffered, but rather conditions in which there is an increased probability, compared to the population at large, that they will be suffered in the future. Individuals with conditions like Huntington disease may suffer no harms for a long period of time, but the harms, when they do appear, may be quite severe. Sometimes, as in Huntington disease, the harms are certain to appear and there is no preventive treatment. Sometimes, as in PKU, the price of forestalling those harms is to employ treatment regimes that themselves involve the suffering of other nontrivial harms. It is for these reasons that it is in accord with common intuitions to consider individuals with nonsymptomatic Huntington disease or those still being treated for PKU to be suffering from genetic maladies.

New genetic discoveries may make available knowledge about genetic conditions that involve being at increased risk of suffering relatively mild future harms. Suppose that a four-year-old boy, because of his particular genetic condition, has a 50% probability of experiencing some mild skin condition in his thirties, annoying but not disfiguring, like eczema of the scalp. He satisfies the definition of a genetic malady; that is, he is at increased risk, compared to the general population, of suffering harms in the future because of a particular genetic condition. If there were no way to prevent those symptoms, it might seem questionable to regard him as currently having a malady at age four. Some may claim that since the harms, even when they occur, are mild, and there is only a 50% probability of those harms occurring and even then not for thirty years, the condition is too trivial to be classified as a malady when he is four years old. However, if a low-cost and low-risk intervention were discovered which would prevent the eczema, we believe people would be much more likely to regard the four-year-old boy as having a genetic malady, albeit a very mild one.

Genetic Maladies and Risk of Occurrence

Whether genetic conditions that, if not treated, involve possible or certain future harms are regarded as genetic maladies seems to be a joint function of several variables. Two seem particularly important: (1) the magnitude of the probability that the malady will occur, and (2) the likely age of the individual when it might occur.

The higher the probability of future occurrence, compared to the population as a whole, the more likely the individual will be regarded, in advance of the harms occurring, as having a malady. Thus a 25-year-old man with a genome indicating he has a 50% chance of developing leukemia before age 60 would probably be regarded as having a malady, but if he were only 2% more likely to develop leukemia than others of his age, he probably would not be. This is consistent with our definition of malady. As discussed earlier, "being at significantly increased risk" in the definition refers to being at significantly increased risk over and above what is normal for the species.

The age of occurrence seems a separate important factor. If, on the basis of his genome, it could be predicted that a 25-year-old man has a 50% chance of developing a serious malady (leukemia, for example) if he survives until his nineties, he would not be regarded at age 25 as having a malady. In fact, even if the likelihood of his developing leukemia approached 100% if he survived to his nineties, he still would not be regarded at 25 as having a genetic malady. Of course, this is based on the assumption that the average life span is in the mid-eighties or lower.

Someone with the Huntington disease gene is regarded by everyone as having a genetic malady, because of the seriousness of the symptoms, the certainty they will occur, and the fact that death will occur prematurely. Although Huntington disease can be accurately diagnosed decades before any symptoms occur, and the individual may feel entirely well during this period, the affected presymptomatic individual is still regarded as having a malady. Even though there is presently no treatment which may postpone or ameliorate its symptoms, if an expensive genetic treatment became available that would prevent the malady from developing symptoms at least 50% of the time, everyone would favor including it in health insurance coverage.

In the future many significant linkages between genes and maladies may be found. Thus the number of individuals who know or could discover at a relatively young age that they have a condition, without a distinct sustaining cause that is associated with a significantly increased risk of suffering serious harms in the future, could increase significantly. For example, the age of occurrence of heart disease and cancer, the two diseases associated with the highest death rates in the United States, will very likely prove to have significant genetic correlates that can be measured at an early age. This could result in one frequently noted ethical problem: the extent to which genetic information about individuals could and should be kept confidential and unavailable to employers and life insurance companies. But it could also result in a large number of young individuals considering themselves and being considered by others as suffering from maladies because of the significantly increased probability they will become seriously symptomatic during middle age.

Being at Higher Risk: Group Membership versus a Condition of an Individual

Some individuals are known to be at increased risk of prematurely developing diseases such as heart disease and cancer because of their family histories. However, as noted earlier, there is a difference between (1) knowing that an individual is at increased risk because he has a particular individual genetic structure associated with a high risk of prematurely suffering a fatal malady, and (2) knowing that he is at increased risk because of being a member of a group, some of whose members will prematurely suffer that malady, while others will not. The two cases must be distinguished, because it is known that the former individual has a malady, whereas it is not known whether the latter has one. This is true even when the objective level of risk is the same.

Consider this example: Jane is born into a family, 25% of whose female members develop breast cancer before the age of 40. It is ordinarily said of Jane, at age 20, that she is at increased risk, compared to other women, of developing a malady, but not that she currently has a malady. Now suppose that Jill is born into a family, none of whose female members has ever, so far as is known, developed breast cancer before the age of 40. However, in mapping Jill's genome it is discovered that she has an aberrant genetic sequence associated with a 25% chance of developing breast cancer before the age of 40. Jill is much more likely to be regarded as having a malady than Jane. Since Jill has a demonstrated aberrant genetic sequence, it is clear she has something wrong with her. It is not yet known whether Jane has something wrong with, for example, one of her genetic sequences, even though her risk is objectively the same. Although Jill now has a genetic malady, it is not yet known whether Jane has one.

Our definition of genetic malady does distinguish between Jane and Jill. "Condition," in the definition, means condition of the individual. Jill is at increased risk because of an aberrant genetic sequence, and this genetic sequence is clearly a condition of the individual. Jane, by contrast, is at the same increased risk, but it is not known if this is because of some condition of her as an individual: being a member of a group (her family) is not what is meant by a condition of the individual. If Jane does develop breast cancer this will almost certainly be because of an aberrant genetic sequence, as is true with Jill, but it is not yet known whether Jane has an aberrant genetic sequence.

We think it is much more likely to be said, of two individuals at equal objective risk of suffering genetically caused harms in the future, that the one with a demonstrable genetic aberrancy has a malady, compared with the other who only may have a genetic aberrancy. If true, this shows the power that the new knowledge of linkages between a person's genome and maladies could have in altering perceptions of individuals' malady status. Thus, discovering genetic conditions of individuals that significantly increase their risk of suffering future maladies will result in many more people knowing they have maladies at much younger ages. By increasing the importance of having a significantly increased risk of suffering harms, it will decrease the close connection between presently suffering symptoms and having a malady. Many more people who have no present symptoms will nevertheless be regarded as having maladies.

Mental Maladies

In our analysis of maladies thus far, we have primarily used as examples physical conditions of the individual. A person is diagnosed as having a physical malady such as cancer, on the basis of accompanying bodily alterations. Even a person who has only an increased risk of a physical malady like cancer, counts as having a malady only after some bodily alteration, such as an aberrant genetic sequence, is discovered. Yet our definition of malady contains no reference to bodily organs or genetic sequences, or to biochemical or physiological processes. The presence or absence of any of these physical conditions or processes does not determine, on our account, whether a condition is considered to be a malady.

Many conditions manifested primarily by psychological symptoms qualify as maladies on our definition. Someone with a severe endogenous depression, for example, is suffering a serious harm (mental pain) which is unrelated to any rational belief or desire, and which exists in the absence of a distinct sustaining cause. Our definition makes no distinction between physical and mental harms because we believe that, in defining maladies, both should be included. Both kinds of harms exist on a continuum of severity. In both physical and mental maladies there can be an increased risk of death as well as other harms suffered. To require of someone suffering psychological harms that an alteration of physical functioning be present before her mental condition is labeled a malady seems ad hoc and unjustifiable.

To illustrate that altered bodily processes are not necessary to establish the existence of a malady, consider the case of schizophrenia. This psychosis is a condition manifested symptomatically primarily by a collection of psychological dysphorias and disabilities. Its etiology is not well understood. Some believe that schizophrenia is caused primarily by certain inherited neurochemical and neuropathological abnormalities; others believe that particular kinds of early psychological experiences play the predominant etiological role; and still others hypothesize that both these factors are conjointly necessary to produce the condition.

Suppose there are three different etiological paths to schizophrenia: (1) some people inherit certain nervous system abnormalities so that schizophrenia develops no matter what the quality of their early psychological experiences; (2) other people have such psychologically traumatic early childhoods that schizophrenia develops even if they initially inherited a normal nervous system; and (3) still other individuals develop schizophrenia only because they have both an inherited central nervous system abnormality and a traumatic childhood.

Suppose further that these groups are phenotypically indistinguishable in terms of the psychological symptoms they manifest, the course of their condition, and the most effective treatment for them. Imagine, however, that with sophisticated neurochemical assays one can detect enzymatic abnormalities in the first and third groups that are not present in the second group. (We assume that cerebral processes are a necessary substrate for the symptoms of the second group but that this group does not show the enzymatic abnormalities.)

If the pathogenesis of schizophrenia turns out to resemble the above model, which it very well could, then those who believe that bodily abnormalities are a necessary condition for malady status would presumably believe that only the first and third groups qualify. We maintain that if the second group manifested the same symptoms, course, response to treatment, and so on, it would be pointless to deny that it shared the same malady status. The patients suffer the same harms, are treated by the same physicians in the same way, and should be covered by the same kind of health insurance coverage. Schizophrenia is a malady regardless of whether some, all, or no schizophrenics are eventually proved to have inherited central nervous system abnormalities. Physical maladies are distinguished from mental maladies in terms of their most salient symptoms, but there is no fundamental difference in cause or severity between physical and mental maladies.

Mental Maladies and Deviancy

Perhaps the most pervasive temptation in past attempts to define mental illness has been to equate behavior that is different with behavior that is a symptom of a mental illness. While it is true that the symptoms of mental maladies are "deviant," in the sense that they are statistically uncommon (relatively few people speak with someone that no one else can see or hear), it is not true that behavior and traits which are statistically uncommon are necessarily symptomatic of a mental illness. Being left-handed, mountain climbing, and wiggling one's ears, are not symptoms of maladies.

Nowhere has the error of equating deviancy with illness been more frequent than in the area of human sexuality. There has frequently been the inclination, on theoretical or other grounds, to believe that normal heterosexual functioning is ideal and healthy, and that engaging in statistically less common kinds of sexual activities is undesirable and sick, independently of whether the individuals involved suffer in any way because of their sexual preferences.

Our definition of malady contains no reference to abnormality or deviancy, except in the auxiliary role of helping to define some of the terms in the definition. The focus is principally on the suffering of harms. If a condition is not associated with the suffering of harms or the increased probability of suffering harms, it cannot be a malady, physical or mental, on our account. Thus if an individual prefers to have sexual experiences with members of his or her own sex, or if a man becomes particularly sexually aroused if he dresses in lingerie, these individuals do not have maladies per se. However, many individuals, and at times the profession of psychiatry itself, have explicitly stated that deviancy alone, even without the suffering of harms, is sufficient to constitute a condition of mental illness.

Mental Maladies and DSM

It is instructive to examine the way in which the American Psychiatric Association, through its series of Diagnostic and Statistical Manuals *(DSM-III, DSM-III-R,* and *DSM-IV)* has defined mental maladies, which the manuals call "mental disorders."

DSM-III was published in 1980. It contained the following definition of a mental disorder:

[A] mental disorder is conceptualized as a clinically significant behavioral or psychologic syndrome or pattern that occurs in an individual and that typically is associated with either a painful symptom (distress) or impairment in one or more important areas of functioning (disability). In addition, there is an inference that there is a behavioral, psychologic, or biologic dysfunction, and that the disturbance is not only in the relationship between the individual and society. When the disturbance is limited to a conflict between an individual and society, this may represent social deviance, which may or may not be commendable, but is not by itself a mental disorder.[11]

In 1982 we critiqued this definition.[12] In part, we applauded it as an improvement over many previous definitions. It captured in a general way the necessary criteria for an adequate definition of a mental malady. In particular, it referred to some (not all) of the harms suffered by individuals with mental maladies, and it incorporated, albeit awkwardly and imprecisely, the notion of a distinct sustaining cause (. . . there is a dysfunction . . . not limited to a conflict between an individual and society.)

One criticism we had of the definition has proved to be of continuing importance: that the word "typically" in the definition was ambiguous. It could mean that an individual who has a malady need not be suffering any evils but only be at increased risk of suffering them. This is in accord with our own definition of malady. But it could also mean that the authors of *DSM-III* were, intentionally or not, leaving open the possibility that an individual could have a mental disorder and not be suffering any psychological harm or even be at increased risk of suffering harm.

This latter interpretation seemed possible in view of the fact that one entire class of disorders in *DSM-III,* the "paraphilias," was defined in a way which did not include the necessity that the individual involved suffer any harms at all. *DSM-III* explicitly states, "The essential feature of disorders in this subclass is that unusual or bizarre imagery or acts are necessary for sexual excitement."[13] In fact, *DSM-III* states on the next page, "Individuals with these disorders tend not to regard themselves as ill, and usually come to the attention of mental health professionals only when their behavior has brought them into conflict with society."[14] But this seems to conflict with *DSM-III*'s own definition of mental disorder, which requires that the individual typically suffer either distress or impairment in functioning, and that his "disturbance" not be limited to a conflict with society.

The appearance of *DSM-III-R* in 1987 made it clear that there was simply an inconsistency between the definition of mental disorder and the criteria given for diagnosing the paraphilias. The *DSM-III-R* definition was as follows:

In DSM-III-R each of the mental disorders is conceptualized as a clinically significant behavioral or psychological syndrome or pattern that occurs in a person and that is associated with present distress (a painful symptom) or disability (impairment in one or more important areas of functioning) or with a significantly increased risk of suffering death, pain, disability, or an important loss of freedom. In addition, this syndrome or pattern must not be merely an expectable response to a particular event, e.g., the death of a loved one. Whatever its original cause, it must currently be considered a manifestation of a behavioral, psychological, or biological dysfunction in the person. Neither deviant behavior, e.g., political, religious, or sexual, nor conflicts that are primarily between the individual and society are mental disorders unless the deviance or conflict is a symptom of a dysfunction in the person, as described above.[15]

This definition is similar to the *DSM-III* definition but there are some small but significant improvements.[16] The word "typically" was removed, making it clear that *all* disorders need to be accompanied by the suffering of psychological harms. Also, a sentence was added ("Neither deviant behavior. . .") making it explicit that deviancy alone does not constitute a disorder. All the more surprising, then, that the *DSM-III-R* criteria for diagnosing several of the paraphilias do not include the necessity of an individual suffering any psychological harms.[17] Thus the apparent inconsistency in *DSM-III* was made clear and explicit in *DSM-III-R:* it was possible to satisfy the criteria for having one of the paraphiliac disorders but not at the same time satisfy the general *DSM-III-R* definition of having a mental disorder.[18]

Finally, in 1994, the American Psychiatric Association came closer to achieving consistency. In *DSM-IV* the definition of a mental disorder is left unchanged from the above *DSM-III-R* definition. However, the definition of all of the paraphilias now contains a "Criterion B," which states: "The fantasies, sexual urges, or behaviors cause clinically significant distress or impairment in social, occupational, or other important areas of functioning." *DSM-IV* further elaborates, when discussing the differential diagnosis of these conditions:

A Paraphilia must be distinguished from the nonpathological use of sexual fantasies, behaviors, or objects as a stimulus for sexual excitement in individuals without a Paraphilia. Fantasies, behaviors, or objects are paraphiliac only when they lead to clinically significant distress or impairment (e.g., are obligatory, result in sexual dysfunction, require participation of nonconsenting individuals, lead to legal complications, interfere with social relationships).[19]

This sentence could be clearer. It seems almost certain that the missing conjunction within the parentheses is "or" and not "and," for the *DSM-IV* authors surely do not intend to require that all five phrases be satisfied before "distress" or "impairment" is present. This presents a problem: it means that Criterion B can be satisfied if the individual's sexual behavior leads (only) to impairment in social relationships, and *DSM-IV* elsewhere states:

Social and sexual relationships may suffer if others find the unusual behavior shameful or repugnant or if the individual's sexual partner refuses to cooperate in the unusual sexual preferences.[20]

But this is much too broad. Suppose a man sometimes dresses in women's lingerie when he is in his own bedroom. The man is not distressed by this behavior in himself; he keeps it secret but it is quite ego-syntonic. However his best friend accidentally discovers that the man engages in this kind of behavior. The best friend is repulsed by the discovery and, as a consequence, severs the relationship. According to the above quotations from *DSM-IV,* the man has a mental disorder. Deviancy, if accompanied by lack of social acceptance, once again seems sufficient to constitute a disorder, despite *DSM-IV*'s general definition that states that it is not.[21]

We think that the authors of *DSM-IV* were simply careless and did not intend the result just described. We believe that they would agree with us and with *DSM-IV*'s own general definition, and regard the man described as not having a mental disorder, but we are not certain. This analysis shows the necessity of being careful in elaborating and following definitional criteria. It also shows the necessity and the power of a good definition. If the authors of *DSM-III-R* had paid strict attention to their own rather good definition, they would not have had these persisting problems with distinguishing between sexual behavior which does and sexual behavior which does not suggest that a mental malady is present.

Borderline and Difficult Cases

Throughout this chapter we have dealt both with clear cases and with less clear cases in the process of developing criteria for a malady. We have been able to show, for example, that some conditions about which there might be dispute, for example phobias and addictions, clearly qualify as maladies on our definition, and that others just as clearly do not: for example, those conditions that are merely abnormal (in the sense of being uncommon), such as many instances of transvestism.

In this section we explicitly address some conditions that may be difficult to classify. This discussion, while making additional clarifications, also functions as a working review, showing how the concept of malady works in some problematic cases.

Menopause

Menopause meets the criteria of a malady, even though it might be welcomed by the individual. It is a condition of the woman that necessarily involves a disability, though the lack of the ability to become pregnant is often not unwanted. The fact that menopause is entirely normal at a certain age does not keep it from being a malady. Similarly, a vasectomy in a man should be regarded as causing a malady, an iatrogenic malady, even if the resulting disability is exactly what is desired. Though it was elected by a male patient and performed by a physician, the result is still a malady since it is a condition of the individual such that not only is he no longer able to do something that he had the ability to do before, but that ability that he once had is an ability characteristic of the human species in its prime.

Menstruation

Menstruation is somewhat more difficult to classify. It has been claimed that prior to the beginnings of civilized society, menstruation was not normally a painful condition. Even now it is not painful for many women. If a particular woman does not suffer, then for her menstruation is clearly not a malady. But to the extent that the condition does cause discomfort and pain, it seems as if it should be considered a malady. It might be less misleading to say that menstruation itself is not a malady, but that it is often accompanied by maladies. On the other hand, the more constant the connection between the occurrence of menstruation and the accompanying harms, the more appropriate it would be to regard menstruation itself as a malady. The strength of the association between menstruation and suffering harms is an empirical matter on which we cannot speak. We are simply pointing out that it could play a role in whether the malady label was to be applied directly to menstruation or only to its accompanying harms.

Premenstrual syndrome (PMS) is clearly a malady, for the very meaning of the term is that the woman is suffering harms. If she is not, then she does not have PMS. PMS is discussed in terms of the harms comprising it, yet it is clear that not every woman experiences it. The harms can be both physical and mental, creating bodily pains as well as volitional disabilities and states of dysphoria.

The phenomenon of teething is in some ways similar to menstruation. Teething is a completely normal occurrence during maturation, yet it often causes a great deal of pain. And in this case, pain is necessarily part of the condition.

Teething is apparently almost always accompanied by some discomfort and pain, and hence for that reason we regard it as a malady, in spite of its being completely normal.

Pregnancy

Pregnancy is also a difficult condition to classify. It is a condition of the individual, other than her rational beliefs or desires, such that she is suffering, especially in the final trimester, some pain, much discomfort, and significant disability, all in the absence of a distinct sustaining cause. Labor and delivery, the inevitable culmination of pregnancies which come to term, are at best uncomfortable and confining, and of course can be extremely painful. Also, throughout pregnancy the woman is at a significantly increased risk of suffering a variety of harms. Thus pregnancy has all the objective features of a malady.

However it does seem counterintuitive to regard pregnancy as a malady. It is not generally regarded as a disease or, for that matter, as a disorder, a trauma, or an injury. None of those terms seem quite right. On the other hand, illness, nausea, and "feeling terrible" are terms frequently associated with pregnancy, and medical insurance pays for their treatment. If there were no child at the end of the process, no one would voluntarily become pregnant.

Despite the objective features that pregnancy shares with other conditions readily labeled as maladies, it is easy to see why the malady label is not easily applied to pregnancy. Malady, and other disease terms, refer to conditions that people avoid unless there is an adequate reason for having them, but many women want to become pregnant. However, there is an adequate reason for becoming pregnant, having a baby, which is an intrinsic feature of the condition. Pregnant women tolerate the malady in order to achieve the desired end.

Our emphasis in discussing malady has been on the harms suffered as a result of the condition of the individual, and pregnancy seems clearly to be a condition of the individual that causes harm. Some might be tempted to regard the fetus as an internal distinct sustaining cause, in which case pregnancy, carrying the fetus to term, is not a malady. Although eventually the fetus becomes distinct, during most of the pregnancy it is not only biologically integrated in the body of the pregnant woman, but it is not easily and quickly removable without special skill, technology, and training. Therefore, according to our criteria, the fetus cannot be an internal distinct sustaining cause.

A bad reason for not labeling pregnancy as "malady" or "disease" is to claim that pregnancy is normal. Though pregnancy is certainly normal, abnormality is only mistakenly taken to be the essence of a disease or disorder. It is a mistake to conclude that since there is nothing abnormal about pregnancy, it therefore cannot be a disease or malady. However, given that there is an adequate reason, intrinsic to this condition, for undergoing the harms involved, some might prefer a slight modification of our definition of malady so that pregnancy is not classified as a malady.

There is a temptation not to call pregnancy, menopause, and menstruation maladies, not only because they are normal, but also and especially because some believe it is insulting and degrading to women to do so.[22] Although some might believe that there is something negative about labeling a condition like pregnancy as a malady, we do not. We believe that labeling pregnancy a malady should not encourage anyone to treat pregnant women worse than they would be treated if they were not regarded as having a malady. Indeed, since we emphasize that an individual who has a malady is suffering some harm, we think applying the term "malady" to a condition should properly lead people to show more empathy toward anyone with that condition.[23] Our account of malady does not support any discrimination against, or valuing less, anyone who has a malady. We resist picking and choosing where the malady label should be applied on the basis of ad hoc and subjective grounds, for in the long run such an arbitrary approach is likely to lead to arbitrary and harmful applications of malady terms.

Shortness of Stature

Shortness of stature is similar to many contenders for the malady label, in that it seems that the physical (or mental) characteristic in question is a disadvantage only in particular social milieus. In a society that values height, shortness is seen as a disadvantage. The disadvantage is most likely be stated in terms of loss of freedom: freedom to play sports, to become a model, or whatever. Certainly there is not necessarily any pain, disability, or increased risk of death. The only problem seems to be falling short of a societal expectation or value by virtue of the condition of the individual. We see no grounds for classifying such conditions as maladies. Of course if the shortness of height is associated, as it often is in severe cases, with disabilities and painful conditions, then the condition would satisfy the definition of a malady.

Earlier we discussed the role of society's reaction to an individual's condition. In the case of shortness, any loss of freedom that is experienced is a direct result of a particular society's reaction. There is no natural, universal human reaction of shock or revulsion to shortness of stature, so there is no malady. There is nothing in the condition of the individual that itself causes harm to the individual; the problem comes about only as that condition interacts with the values and beliefs of particular societies. That may be a social problem, but it is not a malady. Furthermore, whether shortness of stature, which does not involve disabilities, is caused by a deficiency of human growth hormone or simply by genetic inheritance makes no difference as to whether or not it is a malady.

Old Age

On the surface it seems that old age is the epitome of a malady, a condition of the individual such that he suffers pain, disability, loss of freedom or pleasure or is at a significantly increased risk of all those harms in addition to an increased risk of death. However, there are several reasons for not calling old age a malady, even though it is usually accompanied by diverse maladies, but the most important is that age is not a condition of the individual. Cirrhosis of the liver, a broken leg, a colon polyp, a missing clotting factor, being pregnant, and teething are all conditions of the individual. Age alone, the mere passage of time, is not a condition so much as a fact about the organism, a fact like "the individual swam in the river yesterday," or "he has lived through two world wars." Cells of the body change with age and different organs of the body change in a variety of ways, though much depends on the environment that the cells and organs have lived through. Thus it is not helpful to characterize the condition of an individual with respect to age alone. Individual systems, cardiovascular, renal, endocrine, and so forth, may have deteriorated with age, but they may not have, and, in any case, each harmful condition is identifiable and is considered a malady.

Artificial and Transplanted Body Parts

Does the individual who has an artificial or transplanted body part still have a malady? This is not a contentious issue, but it is interesting to test the logic of our account of malady. It is fairly straightforward to apply the malady label. If an individual who had suffered from a chronic malady and, because of available therapy, is now no longer suffering or at increased risk of suffering any harm, then we say that he no longer has a malady. He is suffering nothing. Of course, realistically, if the individual has received a transplanted organ, very likely he is at increased risk of harm, and hence still has a malady. Normally he is at less risk of harm than he was before the transplantation, but the comparison for determining the relative risk, as we have pointed out, is not with his previous condition but with the norm for the species. However, after the transplantation, this individual's malady is normally less serious than his previous malady.

Suppose a woman had hypothyroidism, and physicians were able to implant in her a lifetime supply of completely safe and effective replacement hormone, so that none of the harms of the hypothyroidism were present and there was no increased risk of harm. We say that she has no malady. The same is true of a formerly diabetic patient who now has an indwelling insulin pump, providing that the harms of diabetes were gone and the risks of harm were no greater than normal for the species. An artificial hip and an artificial lens implant in the eye are other examples. However if these artificial or transplanted parts developed problems, the individual does have a malady. Now the individual is suffering a harm or would be at a significantly increased risk of suffering a harm due to a condition of that individual and there is no distinct sustaining cause involved.

Advantages of the Concept of Malady

A subtle benefit of using "malady" in this new technical sense described here is that it is apparently the first explicit term in any language with the appropriately high level of generality. No language that we have investigated (English, French, German, Russian, Chinese, or Hebrew) contains a clearly recognized genus term of which "disease" and "injury" are species terms. Each term in the usual cluster of disease terms has specific connotations which guide and significantly narrow its use. That is as it should be, if specificity is desired and justified. "Disease," "injury," "illness," "dysfunction," and other such terms overlap somewhat, yet each has its own distinct connotations.

The advantage of "malady" comes by way of the term's generality, by way of its including all those conditions whose terms have their own individual, though overlapping, connotations. This by no means makes the old terms irrelevant; rather "malady" is useful precisely in those contexts where generality is important. One such situation is when nothing is known about a patient's condition that justifies the connotations of any of the other terms. All these more specific terms have connotations with respect to what the condition is and how it was caused. Inappropriate use of these terms can lead to wrong expectations and hence lead one temporarily down the wrong path of diagnosis. "Malady" is general and noncommittal with respect to particular connotations. It is useful as a beginning point for labeling a phenomenon. Thus, though it is not as informative as other disease words, it is a useful term when none of these circumstances are known.

The search for a general term initiated the question, what do all the human conditions designated by the various disease terms have in common? This is the question that this chapter has tried to answer, and in doing so, has arrived at an analysis of the variables that enter into the labeling of these various human conditions. Our account of malady led to the recognition that all maladies involve either suffering at least one of the harms, namely, death, pain, disability, loss of freedom or loss of pleasure, or being at a significantly increased risk of suffering them. Because these harms are objective (in the sense that they are avoided by all rational persons unless they have an adequate reason not to), the influence of ideologies, politics, and self-serving goals in manipulating malady labels is considerably diminished. The possibility for some subjectivity does remain, as we have pointed out, but given the above explication of malady, exactly what elements are open to subjective bias can be determined. In short, our definition clarifies what may be causing the disagreement, and hence may facilitate efforts to resolve it.

The concept of malady has values at its core, but the values are universal and objective. Thus, our explication shows the inadequacy of either regarding disease as being totally value-free or as being heavily determined by subjective, cultural, and ideological factors. We have also tried to show how culture influences malady labeling in those few instances in which it does.

An important feature of our account of malady is that it shows that abnormality is neither a necessary nor sufficient definition of disease or related terms. Abnormality becomes important in certain contexts, which we have specified, namely, in the determination of disabilities, distinct sustaining causes, and increased risks, but it does not play the major role that many other definitions have assumed it plays. Labeling a behavior or a condition a malady simply because it is abnormal sometimes leads to unfortunate consequences, as with some paraphilias. All of the various disease terms, such as "disorder" or "dysfunction," require more than abnormality for proper application; all require the suffering, or significantly increased risk of suffering, one or more of the harms. Deviancy is not sufficient for using any disease term and the consequences of so regarding it can be significant. One tendency in the medical-scientific world has been to establish a normal range for this or that (some component of the human body), and, ipso facto, to have "discovered" two new maladies: hyper- and hypo- this or that.[24] Our account makes it clear that this use of abnormality represents a misunderstanding of the concept of malady.

A final advantage of our explication of malady is that its basic elements, concepts, principles, and arguments are the same when applied to mental maladies. The usual bifurcation between mental and physical maladies disappears. As we have seen in numerous examples throughout this chapter, significantly increased risk of premature death, pain, disability, loss of freedom and pleasure, and the absence of distinct sustaining causes are applicable to the mental domain as well as to the physical.

Notes

1. Our introduction of this technical use of "malady" and our earliest treatment of the concept appeared in K. Danner Clouser, Charles M. Culver, and Bernard Gert, "Malady: A New Treatment of Disease." *Hastings Center Report,* 11 (1981), pp. 29–37.

2. This is true in other languages as well; see below.

3. Thomas M. Peery and Frank N. Miller, *Pathology,* 2d ed. (Boston: Little, Brown, 1971).

4. Peter J. Talso and Alexander P. Remenchik, *Internal Medicine* (St. Louis: Mosby, 1968).

5. William A. White, *The Meaning of Disease* (Baltimore: William and Wilkins, 1926).

6. Robert L. Spitzer and Jean Endicott, "Medical and Mental Disorder: Proposed Definition and Criteria," in Robert L. Spitzer and Donald F. Klein, eds., *Critical Issues in Psychiatric Diagnosis* (New York: Raven, 1978), pp. 15–39.

7. Donald W. Goodwin and Samuel B. Guze, *Psychiatric Diagnosis,* 2d ed. (New York: Oxford University Press, 1979).

8. Boston: Butterworth-Heinemann, 1992, p. 14.

9. Another connotation of "having something wrong with oneself" is that something is not going in the way it should be going, that its occurrence is abnormal. We do not intend that connotation, for we believe that a normal condition like teething is a malady (see below).

10. Thus what we call irrational beliefs, psychiatrists refer to as delusions. For a further discussion of the relationship between irrational beliefs, irrational desires, and mental disorders, see Bernard Gert, "Irrationality and the *DSM-III-R* Definition of Mental Disorder," *Analyse & Kritik,* 12 (1990), pp. 34–46.

11. *DSM-III: Diagnostic and Statistical Manual of Mental Disorders* (Washington, D.C.: American Psychiatric Association, 1980).

12. Charles M. Culver and Bernard Gert, *Philosophy in Medicine* (New York: Oxford University Press, 1982), pp. 91–95.

13. *DSM-III,* p. 266. "Paraphilia" is the term currently used by psychiatrists for the conditions that were once called "sexual perversions."

14. Ibid., p. 267.

15. *DSM-III-R: Diagnostic and Statistical Manual of Mental Disorders* (Washington, D.C.: American Psychiatric Association, 1987), p. xxii or p. 401.

16. These improvements are based on the definition of malady proposed in K. Danner Clouser, Charles M. Culver, and Bernard Gert, "Malady: A New Treatment of Disease." Gert served as a consultant for *DSM-III-R,* and his suggestions for improving the *DSM-III* definition were incorporated into the *DSM-III-R* definition.

17. For an extended analysis of *DSM-III-R*'s discussion of the paraphilias, see Bernard Gert, "A Sex-Caused Inconsistency in DSM-III-R: The Definition of Mental Disorder and the Definition of the Paraphilias." *The Journal of Medicine and Philosophy,* 17 (1992), pp. 155–171.

18. "If any proof were needed of the powerful influence that sex has on one's thinking, examination of the inconsistency between the *DSM-III-R* definition of mental disorder and the *DSM-III-R* definition of paraphilias, would provide that proof." (Gert, ibid., p. 155).

19. *DSM-IV: Diagnostic and Statistical Manual of Mental Disorders* (Washington, D.C.: American Psychiatric Association, 1994), p. 525.

20. Ibid., p. 523.

21. In fact many individuals with ego-syntonic homosexuality would satisfy the criteria for having a paraphilia, surely a result the *DSM-IV* authors do not want.

22. Michael Martin, "Malady and Menopause," *The Journal of Medicine and Philosophy,* 10 (1985), pp. 329–337.

23. Bernard Gert, K. Danner Clouser, and Charles M. Culver, "Language and Social Goals." *The Journal of Medicine and Philosophy,* 11 (1986), pp. 257–264.

24. Alan Bailey, David Robinson, and A. M. Dawson, "Does Gilbert's Disease Exist?" *Lancet,* 8018 (1977), pp. 931–933.

6

Competence

There is widespread agreement in ethics and in law that patients must be competent to consent to treatment or else their consent is not valid. There is also a general presumption that if patients are competent, then their consent or refusal of treatment should seldom if ever be overruled. We discuss the concept of competence in this chapter and the more general topic of consent in the next.

Definitions of Competence

The concept of competence, and even more so incompetence, is important in medicine, for it is generally accepted that incompetent patients can at least sometimes be treated over their objections. However, the concept has lacked a precise definition. Its definition, in fact, has been the subject of extensive discussion and theoretical dispute.[1] The lack of an agreed-upon definition is characteristic of law as well as ethics; Alan Stone has written, "Strange to say, there is very little applicable law on the important subject of the capacity to make medical decisions. No legal test of competency commands general acceptance and a search of the state statutes is surprisingly unrewarding."[2] We first review several current and plausible definitions of "competence," and then suggest a new one of our own.

The "Understand and Appreciate" Definition

A traditional way of defining "competence," and the way in which some states have explicitly defined it in either statutory or case law, is in terms of whether a patient can adequately understand and appreciate (U + A) the information given during the consent process. As such, this definition focuses exclusively on intellectual abilities. If a patient does understand and appreciate the information, she is competent; her consent may be and usually is acceded to and her refusal cannot be overruled. If she does not understand or does not appreciate the information, she is not competent: her physician may choose not to accede to her consent, and may decide to overrule her refusal. Should a physician never accept an incompetent patient's consent and always overrule an incompetent patient's refusal? We attempt to answer these questions later in this chapter and in Chapter 10, on the justification of paternalism.

The information which a patient needs to understand and appreciate is the body of information that pertains to the particular treatment being suggested. (In the next chapter we discuss the nature of the information that must be disclosed in order for the information disclosure to be deemed "adequate.") Thus "competence" is specific to the task at hand. This is recognized by not only the U + A definition of competence but by most other definitions. Part of the logic of the term "competence" is that persons are not globally "competent" but rather "competent to do X," where X is some specific physical or mental task. It is true that some persons (for example, the unconscious) are globally "incompetent," in that they do not have the ability to do anything. But there is no one who is globally "competent"; that is, there is no one who has the ability to perform all mental and physical tasks.

Appreciating that competence is always task-specific makes clear that it does not follow from the fact that a person is competent to do X, that the person is also competent to do Y. For example, a somewhat confused person may be competent to eat his breakfast by himself but not be competent to make a decision about having a radical prostatectomy. There are even differential competencies within the realm of consenting to medical treatment: a person may be competent to consent to a treatment with some obvious probable harms and benefits (applying a Band-Aid to a cut finger) but incompetent to consent to a treatment with a complex set of probable harms and benefits (having a radical prostatectomy or a carotid endarterectomy).

The terms "understand" and "appreciate" are usually not defined precisely by those using the U + A definition. Their meanings are not thought to be technical and are made reasonably clear in the definition's applications. "Understand" refers to a patient's general comprehension of the information presented; it is tested, if need be, by asking the patient questions about what she has been told, to ascertain if she can answer them correctly. We take "appreciate" to refer to a patient's knowledge that the information she has "understood" does in fact apply to her in the present situation.

The two cognitive abilities of understanding and appreciating correlate highly with one another. Patients who understand the information given usually realize that in fact it applies to them; clearly, that is the point of their having been given the information in the first place. However, there are rare cases of delusions affecting the consent process in which a patient might understand the information adequately but think it did not apply to her. For example, she might believe she was heaven-blessed and could not be harmed on earth, so that risks pertaining to others had no relevance to her. Therefore although her "understanding" might be intact, her "appreciation" would not be, and her competence to make treatment decisions would be judged faulty.

It is an important feature of the U + A definition, and is seen by many as its strength, that the patient's decision about treatment in a particular case, that is, whether she consents or refuses, does not enter into the determination of competence for making that decision. By divorcing the state of competency from the actual consent or refusal, one can achieve what many see as the highly desirable goal of allowing patients to make any decision they want, provided they are competent. The patient's competence, using this definition, can in fact be determined before the patient has communicated, or has even decided, what her decision will be in a particular case. If, by contrast, the patient's decision in a particular case were allowed to enter into the determination of competency, then some decisions, for example some seriously irrational ones, might be taken as prima facie evidence of incompetence. Thus it would no longer be true that patients who are otherwise competent could make any decision they wished to make. This is regarded by some as an undesirable result.

It seems clear that most courts have carefully avoided including the rationality of a patient's actual treatment choice in the evaluation of competence. The recent extensive empirical study of competence by Appelbaum and Grisso[3] is based on this same assuption: that they measurement of competence has been based by the courts on one of four standards but that the patient's choice itself does not enter into the determination of competency.[4] Appelbaum and Grisso are descriptive and not prescriptive in their approach and it is not clear whether they believe the courts have adequately defined the concept of competence.[5]

A problem with the U + A definition is that it does not always agree with strong moral intuitions that people have about particular cases. There are cases in which a patient who is competent (according to the U + A definition) refuses treatment, even though almost everyone believes that the patient's refusal should be overruled and the patient treated over his objection. We call this the "overruling the competent patient" (OCP) problem.

Two cases illustrate the OCP problem:

CASE 6.1

A man with an unstable cardiac condition is severely depressed. He is anorexic and has lost a great deal of weight. He refuses to eat and refuses therapy for his depression. His doctor believes there is a high likelihood the patient will die from his weakened condition within a few weeks if he does not accept treatment for his depression and begin eating. The patient understands and acknowledges that without treatment he may die and that with treatment he will almost certainly recover. Unlike some depressed patients, he has no "cognitive distortions." Nonetheless, because of his depressed mood, he refuses nourishment and potentially lifesaving treatment because, he states, he wants to die.

CASE 6.2

A depressed woman, phobic about receiving electroconvulsive therapy (ECT), cannot bring herself to consent to the procedure, despite her agreement with her doctors' opinion that she may die without ECT, her avowal that she does not want to die, and her acknowledgment that ECT would likely prevent her death. She understands and appreciates everything her doctors tell her, but she has a fear, which she herself calls "foolish," that prevents her from consenting.

Almost everyone thinks that patients like these two should be treated, and probably they are or would be treated in all clinical settings. However, to treat them goes against the principle of never overruling the refusal of competent patients, if competence is defined strictly in terms of understanding and appreciating information.

One might try to preserve the U + A definition by broadening the meaning of "appreciate" to include factors other than its usual meaning. This usual meaning is limited to the patient's realization that the knowledge given to him about the likely harms and benefits of various treatment options applies to him at the present time. For example, one might invoke additional formal cognitive operations, whose successful performance was stipulated to be necessary in order for patients to "appreciate" information adequately and thus make medical decisions competently. For example one might require that patients show how their decisions are logically consistent with the ends they wish to achieve. Or one might require that patients' decisions be expressed nonimpulsively in a "cool moment" and therefore require that a patient maintain his refusal over a period of time in the face of efforts to persuade him to consent.

No definition of "appreciation" or "competence" comprised solely of formal cognitive operations, however, seems to solve the OCP problem. No matter what formal cognitive operations might be included as necessary, it would still seem possible for a patient to satisfy them, and yet go on to make a seriously irrational decision that all rational persons would agree it would be justified to overrule. For example, a seriously depressed patient could claim, as some do, that her refusal of treatment was logically consistent with her overwhelming desire to die, and she might maintain this refusal over time despite attempts to persuade her otherwise.

One reason for this state of affairs is that affective states, like depression and fear, can significantly influence decision making without necessarily distorting formal cognitive operations. Of course, affective states often do distort formal cognitive operations: under their influence a frightened patient can lose the ability to understand what he is told, or a depressed patient can become delusional about her medical situation. However, formal cognitive distortions are not inevitable in the presence of strong emotions.

On the other hand, if the definition of "appreciation" or "competence" were to move away from formal cognitive operations and be widened sufficiently to include a judgment about the quality of the patient's actual decision to consent or refuse, then it seems inevitable that the concept of irrationality, or some similar concept (for example, that the refusal exposes the patient to danger without an adequate reason) would enter into the definition. This might turn out to be a necessary and desirable move to make. However, among its results would be that some seriously irrational (or "dangerous") refusals would inevitably entail that the patient is incompetent, and it would therefore be morally justified to overrule him. Thus some refusals would never be accepted since the decision itself would be decisive in determining that the patient was incompetent. Therefore competent patients (on the original U + A definition) would not be free to successfully refuse some treatments they wanted to refuse. This is a result many want to avoid. Others, however, including us, think this would not be an undesirable result.

Other Definitions

There have been at least two major attempts to deal with the OCP problem described above. One, apparently initially suggested by Roth, Meisel, and Lidz, then elaborated by Drane, and more recently promoted by Buchanan and Brock, relies on a scheme whereby the definition of competence changes in different clinical situations.[6] According to Drane, in situations in which consent is the patient's only rational choice, competence is defined simply as the patient's saying yes to the suggested treatment. In situations in which it would be rational either to consent or refuse, competence is defined in terms of the patient's understanding and appreciation of the relevant information. Finally, in situations in which refusal appears to be prima facie irrational, competence is defined as the patient's refusal being in fact, after close investigation of the patient's beliefs, including his religious beliefs, a rational one.[7]

We believe that the approach of having a central theoretical term like "competence" take on significantly different meanings in different situations can lead to unacceptable results. What if, for example, two doctors agree about all the facts of a hospitalized patient's situation but disagree about the patient's prognosis: one believes it is serious and the other does not think it is serious. If the patient refuses further diagnostic testing, without explanation, the first doctor would view the patient as incompetent to refuse, while the other doctor would view him as competent to refuse. Their differing views about the patient's competence would be a function not of any objective attributes of the patient's mental state, for they agree about all the objective attributes of the patient's mental state, but a function of their own prognostic speculations. Yet it seems fundamental that competence is an attribute of patients, not of doctor's prognostic disagreements, and that different judgments about competence should covary only with different attributes of the patients toward whom they are applied.

A second approach to the OCP problem was described by Culver and Gert.[8] We suggested that "competence" continue to be defined in terms of a patient's understanding and appreciation of the relevant information, but also argued that it was necessary to employ a second concept—irrationality—in order to account for the agreed-upon moral intuitions about clear cases, including cases like the two described above. "Irrationality," as defined in Chapter 2, is a characteristic of some patient decisions, especially of some treatment refusals, and is conceptually distinct from "competence."

In the writing cited (see note 5), we argued that irrationality, not competence, is the key normative concept which should be used in determining when it is morally justified to overrule some treatment refusals, and we offered a specific decision-making procedure for determining when irrational refusals are sufficiently irrational that overruling them is morally justified. We also argued, unlike all of the above approaches, that it is sometimes justified to overrule patients who are competent on the U + A definition, but who make seriously irrational decisions. We realized that this went against the general legal principle of never overruling competent patients but believed that this legal principle, and its attendant U + A definition of competence, had not been the product of careful argument and, in fact, was often and appropriately ignored by the courts, especially the lower courts, in particular cases. While we believed that our approach had a conceptual consistency missing in other approaches, we acknowledged that, unfortunately, it produced results at variance with the legal tradition.

In what follows we take an approach different from Drane, from Buchanan and Brock, and also different from our earlier position.

A New Definition of Competence

Instead of defining competence and rationality strictly independently of one another, as we have in the past, we now realize that they are conceptually related. We make this relationship explicit in our new definition by saying that competence, in making medical decisions, is the ability to make a rational decision. We pointed out earlier that competence is always task-specific; a person is not simply "competent" but is competent to do some specific task. Our new definition makes explicit that the person's task in the consent situation is to be able to make a rational decision of the kind at hand.

Whether a person has the ability to make a rational decision is important not only in medical situations but in any life situation in which she must decide between different states of affairs, each of which contains different sets of possible harms and benefits. We are particularly likely to raise the issue of a person's competence to make a rational decision whenever, by law or custom, we have some duty to look out for that person's well-being: for example, with respect to our patients, students, clients, or members of our family, especially our children. In such relationships, if we believe the person does not have the ability to make a rational decision of the kind necessary, it is more likely that the moral justification for paternalistic intervention exists than would be the case where we have no such duty; see Chapters 2 and 10.

The Nature of an Ability

The ability to make a rational decision of a certain kind is, like all abilities, usually a relatively stable attribute of a person, not something that quickly comes and goes. Thus if, at a particular time, a person is capable of making a rational decision of a certain kind, or if he has the ability to play tennis or speak Italian, then in normal circumstances the person will still have the ability to play tennis, speak Italian, or make decisions of that kind a day, a week, or a month later.

Of course catastrophic events, such as a gunshot wound to the brain, can quickly bring about the loss of an ability. Although transient circumstances like fatigue or anger may temporarily cause one to perform poorly, they rarely if ever abolish an ability. A championship golfer who is sick and feverish with the flu today may take at least three putts on every green, but we would still say he has the ability to play championship golf. We would not even say that he lost the ability today, merely that he played poorly today. Similarly, a patient who irrationally refuses a treatment because of temporary anger at her doctor may still be correctly described as having the ability to make rational treatment decisions of the kind involved. We acknowledge that her anger has caused her to make an irrational choice, but assume that when her anger subsides she will once again manifest the ability to make rational treatment decisions.

To have an ability is to be able to perform a particular kind of action. An ability manifests itself on particular occasions, but it always involves being able to perform *a kind of action*. A choice must often be made about how narrowly or broadly to describe the kinds of actions that someone does or does not have the ability to perform. Thus it would clearly be correct to say of someone who has defeated five consecutive opponents and thus won a tennis tournament that she has the ability to play tennis. We could also say, without fear of error, that she has the ability to serve tennis balls correctly over the net, because if she did not have that ability she could not have won any matches. Which of these two descriptions we choose depends upon our purposes.

We can often surmise the existence of one ability from the presence of a different but similar one. For example we could surmise, almost always correctly, that someone who has the ability to play tennis well also has the ability to jog two hundred yards without stopping. The two abilities share something in common—the requirement of having a moderate amount of stamina—and would be highly correlated. It might not be impossible to find a good tennis player who lacked the stamina needed to run two hundred yards, but it would be so unusual that we can fairly confidently infer the second ability from the first.

To say of a patient that he appears to have the ability to make a rational treatment decision always means that he appears to have the ability to make a rational decision of a certain kind: the kind represented by the particular treatment decision at hand. Usually we make that judgment based on indirect evidence. That is, we often have no evidence about the patient's ability to make rational decisions about this particular kind of medical treatment; we may, in fact, have no evidence about his ability to make rational medical decisions of any kind. However, we may have abundant evidence about his general ability to make rational life decisions about states of affairs of a similar degree of complexity and seriousness.

Life decisions, including treatment decisions, vary along many dimensions, for example, the complexity of the information about possible harms and benefits that the person must understand, and the amount of anxiety involved in making a decision under a particular set of circumstances. Some persons may be able to make rational life decisions under almost any circumstances, but others may be able to make rational decisions only when the relevant associated information is rather simple but not when it is at all complex. Or, a nine-year-old child may have the ability to make a very broad range of rational decisions, but not have the ability to make rational decisions involving consenting to temporary short-term suffering to avoid later long-term suffering, like consenting to go through a temporarily painful dental procedure.

The Ability to Make a Rational Decision

The ability to make a rational decision of a certain kind is not an undifferentiated, homogeneous ability; it contains several constituent subabilities and also requires the absence of potentially interfering personal characteristics or mental disorders. Among the factors that can interfere with a person's ability to make a rational decision of a certain kind, are:

A. a cognitive disability that prevents the person from understanding the information relevant to making a decision of a particular kind. In the case of medical treatment decisions, this would be the lack of ability to understand the "adequate information" given during the consent process (see Chapter 7).

B. a cognitive disability that prevents appreciating that the relevant information in (A) does indeed apply to one in one's current situation.

C. a cognitive disability that prevents coordinating the information in (A) with one's personal ranking of the various goods and harms associated with the various available options, insofar as one has stable rankings which are relevant.

D. the presence of a mental malady, such as a mood disorder or a volitional disability, that causes one to make irrational decisions.

If either (A), (B), (C), or (D) is present, then the person lacks the ability to make a rational decision of the particular kind involved, which is to say that she is not competent to make a rational decision of that kind. Thus the ability to make a rational decision has intellectual, affective, and volitional components.

Each of the above four factors may interfere with one's ability to make a particular kind of rational decision. We think this list is exhaustive and thus the absence of all four factors is sufficient to insure that the person is competent to make a rational decision of the kind involved. However, each of the factors could be more precisely defined and each factor could itself be separated into constituent subfactors. In addition, a patient may not have the ability to make a rational decision of a particular kind because more than one of the factors may be present; for example, he may have only marginal cognitive ability to understand the relevant information, and also be so depressed that his marginal understanding renders him unable to make a rational decision.

Following are some illustrative cases:

Case 6.3

A patient is mildly demented, and despite what appears to be a sincere effort he cannot understand the information about the harms and benefits which he has been told about a suggested treatment. In the clinical circumstances in which he finds himself, it would be rational either to refuse or to consent. He nods his head pleasantly and says that he will do whatever the doctor suggests, but when asked to repeat or explain the information he has been given, he is unable to do so. It would be correct to say of him that he does not have the ability to make a rational decision of the kind required in this situation. Although it would be rational to consent to the suggested treatment, one cannot say that this patient has made a rational decision at all; to acquiesce ignorantly is not to make a rational decision. (Note that he might have the ability to make other kinds of rational decisions, for example, which kind of cereal to select from a menu for his breakfast.)

CASE 6.4

A patient has the delusion that he is Superman. While he understands all of the information given to him about a treatment choice, he falsely believes that none of the risks apply to him personally, and therefore unhesitatingly consents to a risky operative procedure which is only one of the available rational therapeutic options. We could say of him that while he is able to understand the relevant information, he does not have the ability to appreciate that it applies to him. Thus he does not have the ability to make a rational decision of this kind; even though his particular decision was rational, that was simply a lucky accident. (He too might have the ability to make other kinds of rational decisions, like what to eat for breakfast or whether to have his car fixed.)

CASE 6.5

A patient is mildly demented and confused, so that while he seems to understand the information given to him about treatment alternatives, and seems to appreciate that it applies to him, he nonetheless makes a choice that seems very much at odds with values that he has previously expressed strongly. When this inconsistency is pointed out to him, he acknowledges it, but denies that he has changed his mind about any of the issues that confront him. He says he is now confused about what he should do. We could say that he has the ability to understand the relevant information and appreciate that it applies to him, but that he does not seem to have the ability to coordinate this information with personal values which he acknowledges apply to him, and thus does not have the ability to make a rational decision of this kind. We call such a decision "unreasonable" rather than "irrational," but most of what we say about irrational decisions also applies to unreasonable ones.[9]

The following are slight expansions of two cases mentioned earlier:

CASE 6.6

A severely depressed man, weakened by a cardiac disorder, refuses lifesaving treatment for his potentially reversible condition. Unlike some depressed patients, he manifests no cognitive distortions; he seems to understand the relevant information and appreciates that it applies to him. He refuses treatment and nutrition because he wants to die. He gives, and apparently has, no reason to refuse other than his depressed mood, and there is no reason to think that his life would not be satisfactory and enjoyable to him if he were to recover from his current condition. We could say his mood disorder has interfered with his ability to make rational medical treatment decisions of the kind at hand.[10]

CASE 6.7

A depressed patient, phobic about electroconvulsive treatment (ECT), cannot bring herself to consent to the procedure: Despite her agreement with her doctors' opinion that she may die without ECT, her avowal that she does not want to die, and her acknowledgment that ECT would likely prevent her death she still cannot bring herself to consent. She did consent to have ECT when she was similarly depressed several years earlier, and she remembers that ECT quickly alleviated her depression. She understands and appreciates everything her doctors have told her, but she has an irrational fear (which she herself calls foolish) that prevents her from consenting to ECT. We could say of her that her phobia about ECT is a mental disorder which has interfered with her ability to make rational treatment decisions of a particular kind. The "particular kind" might be those treatment decisions involving the use of ECT; she might, for example, be able to make rational decisions about most or all other treatment modalities, for depression or for other physical or mental maladies.

On the U + A definition of competence, patients 6.3 and 6.4 would be labeled incompetent, 6.5 would probably be competent, while 6.6 and 6.7 would be competent. If competence is defined, as we now suggest, as the ability to make a rational decision of a certain kind, then all five patients would be labeled as incompetent to make the relevant medical decision.

Irrational Decisions and Incompetence

It is likely true that the vast majority of patients who make irrational treatment decisions are not competent to make rational decisions of the kind involved. With regard to seriously irrational treatment decisions, even those that are temporary, it is quite likely that almost all are made by those who are not competent to make that kind of decision. Persistent seriously irrational decisions of a given kind show that the person is not competent to make that kind of decision.

For example, consider a middle-aged patient, in otherwise good health, who refuses to have an appendectomy for his acute appendicitis, which is in danger of rupturing and causing a possibly fatal peritonitis. It almost always is the case that: (1) patients of this kind do not have the cognitive ability to understand their situation; or (2) do not have the volitional ability to consent, because of, say, a fear of general anesthesia; or (3) are so depressed because of their situation that, despite their accurate cognitive understanding, they do not have the ability to make this kind of rational decision. Thus this man will almost certainly be found to be incompetent to refuse surgery. Seriously irrational decisions, in the medical arena or elsewhere, are seldom made by persons who have the ability to make rational decisions. By definition, seriously irrational decisions are those that will almost certainly lead to the person experiencing significant harm for no adequate reason, and all rational persons avoid suffering point-less harm.

However, less seriously irrational decisions are sometimes made by patients who have the ability to make rational decisions. Consider a man who has a wart on the sole of his foot. He is suffering from mild to moderate chronic pain and disability, that is, he limps. The condition can almost always be totally reversed by one or another podiatric procedure, such as blunt excision, that causes only mild brief pain and is essentially risk free. Nonetheless the man suffers from the condition for weeks or months, despite his accurate knowledge of the above facts, despite having no adequate reason for delaying the treatment, and despite having no mental disorder which interferes with his ability to choose rationally. Thus we could say of him that he is competent, that he has the ability to choose rationally, but he has made an irrational choice.

Determining Competence

Only occasionally in clinical practice does the issue arise of a patient's competence to consent to or refuse treatment. It obviously arises whenever a patient is so cognitively impaired that he is unable to consent or refuse; in these cases the patient is unhesitantly thought to be incompetent and a surrogate decision-making agent is usually found.

Naturally, the issue of competence seldom arises when patients consent to treatment, because doctors almost always recommend treatments that it would be rational for patients to choose. Thus a patient's consent, even if the patient cannot, for example, adequately understand and appreciate the relevant infor-mation, will expose him at worst to a treatment that it would be rational for him to choose if he were competent. In those situations in which the treatment recommended is the only rational option (that is, there are no rational alterna-tive treatments and refusal of the treatment would be irrational), it is often of no great moment if the patient does not fully understand and appreciate the rele-vant information. Were he able to understand and appreciate the information, he would consent to the treatment.

However if a patient consents to a treatment when there are alternative ratio-nal treatments, or if refusing the recommended treatment is not irrational, then it is important to make certain that the patient is competent to consent. If the patient is not competent then he may be "consenting" to a treatment that, though it may be a rational option, could be unreasonable for him to choose. His own ranking of the different harms and benefits of the available options might lead him, were he competent, to choose another option than the one he has chosen.

It is in cases of treatment refusals, especially those that appear to be irra-tional, that the question of a patient's competence most frequently and appropriately arises. How can one determine whether a patient who makes an irrational treatment refusal is competent, that is, whether he has the ability to make a rational decision of the kind at hand? This determination is usually based on two kinds of evidence. The first is whether there is positive evidence that the person has usually shown the ability to make rational decisions in his life—perhaps even medical decisions—of this level of complexity and seriousness. The second and more important is whether there is evidence of the presence of cognitive disabilities or of mental maladies that would, under the current circumstances, make him unable to make rational decisions of the kind involved.

Persons who do and persons who do not have the ability to decide rationally should be regarded and treated differently. If a patient lacks the ability to decide rationally and decides irrationally, it is usually unfruitful to try to persuade him to change his mind. For example, suppose the man with the wart on his foot has a phobia about being injected by needles and on that basis refuses extirpative surgery for his wart (it is usually necessary that the skin surrounding the wart be anesthetized with an injection of an anesthetic prior to the extirpative procedure). One can rarely persuade people not to experience phobic anxiety, so any efforts to help him would need to take other forms (for instance, suggesting that his needle phobia be treated with behavioral techniques, usually a successful and rapid procedure). On the other hand, if we judge the person has the ability to decide rationally, we may, if he is willing to discuss the matter with us, confront him directly with what appears to be his pointless and needless suffering of harm, and argue with him that he should change his mind. We regard him as responsible for his decision, and capable of changing it, in a way we do not regard the phobic man.

Can a patient's competence be determined before knowing whether the patient consents or refuses? This key question must be addressed by any account of competence. On the account we are giving here, competence usually can be determined without yet knowing the patient's decision. Some patients, for example, have sufficiently prominent cognitive disabilities—for example, they do not understand at all, or only very slightly, the information they have been given—that they clearly do not have the ability to make rational decisions of the kind involved. Other patients, the vast majority of all patients, evidence such clear understanding during the consent process of the issues involved in making a decision that it is clear that they have the necessary cognitive abilities to make a rational decision.

However, the situation of patients with mental maladies which might interfere with the consent process is sometimes different. These patients may have a cognitive disability due to a delusion that renders them unable to appreciate that the information applies to them. Or they may have no cognitive disabilities: like Cases 6.6 and 6.7 above, they may understand and appreciate the information adequately. Patients who irrationally refuse treatment because of their mental malady indicate that they lack the ability to decide rationally in situations of this kind. However, there may be no way to know whether the patient has the ability to decide rationally until the patient makes a decision. In either the 6.6 or 6.7 case, if the patient had consented to treatment when it was initially suggested, it would have indicated that he or she was competent to make that kind of rational decision, and very likely the issue of competence would never have arisen.

We agree with Buchanan and Brock that in some clinical situations that involve patients whose mental maladies interfere with their ability to make a rational decision, consent and refusal may be "asymmetrical."[11] With delusions, the asymmetry can go both ways, it depends on the delusion and how it affects the appreciation of the information. With volitional disabilities, the patient's consent to treatment would show she was competent to consent, while her refusal would show she was not competent to refuse. Thus for us the symmetry of consent and refusal depends on the kind of incompetence involved. In cases of cognitive incompetence not due to delusions, consent and refusal are symmetrical: such a patient who is cognitively incompetent to refuse is also incompetent to consent, because consent and refusal are based on the same information and she does not have the ability to understand that information. However, both cognitive incompetence due to delusions that affect adequate appreciation of the information, and volitional incompetence, can result in someone being competent to consent but not competent to refuse. The distinction between different kinds of cognitive incompetence and volitional incompetence, and its implications for overruling some patient refusals, is discussed further in Chapter 9.

Advantages of the New Definition

Different definitions of competence (in the context of a patient's decision making) vary in the way in which they articulate the concepts of "competence" and "rationality." In our earlier accounts, we sharply distinguished between competence to make a decision, defined according to U + A criteria, and the rationality or irrationality of the decision once made.[12] By contrast, both Drane and Buchanan and Brock, include irrationality as part of their shifting definitions of competence. They specify that treatment refusals in high-risk clinical situations must be rational before the person can be called competent to make them, but they do not require rational decisions in less risky settings in order to classify patients as competent.[13]

We now reject both of the above approaches and suggest a third approach. We say that a patient is competent to make a particular medical decision if and only if he has the ability to make a rational decision of a certain kind. The ability to make a rational decision of a particular kind has constituent cognitive, volitional, and affective components.

We believe our new account has certain advantages:

(**1**) Everyone agrees that competence is task-specific, but we have provided the first explicit statement of the kind of task that competent patients must be able to perform. Defining competence as the ability to make a rational decision explains why the degree of irrationality of patients' decisions is a major factor in determining the competence of patients and thus in justifying paternalistic intervention of incompetent patients.[14] Irrationality, as a criterion for overriding patients' decisions, is much more closely related to the justification of paternalistic behavior than is competence defined in terms of understanding and appreciating information alone.[15] By continuing to distinguish between the competence of a person and the rationality of a particular decision, we make clear that determining competence and justifying paternalistic intervention are separate and distinct. Other approaches, which simply sort patients into two groups, the competent and the incompetent, do not seem to consider that further justification is needed for determining when to overrule the refusals of incompetent patients. And further justification is necessary: for example, if a demented man refuses to have a Band-Aid put on a small scratch on his arm, it would rarely be morally justified to force the Band-Aid on him, despite the fact that he is not competent to refuse. Competence is not determined by the seriousness of a patient's situation, but the justification for overruling a refusal is.

(**2**) By defining competence as the ability to make a rational decision, we allow all or nearly all of the persons who make seriously irrational decisions to be designated as incompetent, and thus we are more in line with the legal tradition than in our earlier account. The fact that we define competence as something other than the understanding and appreciation of information does not put us at odds with the legal tradition, since, as noted earlier, competence has not been defined at all in many states, and only imprecisely in others. In fact, in a well-known New York Court of Appeals case, one of the few cases which straightforwardly and explicitly addresses the problem of defining competence, the court suggests that "competence" be defined according to a host of "factors," including "the absence of any interfering emotional state," and "the absence of any interfering pathologic motivational pressure."[16] These two factors seem closely related to our own notion that no mood disorder or volitional disability be present that would interfere with a patient's ability to make a rational decision. Thus our account fits comfortably with the present legal guidelines in the state of New York.

Although we define competence as the ability to make a rational decision, the incompetence of a person to make a kind of medical decision is never determined simply by the irrationality of their decision in the present case. A person is competent to make a rational decision if the following is true: she does not have a cognitive disability preventing her from understanding and appreciating the relevant information or coordinating that information with her own stable values, and she does not have a mental malady involving a volitional disability that interferes with her ability to make a rational decision. If none of these disabilities, including a relevant mental malady, is present, she is competent to make a rational decision, even if she is presently making an irrational decision. Of course, persistent seriously irrational decisions would show that the patient is incompetent to make that kind of decision, but if a person overcomes her volitional disability, say, her phobia of ECT, and consents, then she is competent to make that kind of decision.

(3) We believe that "the ability to make a rational decision of a certain kind" is what people have always had in mind when they accorded "competence" the primacy it has in the consent process. They did not simply have in mind the bare-boned understanding and appreciation of the information presented. Our account thus simply makes explicit what we believe people already hold. It is understandable that "understanding and appreciation" were initially selected as the criteria for determining competence; they are fairly easily assessed, and they usually do agree with our intuitions about particular cases. This is because the majority of patients who lack the ability to make a rational decision lack it because they do not understand and appreciate the relevant information. However, cases like 6.6 and 6.7 force us to see that understanding and appreciation are only markers of the ability to make a rational decision, and do not capture the entire meaning of that concept.

The woman in Case 6.7 is especially instructive in that she possesses not only the ability to understand and appreciate the relevant information, she also possesses the cognitive ability to understand that she is making an irrational decision. However, because of her phobia about ECT, she does not have the volitional ability to consent and thus does not have the ability to make the kind of rational decision involved. We think this woman would and should be given ECT in any clinical setting, despite her refusal to consent. If, through extensive talks with her doctors, she lost much of her phobic anxiety about ECT and subsequently consented, it would seem impossible to regard her as anything but competent to consent.

If one wants to hold that only incompetent patients should be treated against their wishes, then one must have an account of competence such that this woman, when refusing ECT, is labeled as incompetent. Such an account would have to include more than formal cognitive operations, and would have to acknowledge that a patient's competence can not always be determined before knowing what the patient's treatment decision is.[17]

We believe that this new account of competence provides the correct articulation between the related but distinct concepts of (1) a patient's understanding and appreciation of the information relevant to a suggested treatment, and (2) the rationality or irrationality of the patient's eventual treatment choice. These two concepts are different, and neither by itself provides an adequate explanation of the meaning of competence. We believe that combining the two concepts in the way we have provides a definition of competence that accords with persons' intuitions about what should be done in particular cases, is linked with a coherent theory about the paternalistic justification of overriding patients' treatment decisions, and is not inconsistent with the prevailing legal account.

Notes

1. James F. Drane, "The Many Faces of Competency," *Hastings Center Report,* 15 (1985), pp. 17–21. Allan B. Buchanan and Dan W. Brock, *Deciding for Others. The Ethics of Surrogate Decision-Making* (New York: Cambridge University Press, 1989). Charles M. Culver and Bernard Gert, "The Inadequacy of Incompetence," *Milbank Quarterly,* 68 (1990), pp. 619–643.

2. Alan A. Stone, "Iatrogenic Ethical Problems: Commentary on 'Can a Patient Refuse a Psychiatric Consultation to Evaluate Decision-Making Capacity?'" *Journal of Clinical Ethics,* 5 (1994), pp. 234–237.

3. Paul S. Appelbaum and Thomas Grisso, "The MacArthur Treatment Competence Study. I. Mental Illness and Competence to Consent to Treatment," *Law and Human Behavior,* 19 (1995), pp. 105–126. See also by the same authors: "Assessing Patients' Capacities to Consent to Treatment," *New England Journal of Medicine,* (1988), pp. 319, 1635–1638.

4. The first three of the four standards they elaborate are consistent with what we have called the U + A definition of competence. Their fourth standard is "whether patients manipulate information rationally." They mean by "rational" something different from what we mean: namely, whether patients are able "to reach conclusions that are logically consistent with starting premises" (1988, p. 1636). They explicitly state, in describing this fourth standard, ". . . . the 'irrationality' to which this standard properly refers pertains to illogic in the processing of information, not the choice that is eventually made" (1995, p. 110). Thus a severely depressed patient with no delusional thinking who refuses treatment because he wishes to die (see Cases 6.1 and 6.6, pages 134 and 140) could clearly be competent on the first three standards and also on the fourth, in that his refusal of treatment is a "conclusion" logically consistent with his "starting premise" that he wishes to die.

5. Appelbaum and Grisso do make the following summary statement about competence, which they neither explain nor elaborate (1995, p. 169): "Conclusions about legal competence are assisted by empirical observations, but they are ultimately moral in nature. They require judgments about patients' interests based on applications of the values of autonomy and beneficence." This suggests they do not distinguish between deciding that a patient is incompetent and deciding whether it is justified to override the patient's refusal. They conflate the two. We believe the two are closely related but that it is important to distinguish between them, as we elaborate below.

5. Loren Roth, Alan Meisel, and Charles Lidz, "Tests of Competency to Consent to Treatment," *American Journal of Psychiatry,* 134 (1977), pp. 279–284. James F. Drane, op. cit; see also James F. Drane, *Clinical Bioethics* (Kansas City: Sheed & Ward, 1994), pp. 152–157. Alan E. Buchanan, and Dan W. Brock, op. cit.

7. This summary does not do full justice to the well-elaborated discussion of these three levels by Drane, and by Buchanan and Brock, but it captures their general approach adequately for our purposes here.

8. Culver and Gert, 1982, *Philosophy in Medicine*, 1990, op. cit.

9. See Chapter 2 for a definition and discussion of the concept of an "unreasonable" decision.

10. Note that this case is different from the case of the woman, previously mentioned, whose transient anger caused her to make an irrational treatment choice but of whom we do not say that she has lost the ability to make rational treatment decisions of the kind involved. In the case of mood disorders, the condition usually persists over a lengthy period of time so that it seems accurate to say that some patients indeed have lost the ability to make rational treatment decisions of this kind, although of course almost never have they lost the ability permanently. However, in emergency situations, seriously irrational decisions may justifiably be overruled even if the person is not incompetent.

11. Buchanan and Brock, op. cit.

12. Culver and Gert, 1982, 1990, op. cit.

13. Drane uses the term "irrational," and in fact references our work in explaining that concept. Although Buchanan and Brock do not use the term "irrational," they employ essentially the same concept.

14. See Chapter 10, "Justification."

15. A point apparently agreed to even by Buchanan and Brock (op. cit.), who are critical of our earlier approach, principally because our approach was at variance with the legal tradition referred to above.

16. *Rivers v Katz,* NY52d 74 (1986).

17. In the case of patients who make only mildly irrational decisions but are judged on our account to be competent to make rational decisions (like the man with the wart on his foot), our account would give the same results as the traditional U + A legal account. We would explain the lack of forced treatment differently from the law. The law would say one could not interfere because the patient was competent (that is, he demonstrated understanding and appreciation of the relevant information). We would agree but would note that the patient had made a (mildly) irrational decision. Our definition of competence would differ from the law, but on both accounts the patient would be competent and his refusal could not be overridden.

7

Consent

It is commonly acknowledged that valid consent, or informed consent, is a central concept in medical ethics, but there may be insufficient appreciation of its true conceptual foundations and hence of its conceptual power. To uncover its foundations we explore the close relationship between the consent process and certain elements of our account of morality, summarized in Chapter 2. Both the breadth and the power of the concept, we hope, will become evident in this chapter.

Morality and the Consent Process

The process of obtaining a patient's valid consent has many facets.[1] It involves the doctor's presenting information to the patient as well as appraising and evaluating the patient's response to the presentation. Certain minimal criteria must be met during this process in order for the patient's consent, if it is forthcoming, to be considered valid. A physician who suggests a treatment to a patient is morally required, except in unusual circumstances, to attempt to obtain a valid consent from that patient in order to proceed with treatment.[2]

In addition, there are further steps the physician can take to maximize the patient's participation in the consent process. These further steps, we believe, are morally desirable but not morally required. If these steps are taken, then, as discussed below, we say that not only a *valid* but an *ideal* consent has been obtained. The distinction between what is morally required and morally encouraged in the consent process rests on the distinction between moral rules and moral ideals.

Moral Rules and Moral Ideals

In Chapter 2 we discussed the difference between moral rules and moral ideals. The moral rules prohibit people from causing harm or performing those kinds of actions which increase the risk of harm being done to others. Everyone is required to impartially obey the moral rules all of the time, and people are liable to punishment when they do not do so. Morality also includes moral ideals, which encourage people to take positive action to prevent or relieve the harms suffered by others. Moral ideals differ in character from moral rules in that adherence to them is encouraged but is not morally required. It would be impossible to require persons to impartially follow the moral ideals all of the time: to do so would require everyone to spend every available minute of their time helping others, and even then one could not impartially help everyone. People are therefore usually praised for following the moral ideals, but it is not legitimate to punish people for failing to follow them.

The Duties and the Goals of a Profession

Professions formulate codes of ethics which are intended to govern the behavior of their members. As discussed in Chapter 3, these codes of ethics stipulate duties that all members of the profession are required to follow, and also often describe goals which all members of the profession are encouraged to pursue.

The goals of a profession are always particular expressions of the moral ideals. They encourage members of the profession to carry out activities that prevent or decrease the amount of harm and suffering in the population, usually in the area of life with which the profession is concerned. Many required duties of a profession, by contrast, are often specifications of the general moral rules, and represent particular explications of them. For example, there are general moral rules prohibiting causing pain or disability. A medical code of ethics may specifically state that a doctor should cause no harm to a patient without his consent and with no compensating benefit to the patient, but that is a moral rule that applies to everyone, not only to physicians. Everyone is morally prohibited from causing harm to another person without his consent and for no compensating benefit to that person.

But professional duties are sometimes specifications of moral ideals; that is, a kind of behavior that would be a moral ideal for the ordinary person is explicitly changed into a duty for members of the profession, at least in some circumstances. Violating that duty, then, counts as a violation of the moral rule "Do your duty," as discussed in Chapter 3. For example, an ordinary person waiting for a friend in an emergency room has no duty to help other people there who are suffering pain, although it might be following a moral ideal to do so. However, a physician in an emergency room who neglects a patient in pain, absent special mitigating circumstances, is failing to carry out her professional duty, is thereby acting immorally, and may be liable for professional and legal sanction. The medical code of conduct has changed what would otherwise be a moral ideal into a moral rule, by converting the action in question from one that is morally encouraged to one that is morally required, because it has become a duty.

When a moral ideal is converted into a moral rule, however, the scope of the behavior in question is narrowed considerably. Thus physicians who work in emergency rooms have no more duty than anyone else to help people who are suffering pain in foreign countries. They would be following one of the highest moral ideals of their profession if they did so, but they have not acted immorally (they have not violated a moral rule) if they do not. With the above theoretical background in mind, we now discuss various aspects of the process of consent.

Valid Consent

The duties that underlie the procuring of a valid consent are all particular expressions of general moral rules which the physician is required to follow, unless a violation can be publicly allowed.[3] Thus there is nothing special or ad hoc about the moral requirements of valid consent; they represent simply the ordinary requirements of morality in the consent situation. It is important to be clear about this, otherwise any who chafe under the requirements to obtain a valid consent might be tempted to claim that these requirements have been imposed arbitrarily and needlessly by judges, legislators, or others outside of the medical profession. But this is false: if all the judges, legislators, and relevant law in the country ceased to exist overnight, physicians would still be morally required to satisfy the criteria for a valid consent before proceeding with treatment. These criteria are:

1. *A physician is morally required to provide a patient with adequate information* concerning any suggested treatment, because to do otherwise would count as violating the moral rule against deception. Not telling someone something is deceptive only when one has a duty to tell the person that thing, but there is a duty to tell patients information about suggested treatments, a duty now explicitly contained in medical codes of ethics.[4] But having stipulated that there is a duty not to withhold information, all the "adequate information" requirement amounts to is reminding physicians not to deceive, a moral rule that applies to everyone in all situations. At its root, it is a very simple notion.

2. *A physician may not coerce a patient into consenting,* because to do so would be a violation of the general moral rule prohibiting depriving persons of freedom. Again, there is nothing special about the medical situation: stating that coercion is unethical simply reminds the physician that it is as unethical to coerce in the medical situation as it is in all situations.

3. *A physician must assess a patient's competence* before administering a treatment to which the patient has consented, *because a patient must be fully competent* (must have the ability to make a rational medical decision of the kind involved) *before a physician can act on the patient's consent.* To do otherwise would count as causing or increasing the risk of causing harm (for example, pain or loss of freedom) to the patient when the patient is not competent to consent to the harm being caused. Again, there is nothing ad hoc about this moral requirement: it is morally unacceptable for anyone to cause pain to another person without that person's valid consent.

It is similarly required that the physician assess the competence of a patient who refuses a treatment, because if the patient is not competent it may be morally required to overrule the patient's refusal, while if the patient is competent it is not morally allowed to do so. Here, a special duty is widely acknowledged if seldom explicitly formulated: that physicians have the duty to treat some incompetent patients who refuse treatment. When an incompetent patient would suffer significant harm if not treated, it is a dereliction of duty for physicians not to force treatment. The general moral rule "Do your duty" becomes specific when applied to a particular professional circumstance.

A physician who provides adequate information, who does not coerce, who adequately assesses a patient's competence, and then who acts appropriately, has carried out the basic duties of obtaining a valid consent. Although the three criteria for determining that a consent is valid are reasonably clear in their meaning and significance, it is important to elaborate how each criterion is manifested in medical practice. We discussed the meaning and the clinical assessment of competence in the prior chapter; in this chapter we discuss the topics of adequate information and coercion.

The Criteria for Valid Consent

Adequate Information

Patients must be given adequate information about a proposed treatment before their consent to that treatment is valid. For a physician to withhold adequate information from a patient, without the patient's consent, would count as deception and thus need moral justification. But what kind of information passes the test of "adequacy"? An accurate but too-general answer is, that information that any rational person would want to know before making a decision. But what information is that?

Alternative rational treatment choices. Rational persons, if they were to examine the consent process closely, would realize that the following descriptions are true:

1. There are many clinical situations in which patients face only one rational choice. A patient may have a serious pneumococcal pneumonia which will probably kill her unless she takes an appropriate antibiotic. The patient wants to live. Thus taking the drug is her only rational option. However, there are also a great many clinical situations which permit more than one rational choice. For example, for many men with a moderate degree of prostatism, both extirpative prostate surgery and medically monitored "watchful waiting" are rational treatment options.
2. Each rational choice contains within it a particular estimated probability of suffering some harms and preventing or relieving others. For example, prostate surgery usually leads to a rapid relief of symptoms but has a small risk of causing incontinence or impotence; "watchful waiting" is rarely associated with these latter side effects but neither will it relieve the patient's symptoms of prostatism. Patients must depend upon their physicians to give them this kind of comparative information and to convey it in an understandable fashion.
3. Rational persons vary among themselves with regard to how they rank the harms contained within different rational choices, and different individuals therefore make different rational choices. Well-informed men with essentially identical clinical pictures do differ in their choice of prostate treatment; some choose surgery and others choose watchful waiting.
4. If a person does rank the alternative choices significantly differently, it would be unreasonable for him not to make that choice which reflects most accurately his own ranking of the harms associated with the different alternatives.[5] To do otherwise would increase the chance that he would experience an outcome that he desired less than some other outcome. For example, one elderly man might dread the possible surgical side effect of impotence; to another, no longer sexually active, impotence might be of much less or of practically no concern. For the second man to refuse surgery, given his ranking of the harms involved, might well be unreasonable.

Many rational persons may never have considered the issues involved in ranking alternative treatments closely and upon first being confronted with two or more rational treatment options may not have applicable sets of rankings of harms ready to apply. Even after considerable thought, a person may be puzzled about which available rational option suits him best. Nonetheless, it seems likely that a great number of persons, given time for reflection, will have distinct preferences when confronted with alternative treatment options. Thus not to inform a patient fully about the details of those options that do exist is to deprive the patient of the opportunity to decide whether he does have a clear preference he would like to exercise.

It is important to emphasize that even when there are two or more rational treatment options available, it might be unreasonable for a patient to select one of them. This is because, as discussed above, a choice can be objectively rational but still unreasonable for a particular person to make. Consider a patient whose essential hypertension is of such severity that both she and her doctor believe a beta-blocking drug treatment should be used. There is a range of drugs available, all with roughly equal efficacy, but they differ among themselves in incidence of side effects, ease of administration (for example, how many times a day a pill must be taken), and financial cost. The drugs with greater ease of administration and, for most patients, fewer side effects cost considerably more; those with lesser ease of administration and, often, more bothersome side effects are considerably cheaper.

Both classes of drugs are objectively rational for patients to take; both offer the promise of significant control of blood pressure at no great risk of permanent harm. If either kind of drug were the only kind available it would be entirely rational for the woman to agree to take it. However consider a woman who is rather poor and for whom the cost of the higher-priced medication would, month-in and month-out, represent a significant financial drain. Suppose further that she is also rather stoic and less bothered than many patients by the kinds of side effects the less expensive drugs can cause. Given her ranking of the harms associated with expensive and with cheaper drugs, she would much prefer to take a cheaper drug, or at least begin by taking a cheaper drug and determine in fact how troublesome the side effects prove to be. For her to start by taking one of the expensive drugs would be unreasonable: she would be subjecting herself to what she considers a significant harm, loss of money, without what she considers an adequate reason for doing so.

Suppose this patient had a physician who told her only about one of the expensive drugs. The woman would not know there was a less expensive, equally efficacious option for controlling blood pressure, which could be used in her circumstances. It would not be unreasonable for her, half-informed, to agree to take the expensive drug, even though, if she knew of both options, the choice of the expensive drug would be unreasonable for her to make.[6]

These considerations make it important for rational persons to have full relevant information about the likely harms associated with all existing rational treatment choices. To have less than full information introduces the possibility that patients will make some choice other than the one closest to their own ranking of harms, either because they do not even know a choice closer to their ranking exists, or they do not know sufficient detail about the harms associated with the choices of which they are aware. It would be unreasonable for a patient who has clear rankings of the harms involved not to make that choice which is closest to her rankings, *even if the choice the patient does make is, objectively, a rational choice.* Thus partial disclosure can, from the patient's point of view, cause significant avoidable harm, which explains why less than full disclosure on the part of physicians is deceptive and morally unacceptable.

Patients should be told about all rational alternative treatments which can be given for their malady. Of course, a physician can only tell about those rational alternative treatments of which she is aware. However, except in emergency situations, a physician is not competent to treat a particular malady unless she is able to give her patients full and adequate information (as described in this chapter) about a minimum number of rational alternative treatments. (What treatments a competent physician must know about should be determined in the same manner as competency is determined for other aspects of medical practice.) To treat a malady without being aware of and able to describe the available rational alternatives is to deprive one's patients of the opportunity to make fully informed choices. Consent under these conditions is not fully valid. A physician who is tempted to undertake a treatment without sufficient knowledge of the rational alternatives should at least inform the patient about her state of relative ignorance. Thus the requirements of informed consent provide strong reasons for physicians to learn about available rational alternative treatments.

Although a physician may believe that, for a given patient, one of the alternative treatments is best, patients should nonetheless be informed about all the available rational options. One test of whether an alternative treatment is rational is for a physician to ask herself whether some other competent physicians might recommend a treatment other than the one she is about to recommend. For example, if a patient has a tumor which the physician believes should initially be treated with radiotherapy, but the physician knows that some other competent physicians would recommend immediate surgery in this setting, the patient should be told about the surgical option and the reason some physicians think it preferable.

A woman with Stage I breast cancer should be told of the different surgical and radiologic treatment options open to her. She should be given the latest morbidity and mortality information associated with each. The law in several states now mandates what has been morally required all along, that physicians present information about all rational treatment alternatives to breast cancer patients. Laws of this kind may be useful, if in fact physicians will not disclose relevant information to patients without a law being in place, but of course there is no reason that sufferers from breast cancer are more entitled to relevant information than sufferers from any other kind of cancer or, for that matter, sufferers from scalp eczema or carpal tunnel syndrome.

Alternative treatments should be presented in a fair manner. To describe a rational treatment alternative that one does not personally favor in a belittling or sarcastic way makes it difficult for many patients to inquire more fully into it or to decide in favor of it. It is particularly important that a physician not overemphasize the attractiveness of a treatment which she can provide, and thus would profit from, in comparison with an alternative treatment that would necessitate the patient's being treated by another practitioner.[7] An internist should describe surgical alternatives in an unbiased fashion, as should surgeons describe medical treatment alternatives. One mental test in which a practitioner might engage is to imagine that her presentation of alternative treatment options were being tape-recorded: ideally she should present the options in such a manner that a panel of judges would be unable to guess which of the treatments she herself performs.

We are not suggesting that physicians not argue in favor of one or more of the available options. If the physician has good reason to believe, from what she knows of the patient's own ranking of the harms involved in the various options, that one should be clearly preferable from the patient's standpoint, then she should present her argument in a straightforward fashion. Not to argue in such circumstances would usually be, as we discuss below, a kind of misguided nondirectiveness.

Consent for diagnostic tests. The same arguments apply no less to suggested diagnostic tests than to suggested treatments. Tests, like treatments, are associated with possible harms and possible benefits, and patients should be told about them. It is often true that it would be irrational for a patient not to consent to a particular test, even one that is associated with nontrivial possibilities of harm, because of the great benefit that might accrue to the patient through a correct diagnosis. By contrast, in our experience, doctors occasionally order nonharmful tests, which may inconvenience a patient considerably, for "academic interest," without telling the patient that the test is being done primarily to satisfy the doctor's intellectual curiosity and not because of any direct benefit that is likely to come to the patient.

It is not only the possible direct harm associated with a test (pain, financial cost, temporary disability, and so forth) that should be disclosed, but also the likely utility of the information obtained. One important example of a test that should not be performed without disclosing the test's questionable utility is the blood test for prostate-specific antigen (PSA). While the PSA test is said to detect the presence of prostate cancers years before they become symptomatic, there is no better than equivocal evidence that early detection and surgical treatment of this cancer has any effect on the life span of the men treated. Since the operation itself often causes impotence and some degree of urinary incontinence, it would be entirely rational for an affected patient to choose not to undergo surgery. Thus whether to do the PSA test in the first place is also a matter for rational choice. Physicians are currently divided about whether to recommend the PSA to their patients.[8] As in any instance where there is professional disagreement, patients should be told the nature of this disagreement and then be allowed to decide for themselves how to proceed.

Another kind of possible harm associated with almost any diagnostic test is the production of false positive or false negative results, and patients should know about the likelihood and the implications of such test results before consenting to be tested. A false negative result occurs when a test indicates that no malady or problem is present, when in fact it is; thus the test result is incorrect and misleading. False negative results can give both patient and physician false reassurance about the patient's condition.

False positive results occur when the test indicates that a malady or problem is present when in fact it is not. This kind of test error can cause both needless aprehension and needless treatment.[9]

False positives are particularly likely to occur in settings where the condition being tested for has a low base rate of occurrence. This is true even if the test itself is "accurate," in the sense that, say, 95% or more of afflicted individuals have a positive test result.[10] An example of this phenomenon is testing for HIV + status in a low-risk population, like applicants for a marriage license, or patients admitted to a general hospital.

"Medical" and "nonmedical" decisions. It is frequently said that some kinds of decisions that doctors make are "purely medical," while others are not, and that "purely medical" decisions need not be communicated or explained to the patients involved. We agree that not all decisions that doctors make need to be communicated to the patients involved, but disagree that it is because these decisions are "purely medical."

Those who advance the distinction between "medical" and "nonmedical" decisions seem to believe that some decisions made by doctors involve only purely technical matters about which patients would have neither interest nor expertise. We believe there are few if any decisions of this kind in medical practice. Doctors who are said to be making "purely medical" decisions are usually choosing between two or more treatments, drugs, tests, surgical approaches, scheduled frequencies of outpatient visits, and so forth, whose expected results are rather similar but which are thought to differ only in some technical aspect. For example, a psychiatrist may be deciding which antidepressant drug to prescribe; an internist, whether to tell a patient to return to have his blood pressure checked in one week or one month; or a surgeon, which operative approach to use to expose a particular underlying structure. The aspects in which two or more options differ are in part technical; for example, the chemical structures of different drugs always differ from one another. However, the technical differences are not important in and of themselves. It is the fact that these technical differences are associated with different harms and benefits that leads the physician to consider them for comparative analysis in the first place.

For example, one antidepressant drug may usually cause more anticholinergic side effects, including sedation, than another drug, and sedation may or may not seem to be a desirable side effect for a particular patient. Or one surgical approach may afford quicker access but also carry a slightly greater risk than an alternative approach. However, information of this kind about the likely different harms and benefits of different options is not purely technical and is potentially always of interest to rational persons.

To see that this is true, consider the following statement by a physician:

"While I would usually consult patients about some kinds of decisions, I would almost never ask a patient whether she thought I should choose X or Y, because that is a purely medical decision."

Now let X and Y be any two alternatives about which a physician might make such a claim, and ask in what ways the two alternatives differ from one another. Of course they are associated with different technical details (like the different chemical structures of two drugs, or the different anatomical structures surrounding two surgical approaches), but the reason that the physician is considering the alternatives in the first place is that they may differ in their potential benefits, harms, side effects, financial cost, or in some dimension that is highly correlated with one of these factors. For example, one surgical approach may be manually easier than another, but that in turn will almost always make it quicker, and thus more risky or less risky, depending on the facts of the case, than a more manually difficult approach. But all of these factors associated with different "purely medical" decisions are ones in which rational patients potentially have a great interest.

Although we do not maintain that doctors should consult patients about every individual decision they make, this is not because these decisions are purely medical. It is because individual decisions are frequently nested within broader treatment approaches and patients have often, appropriately, given consent for the broader treatment approach with its attendant probable harms and benefits. Thus patients need not always be consulted about every individual turn of the road that occurs during their treatment. We will refer to this phenomenon of patients' giving a single valid consent to a multifaceted treatment intervention as *total treatment consent.*

Total treatment consent. Some medical treatments are simple and discrete: taking two aspirin to relieve a headache, for example. The aspirin are taken on a particular occasion, the possible and probable harms and benefits associated with the drug either materialize or they do not, but several hours later the treatment episode is usually over. Other medical treatments, however, are structurally more complex: for example, the interventions employed during the first few hours of treating an acute myocardial infarction. The total treatment consists of a series of individual treatments that occur over many hours or days. Some of these individual treatments typically occur in the early hours of the episode, others occur later.

Sometimes administering even one treatment is not done on one discrete occasion. For example, a patient withdrawing from longstanding alcohol intoxication is usually given, along with other medications, some sedative drug like Librium so that the alcohol withdrawal can be accomplished without the patient experiencing a possibly dangerous rebound excitation of his central nervous system (delirium tremens). Typically, the Librium is given several times daily in gradually decreasing amounts, the rate of decrease determined by constantly measuring the patient's level of nervous system excitation. Depending on the magnitude of the measured signs of nervous system excitation, the Librium dosage can be increased, decreased, or kept constant on each ensuing occasion of medication. Consent for this withdrawal process is usually and appropriately obtained on only one occasion, before beginning the withdrawal protocol, and is not reobtained every time that nervous system excitation is measured and another particular dosage of Librium is administered.

This kind of anticipatory total treatment consent can be and usually is obtained even for treatment regimens that are structurally more complex than is withdrawal from alcohol intoxication. For example, a patient admitted with an early myocardial infarction can give consent to a battery or cluster of interventions, all designed to try to save his life and preserve maximal cardiac function. These may include such diverse treatments as morphine for pain, oxygen for increased oxygenation of bodily tissues, and one or more antidysrhythmic drugs intended to stabilize cardiac function. The patient should be told at the outset about the overall likely benefits and harms of the treatment regimen, but need not give consent individually to each new intervention, nor each increase or decrease in dose of an intervention already in place.

On the other hand, there often occur distinct forks in the road in administering a battery or a sequence of treatments. For example, the choice may arise of whether to attempt to recanalize an occluded coronary artery with drugs or with surgical laminoplasty, each with its own spectrum of likely harms and benefits. Or a schizophrenic patient who has not responded well to several neuroleptic drugs may appear to be a candidate for Clozapine, an often beneficial drug which unfortunately carries some risk of interfering, occasionally permanently, with the body's ability to make white blood cells. In such cases, earmarked by the presence of a new and significant set of possible harms and benefits not covered by previous total treatment consents, the consent process must be reopened.

The critical question at each new juncture point is whether the patient's previous total treatment consent clearly covers the possible harms and benefits of the new treatment action. A "new treatment action" can either be an entirely new treatment or a previous treatment administered in a different way. For example, consider the following case, described in an article by Piper:[11]

> At 11:45 P.M., Mr. Smith, being treated with intravenous medications in the hospital, develops mild diarrhea—an early sign of toxicity—from a drug that is clearly benefiting him. The nurse notifies the attending physician at home. The doctor decides to lower the dose of the medicine, thereby risking worsening the underlying disorder. Does the doctor require Mr. Smith's informed consent?

Piper clearly believes the doctor does not need to obtain Mr. Smith's informed consent; the example is included as illustrative of the absurdity of requiring patients to consent to each new intervention that doctors carry out.

Our view is that whether the doctor needs to obtain Mr. Smith's consent for the reduced dosage depends upon important facts about the case that are not specified in the article. If, without lowering the dosage, the toxicity would almost certainly progress to a dangerous state, and if the risk of worsening the underlying disorder (whose seriousness Piper does not mention) with a dosage decrease is low, then it is probably not necessary to obtain consent at 11:45 PM: the total treatment consent presumably given earlier by Mr. Smith should cover these kinds of dosage adjustments. On the other hand, if the risk of worsening a serious underlying disorder by lowering the dosage were great, and the toxicity might well amount to nothing more than mild diarrhea, then the dosage should not be lowered without consulting with Mr. Smith. Even if Mr. Smith's late-night consent is, justifiably, not sought, it would seem appropriate for the doctor to ask the nurse to explain the situation to Mr. Smith until the doctor can see him the next day.

Scientifically unvalidated treatments. Physicians have no duty to inform patients about treatment options that have not been shown to have any scientific support. For example, there have been and doubtless will continue to be many touted but unproven treatments for cancer, such as Laetrile and megavitamin therapy. Rational persons, however, usually have no desire to consider ineffective or almost certainly ineffective treatments as viable alternatives, and a physician has no duty to present such treatments as options.

Treatment at different sites and with different physicians. If the physician has good reason to believe that a recommended treatment can be carried out with significantly reduced morbidity or mortality at one rather than another medical center, or by one rather than another physician, patients should be given that information.[12] Any rational person, in deciding where and by whom to be treated, would want to have access to data of these kinds. This seems confirmed by the fact that, in our experience, physicians frequently share this kind of information among themselves when they become seriously ill and need treatment.

One example of differential success rates is that, for at least some kinds of surgery, better outcomes are often produced by hospitals which perform the surgery more frequently. Thus Gordon, Burleyson, Tielsch, and Cameron note, "The relationship between volume of surgical services performed by surgeons and hospitals, and positive outcomes of care, has been well documented."[13] These authors in their study examined the outcomes of all 501 Whipple procedures (pancreatico-duodenectomies, a complex, fairly high-risk operation) performed in the state of Maryland from 1988 through the first half of 1993. More than half of these procedures (271, or 54.1%) had been performed at the Johns Hopkins Hospital while the remainder (230, or 45.9%) were performed at 38 other hospitals in the state, no one of which performed more than 20.

The outcome of the procedure was significantly different between the two groups (that is, Johns Hopkins versus all the other hospitals combined), even after the two patient groups were matched statistically for age, gender, race, source of payment, source of admission, and extent of comorbid processes. Hospital mortality was more than six times higher at the low-volume hospitals than at Johns Hopkins (13.5% versus 2.2%, $p<.001$).

Even among the low-volume hospitals there was a significant linear monotonic relationship between volume and mortality. When the 38 low-volume hospitals were divided into four groups that performed, respectively, 1–5 procedures (20 hospitals), 6–10 (9 hospitals), 11–15 (6 hospitals), or 16–20 (3 hospitals), the associated mortalities were: 19.1%, 14.3%, 13.0%, and 8.9%. Thus, among the 20 hospitals in Maryland (more than half the total number of hospitals) that performed only between one and five procedures, the chance of dying in the hospital was almost nine times greater than at Johns Hopkins (19.1% versus 2.2%). This represents almost a one-in-five versus a one-in-fifty chance of dying. Even at the three hospitals that performed 16–20 procedures, the chance of dying was four times greater than at Johns Hopkins (8.9% versus 2.2%).

These are clearly substantial differences, not merely statistically significant differences of limited practical importance. Any rational person confronted with this information would choose, everything else being equal, to have her surgery performed at Johns Hopkins. In fact under most circumstances it would be seriously irrational to choose otherwise, that is, to expose oneself, without any compensating benefit, to a one-in-five rather than a one-in-fifty chance of dying while in the hospital. Now that this information is available, physicians in Maryland have a duty to disclose it to any patient for whom a Whipple procedure is recommended to be carried out at any hospital other than Johns Hopkins.

However these data have significance beyond the state of Maryland. There is no reason to believe that the Whipple volume-outcome relationship is different in

Maryland than it is in other states. Thus we believe that all patients everywhere for whom a Whipple procedure is recommended should be told that there is now compelling evidence that their chance of dying from the operation depends significantly on where it is performed; that in large, high-volume hospitals the death rate may be about 2%, but in small, low-volume hospitals it is probably four to nine times greater. These data can be as or more important than conventional harm-and-benefit data in influencing patients' treatment decisions.

Information about differential success rates in different hospitals, as it becomes increasingly known and available, should be routinely communicated during the valid consent process.[14] Of course patients given data about differential outcomes may not always decide to go for treatment to the site with the very best results. In the case of some treatments, for example, the possible improvement in outcome may not seem to the patient to be great enough to justify the increased expense and bother of traveling to a more distant medical center. Also, the patient's ability to travel may be limited by physical factors, or he may be a member of a prepaid health plan under which choosing to be treated elsewhere would involve a much greater, perhaps an impossible expense. Thus it may not always be irrational for a patient to choose to be treated closer to home, even if the outcome statistics are less favorable. The critical point is that the patient should not be deprived of the opportunity to know the facts or to make the decision.

Patients in HMOs and other managed-care plans should be given just as much information about significant site-specific differential outcomes as should patients in private insurance plans who are relatively free to obtain treatment wherever they wish. HMO patients can then decide for themselves whether to attempt to obtain therapy elsewhere. Not to disclose data to such patients seems to be acting on the faulty principle that data about differential outcomes should be given only to patients wealthy enough or otherwise fortunate enough to do something about it.

Harms and benefits. The information that rational persons want to know, at a minimum, consists of the probable significant harms and benefits associated with a suggested treatment, with any rational alternative treatments, and with no treatment at all. One of the "harms" that should be described routinely is the treatment's likely financial cost to the patient. Financial cost is a "harm" because it deprives persons of the opportunity to spend their money in other ways than on medical treatment.[15] Thus rational persons desire to factor cost into a treatment decision, just as they factor in harms like pain, disability, and the possibility of dying.

Some physicians have objected that accurately conveying information about significant harms and benefits is all but impossible, because to do so would require giving patients a medical education. That is not true. The language and level of specificity in which rational patients want harms and benefits explained is in terms of the significant harms that will likely be eliminated, diminished, or caused by any available rational treatment. The basic harms which concern rational persons are: death, pain (psychological as well as physical), disabilities (both mental and physical), and loss of freedom or pleasure (see Chapter 2). Patients almost never care about, say, the chemical structure of a chemotherapeutic agent, or about its postulated mechanism of interference with the metabolism of neoplastic cells. They do care about pain, nausea, weakness, and hair loss—about how likely these are to occur, how severe they are apt to be, and how long they may be expected to last. Technical language is not only not necessary, it is often counterproductive, resulting in patients understanding less of the information they really want to know. Unless well-informed patients specifically request technical details, they should not be given.

How probable must it be that a harm will occur in conjunction with a treatment before a patient should be told about it? That is a joint function of the severity of the harm and the probability of its occurrence. Any risk of death sufficiently large that at least some rational persons would take account of that risk in deciding whether to consent to the treatment should be told. Death is such a serious, irreversible harm that rational persons are likely to factor its risk of occurrence into their decision making unless the risk is extremely low, perhaps on the order of 1 in 100,000 or less.[16]

Less serious harms of a low probability of occurrence often need not be told, but any serious harm that is likely to occur should be. Thus a 5% chance of mild pain may not need to be disclosed, while a 5% chance of moderate pain usually should be. The test, not arbitrary but with frequent borderline cases, should always be: would a rational person want to know this information before making a decision? That is the test dictated not only by morality, but also by some state laws in specifying the medical standard of care to which a physician will be held if the scope of information disclosure is later challenged by the patient in a tort action.

We believe that information about risks should usually be given in numerical form. Rather than using terms and explanations like "common," "rare," or "it hardly ever happens," physicians should give reasonably precise numerical information, like "this drug is very good in cases like yours at lowering blood pressure about 80% of the time," or "about 1 in 200 times this operation, even when it's performed technically perfectly, causes a person to become paralyzed from the waist down." The problem with words like "most" or "hardly ever" is that they are vague and mean different things to different people. It is now well documented that physicians who use such words in talking with patients attach different numerical meanings to them: one doctor may use "most" whenever something occurs 51% of the time or more, another doctor may use it only if something occurs 80–90% of the time. In many situations the difference between these two different interpretations could critically influence a patient's decision about whether to consent.

It is often useful to express probabilities in terms of events with which the patient has some personal acquaintance. This seems particularly true with risks of low probability, because most persons are unaccustomed to thinking about and weighing fractions like "1 in 2,000," or even "1 in 500." For example, one might say, "There is a risk of death with this operation, but it is small: about the same as if you drove your car between New York and Boston." Or, "This thyroid test exposes your body to some slight nuclear radiation, about the same as the increased radiation you'd be exposed to if you flew on a airplane between New York and London."

One technique of disclosing risks is to first tell the patient about those risks that one believes any rational person would want to have disclosed. Then one can say, "There are other, less likely risks that can occur with this treatment that I'd be happy to discuss with you if you'd like." One can then proceed according to the patient's expressed wishes.

No treatment. It is important that patients know the probable outcome of their malady if they choose to have no treatment at all. It is nearly impossible to make a rational choice about accepting or refusing a treatment without having this information, since the rationality of a treatment decision involves comparing the probable harms and benefits of a suggested treatment with those of any alternative treatments, and those of no treatment at all. This point is especially important in situations where electing to have no treatment is a rational option. Two such situations often occur. One is when the malady itself is only mild to moderate in its severity and the treatment may itself be associated with significant harms or be financially costly, for example, prostatectomy surgery for moderate prostatism, or prolonged psychotherapy for mild chronic depression. The other situation is when the malady is grave and the treatments usually help only moderately: many treatments for advanced cancer, for example, though they may prolong life for a period of time, have a high probability of being accompanied by significant harms, and in many situations it is quite rational for a patient to refuse treatment even if he thereby increases the likelihood that he will die sooner.

It is often claimed that some physicians value the mere extension of life, even life of very poor quality, more than do many of their patients. These physicians are said to urge their terminally ill patients to continue treatment longer than most patients would desire if they knew all the facts. We do not know the extent to which these claims are true. However, the best way to combat any such tendency is to make certain that patients are supplied with accurate knowledge at all times about the likely outcome of the available rational treatment options (including, when rational, no treatment at all) and that patients know that they always have the option of stopping treatment if that is their desire.

Alternative ways of presenting information. Rational persons desire to make treatment decisions consistent with their own stable long-term values. It is in their interest for information about harms and benefits to be presented in a way which does not interfere with their ability to make an informed medical decision.

There is often more than one way of presenting even objective information. Information can sometimes be presented in a way that leads most people to have a particular impression about the information's import, but that impression can be modified if the information is presented in another way. Though the two ways of presenting the information may lead to different impressions, neither way is false. When impressions differ solely as a function of the way in which information is presented, these differences are often referred to as "framing effects."[17]

Sometimes the alternative descriptions of information are related to one another in a completely straightforward manner; neither contains any information not present in the other. For example, a surgical procedure can be described either as having a 5% death rate, or a 95% survival rate. Both the "5%" and the "95%" description are completely equivalent to one another. Yet psychologists studying decision making have shown that significantly more persons will consent to have the procedure when the survival rate is mentioned than when the death rate is mentioned.[18]

Other alternative descriptions are related to each other in a more complex way. For example a patient might be correctly told that a particular drug, though it is expensive and is accompanied 85% of the time with certain quite unpleasant side effects, will decrease her chance of having a heart attack by 50%. Rational persons essentially never want to have heart attacks, and thus she might rank the diminution of the risk of death much more highly than the harms associated with taking the drug. However, if her physician tells her, equally correctly, that the drug would, in fact, decrease her chance of having a heart attack from 1/100 to 1/200, her choice might change. She might consider the difference in absolute magnitude between the two risks to be trivial, and hardly worth enduring any avoidable harms associated with the drug. Another patient in the same situation might decide differently because he prefers to endure the costs and the side effects of the drug even though he realizes that the difference between 1/200 and 1/100 is small.

What seems to be true is that if one hears only the "50% reduction" description, one may incorrectly assume that one's chance of having a heart attack is

100%, or some other high number, and that the drug will reduce that figure to around 50%. If that were true, then unless the side effects were extremely severe, almost any rational person would choose to take the drug.

One easily calculated statistic which is useful in assessing the relative harms and benefits of treatments is called the "number needed to be treated" (NNTT).[19] This number tells how many persons need to subject themselves to the possible harms of a treatment before, on average, one person is helped who would not otherwise be helped.

In some cases the NNTT is gratifyingly low. It has its lowest value, 1, in those occasional treatments which help all patients who would not otherwise be helped, since in that case only one person needs to be treated before one person is helped who would otherwise not have been. Other treatments which are highly but not universally effective have somewhat higher values. For example, a particular antidepressant drug may significantly help two out of three patients who take it, though one out of six patients will improve without it. Thus if 100 patients take the drug, 67 will improve; if 100 patients are given no drug, 17 will improve. Therefore, treating 100 patients will benefit 50 who would not otherwise have benefited (67 minus 17); thus two patients, on average, need to be treated to benefit one who would not otherwise have been benefited. The NNTT = 100/50 = 2.

However, unfortunately, the NNTT is often quite high. This is true for many treatments which are given over a long period of time in order to lessen the risk of some adverse event occurring. It is frequently true that the probability of the adverse event, even in a "high-risk" population, is fairly low, so that even if the treatment results in a large relative risk reduction, the NNTT is nonetheless rather high.

The following example from Laupacis, et al. illustrates this phenomenon.[20] In a particular study, 201 male patients under 50 years of age with elevated blood pressure (diastolic = 90 to 114 mmHg), but without target organ damage, were treated either with antihypertensive drugs or with a placebo for three years. The outcome measure was whether by the end of the three years any significant adverse cardiovascular event (stroke or myocardial infarction) had occurred. The rate of significant adverse events of this kind was as follows:

With antihypertensive drugs	4.0%
With placebo	9.8%

Thus the relative risk reduction was rather high: the difference between 9.8% and 4.0% represents a 59% reduction. Therefore one could say, correctly, to a patient that taking these drugs might decrease by 59% his chance of suffering a significant adverse event within the next three years.

However because the likelihood of an adverse event occurring even without treatment was rather low (9.8%), the NNTT was 17. That is, if 100 patients were treated for three years with drugs, 4 would have an adverse event; if 100 were given no drugs, 10 would have an adverse event. Thus treatment would prevent 6 adverse events. Thus 17 patients (100/6) would need to subject themselves to the cost and side effects of antihypertensive drugs for three years in order for one of them to forestall an adverse event that otherwise would have occurred. For the other 16 of the 17 patients, either no adverse event would occur, with or without treatment, or an adverse event would occur even with treatment. When the data are understood in this way, some patients may choose to have the treatment while others may not.

It is useful to point out and explain the NNTT concept to patients because the result that this concept yields is quite counterintuitive for most people. That is, "this drug is associated with a 59% smaller chance of suffering an adverse event" does not sound consistent with "only 1 in 17 people who take this drug will be directly benefited by taking it." Yet both statements are true.

It is true, in fact, that the vast majority of patients treated by many risk-reducing interventions will not themselves benefit from the intervention. Many NNTTs are much higher than the 17 produced by the above data. This applies not only to drug treatments but to such life-style changes as adopting a vigorous exercise program or eating a very low fat diet.[21] Many of these interventions do lead to a noticeable *relative* risk reduction but, because the *absolute* risk reduction is small, they forestall illness only for occasional persons who undertake them.

An exercise program may confer benefits other than a lessened risk of illness, but drug treatments for mild hypertension or hypercholesterolemia usually do not. Except for the patient who feels better psychologically simply because he is taking medication regularly, taking these treatments everyday for many years is, for the great majority of patients, all loss and no gain. Considering the small chance that the treatments will benefit any individual patient, the certainty that they will cost money, and the near-certainty that they will cause noxious side effects, it can be entirely rational to decide not to take them. Of course for the one patient in 17 who avoids having a stroke the benefit is great, so that it is also entirely rational to choose to take the medicine. When there are two ways of presenting data, each likely to lead to a different impression in many persons, it is clearly in a patient's interest to have data presented in both ways.

The choices involved in many clinical scenarios are clearly important ones. Significant harms and benefits may be involved, including whether one lives or dies, depending on whether one consents to treatment or not. Any rational person facing such an important decision and knowing that there was a one-in-seven chance she would make a different treatment decision with information presented in both ways rather than with information presented in only one way, would choose to have information in both ways.

Does it follow that physicians are morally required to describe outcome data in all of the various ways possible? That would be too strong a requirement.

However, we believe that to present only relative risk data, such as "This drug will lower your chance of having a stroke by 59%." seems misleading and deceptive and thus morally unacceptable. At the very least, absolute risk reduction data should be presented at the same time. We think that presenting NNTT data should be morally encouraged but not morally required. We explain more fully below the distinction between what is morally required and what is morally encouraged in the consent process.

The process of giving information to patients. The length of time required for the consent process varies from situation to situation. The process can be short and straightforward; for example, in a situation where the patient's malady is dangerous or very unpleasant, the patient wants to have the malady treated, there is one clearly best drug or procedure available to treat it, and the drug or procedure is effective and relatively safe. In this setting it is not only rational for the patient to consent to treatment, it would be irrational for her to refuse it. The patient should nonetheless be told the likely harms and benefits of treatment versus no treatment, but since only one rational choice is available, little weighing of information is usually necessary.

At other times the information about possible harms and benefits is more complex and takes longer to present, even to intelligent and competent patients. One example is a patient with carotid artery arteriosclerosis and accompanying very mild transient ischemic attacks who is faced with the question of whether to have carotid artery surgery. In this situation there are significant harms and benefits associated with either having carotid artery surgery or with not having it; in addition, the possible harms associated with surgery are more likely to occur perioperatively, while those associated with medical treatment are apt to occur over ensuing months and years. The difference between the two kinds of treatment is significant but somewhat subtle, so making a choice requires good information and careful thought. Whenever there is more than one rational choice, including the choice of having no treatment, the data about the likely harms and benefits of each choice are apt to be statistical and complex and it may take time to present them in an understandable fashion.

One way of managing this situation is for doctors not to depend entirely on themselves to present the needed information. Health care professionals other than physicians can be used to give information to patients about treatment alternatives. With adequate training, many nurses and physician assistants should be competent to play that role. But this requires improving communication between members of the health care team, so that everyone will know what the patient has been told.

In addition there are now available printed brochures which describe many common maladies and the likely benefits and harms of the drug therapies and the surgical procedures most often used to treat them. Doctors can give a brief verbal summary of this information to patients, then encourage them to take printed material home for further study, discussion with their family, and so forth. For example, the American Psychiatric Association has published a series of pamphlets describing the nature of several of the common psychiatric maladies and the possible benefits and harms of the usual treatments suggested. For a number of maladies there now exist videotaped presentations of information about the disorder and its treatments. Videotapes about other disorders will be available within the next few years. Increasingly, useful and detailed medical information is available on the Internet. Patients without home computers with modem access to the Internet can often use terminals in public libraries and, increasingly, in hospitals.

If patients have further questions, after studying written, videotaped, or online material, they can talk with the doctor in person or by phone. The use of this kind of material not only saves physicians' time, it seems desirable from the patient's point of view as well. It can be difficult for any patient, soon after learning that he has a serious malady, to remember all that he is told about the harms and benefits of alternative treatment options. Treatments often have many significant side effects, some of which may not appear until some time after the treatment begins. In our experience, patients seldom take notes about what doctors tell them, nor do doctors encourage them to do so. Studies have shown that some patients remember little of what they have been told during the consent process. Rather than conclude from these studies that the consent process is of limited usefulness, we believe it is better to change the process so that interested patients are better able to retain and use the information they have been given.

How much do physicians know? Much of the above discussion has been predicated on two assumptions: (1) that a reasonably precise and useful body of knowledge exists about the comparative harms and benefits of alternative treatments in particular medical situations, and (2) that individual physicians are knowledgeable about this data-base and therefore able to present relevant portions of it to their patients. It is becoming increasingly clear that both of these assumptions may be less than totally accurate.[22]

While there is no denying that most medical treatments are at least somewhat effective, only a minority of them have been tested in valid randomized clinical trials. When such trials are conducted, it is not unusual for previously touted treatments to be discovered to be less effective than had previously been assumed.

Large geographical practice variations are commonly found in the utilization of most diagnostic and therapeutic interventions, suggesting the absence of any widespread professional consensus about when the tests and treatments are best employed.

Study after study of particular medical procedures has discovered a high incidence of care deemed inappropriate by panels of experts. It is common for one fourth of the surveyed instances of treatment to be labeled as "clearly inappropriate," and another fourth to be labeled as "equivocal." When physicians are questioned, it is common to discover a great range in their opinions about problems such as the frequency with which, within their specialty, a particular harmful outcome is associated with a particular medical procedure. Incidence estimates by individual physicians ranging from 0% to 100% have been reported, and ranges only slightly less extreme are common.

What implications do these findings, about which there seems to be little dispute, have for the process of valid consent? We believe there are two important implications. The first is that physicians, in order to perform their professional duty of transmitting adequate information, must be certain they are aware of whatever valid information does exist. To describe a suggested treatment to a patient, without knowing and disclosing the best current information available about what harms the suggested treatment might cause, is a breach of professional duty and is unethical.

The second implication concerns those situations, of which there are a great many, where the available information about harms and benefits is uncertain, conflicting or in some way inadequate. When information is uncertain, patients should be told it is uncertain. If there is disagreement in the literature about the value of different treatment alternatives, patients should be told about that disagreement. If two competent physicians might reasonably disagree about what should be done in a particular situation, the patient should know about that disagreement and the reasons behind it.

Some may object that patients want to believe that their doctors know at all times what the best treatment is, and also that it is difficult to convey uncertain information. We agree that patients want to have confidence in their doctors, but we think that they want that confidence to be justified confidence, not the blind confidence that little children have in their parents. If doctors do not know with precision the harms and benefits associated with alternative choices, whether because of personal ignorance or because of knowledge lacunae in the field, they should sensitively but honestly tell their patients about their uncertainty. The claim that doctors whose knowledge is uncertain cannot convey that uncertainty to patients has little force. A physician who puts it forward is subject to the following dilemma: if knowledge is this inexact, then how can the physician rationally decide which of the various alternative treatments to recommend? Whatever estimates the physician makes of the harms and benefits involved, including their uncertainty, can be described to the patient. Unless one wants to defend purely intuitive judgments that cannot be rationally justified even to colleagues, then it must be possible to convey the grounds of one's judgment in language understandable to the patient.

Patients who do not want to be told information. Occasionally patients say they do not want to know information of the kind detailed above and that they prefer that their doctor or their family decide what should be done for them. In a variant of this situation, family members may request that the family be allowed to make treatment decisions for the patient and that the physician not even disclose information about diagnosis or treatment alternatives to the patient. It is even said that there are some entire societies, for example in Latin America, where patients prefer not to know information about diagnosis and treatments, especially about serious illnesses, and desire instead that their doctor or their family make decisions for them.

Is it unreasonable for a patient to allow others to decide for him? That depends on a number of factors. Consider first a patient who generally wants to know information about his condition and wants to make his own treatment decisions. Although he is interested in knowing what his family or his doctor think he should do, he generally wants to make his own final decision. It is usually unreasonable for this kind of patient to allow others to decide for him. This is because whenever he is faced with a choice between two or more options, though each may be rational, it is possible that because of his own ranking of harms and benefits it would be unreasonable for him to choose one or another of the available options. Unless he is certain that his family or his doctor will not make decisions contrary to his personal values, there is a chance that the choice they make for him would be one that, were he to know all the relevant information, he would regard as unreasonable.

For example, a patient gravely ill with metastatic cancer is faced with the option of one or two types of treatment but also with the option of no treatment, and all of these choices are rational. If a particular patient, given adequate information, strongly favors the option of no treatment, preferring an earlier death to the pain of continued life, then for him to choose continued treatment is unreasonable. Thus it is unreasonable for him to decide what to do by flipping a coin, because there is a significant possibility that by chance he would be subjected to further treatment and he does not want further treatment. To let someone else make his decision is like flipping a coin; there is a significant possibility that a choice will be made for him that, given adequate information, he would regard as unreasonable. Therefore, unless he has an adequate reason, for instance the anxiety that he suffers when forced to make a significant medical decision, for allowing someone other than himself to make the medical decision, it would be unreasonable for him to do so.

We believe that there are patients who suffer considerable anxiety when forced to make a significant medical decision, although our impression is that people much more frequently assert that claim on behalf of others than profess it for themselves. It is also true that some research shows that the overwhelming majority of persons say they would like to be given extensive information about their condition and also be involved in making treatment decisions.[23] Thus it seems that in the United States only a small minority of patients prefer to be uninformed and to allow others to make decisions for them.

If it would be unreasonable, a significant percentage of the time, for a patient to allow others to make decisions for her, and if, in fact, most patients, when asked, state that they want to have information about their conditions and would want to participate in making choices among the rational alternatives, then we believe that the physician has the duty with every patient to determine whether that patient wishes to be informed. To assume without asking that a patient does not want to be informed, or not to inform a patient at the family's request, seems unwarranted. We do not argue that the doctor has the duty to inform every patient; we do argue that the doctor has the duty to ask the patient in every case if he wishes to be informed.

Obtaining consent for the process of consent. Because there are rare occasions when the consent process itself might cause a patient more harm than it prevents, it is useful to consider the consent process itself as a medical intervention for which consent should be obtained. Of course it is often abundantly clear, at least in the United States, from the way in which patients present their complaints and ask questions about them, that they want full information about the alternatives they face.

But on some occasions in some cultures, it is unclear just how much patients want to be involved in the consent process. Physicians, however, can usually determine this without a great deal of difficulty if they structure their discussions with patients properly. For example, after a patient has described her complaints, a physician might say,

> "It seems to me from what you've said that there are a couple of possibilities which might exist."

Or,

> "It seems to me that what is probably wrong is this: . . . " or "I think there are two approaches we might take: . . . "

Or,

> "At this point we should probably do a few tests to look more closely at a couple of things."

Then he can add,

> "Are you interested in my telling you how it looks to me at this point?"

Or, if relevant,

"There are one or two choices that need to be made here and I'd like to have your opinion about them if you'd like to give it to me, after I've told you what I'm thinking."

If the patient indicates at this point that he does not want to hear information, or be involved in decision making, then the physician can ask him under what circumstances he would want to be informed, and so forth, and discuss directly with him his wishes about the consent process. As the discussion develops, statements like the following might be appropriate:

"We'll be doing a lot of studies to try to find out exactly what's wrong. Some patients want to know the results of the studies and to have full information, but others don't. How much would you like to know?"

Or,

"What turns out to be wrong might be serious or it might not be serious. Some patients want to know all the facts, others prefer just to be generally told what's going on, but let the doctor or their family worry about the details. How do you feel?"

Or,

"At this point we need to make some decisions about what kind of treatment to use. If you like, I can give you all the important details about what needs to be decided and you can help make a choice. Some patients want to do that, others prefer that their doctors and their families make those decisions. What do you prefer?"

To determine if a patient wishes to be informed about her condition after a serious illness has developed can be more difficult than to determine the patient's wishes about these matters ahead of time. Physicians, especially primary care physicians, should discuss these issues with patients early in the doctor-patient relationship, so that the doctor knows each patient's general desires. Also, the earlier in a disease's progression that these matters are discussed, the better. To wait until after the diagnostic studies have been done, or after the exploratory surgery has been carried out, may, if the results are serious, make the conversations more difficult. However, even though the patient will know that he has a serious problem, the practice can still be followed of determining how much a patient wants to know and to what extent he wants to participate in decision making:

"We now have a pretty good idea of what's wrong. In my experience some people want to know the details themselves, and then help decide what to do. Others prefer to let their family or their doctors handle things. What would you like to do?"

Many patients will then ask, "Is it serious?" to which the reply should almost always be, truthfully, "Yes," or "It could be." One can then proceed according to the patient's expressed wishes.

Lack of Coercion

Valid consent requires the absence of any coercion by the doctor or the medical staff. Coercion involves a threat of sufficient evil or harm that "it would be unreasonable to expect any rational man in that situation not to act on it."[24] A threat of this kind means that the person being threatened has been deprived of her freedom to choose, which is morally prohibited. Strong recommendations, even forcefully given, are not coercive. To extend the term "coercion" to include any pressure by a doctor on a patient to change a treatment decision, and hence to require that the pressure be morally justified, seems to us undesirable. In fact, as explained below, we think that sometimes it is morally praiseworthy for a physician to put pressure on a patient during the consent process.

On occasion, patients are coerced to choose or reject a treatment option not by the health care team, but by their family or friends. If, as is sometimes the case, the patient has not been given adequate information, or if the patient is not fully competent to make a rational choice, then on those grounds the coerced consent would not be valid. Sometimes, however, the patient has been given adequate information and is fully competent, but nonetheless consents only because of coercion from a family member.

Consider the following case: Mrs. R is a 61-year-old, legally blind and chronically physically ill woman who is admitted to an inpatient psychiatry unit for treatment of a severe depression which had been poorly responsive to a series of antidepressant medications. She has had three other episodes of depression during the past 10 years, each of which has similarly been poorly responsive to medication but in each case has subsequently resolved quickly with electroconvulsive therapy (ECT).

On admission to the unit, Mrs. R is reluctantly agreeable to receiving ECT. However, two days after admission she tells her psychiatrist, Dr. B, that she is actually very frightened of having ECT and is consenting only because of threats from her husband. Her husband had threatened her at the time of admission by telling her that he would not help to care for her at home if she returned without having had ECT. Because of her blindness and her compromised physical condition, she requires much assistance at home for such basic physical needs as personal hygiene, and clothing and feeding herself. There is no one on whom she can depend other than her husband. Numerous attempts by various health care professionals to contact Mr. R over the next week prove unsuccessful, but Mr. R tells his wife by telephone that he refuses to come to the hospital or talk to any staff member until she has ECT. Mrs. R asks the staff to stop trying to reach her husband. She says that she is willing to give permission for

ECT, and sign a consent form, though she continues to insist to the staff that if it were up to her alone, she would not consent.

The treatment staff is unsure what to do. Mrs. R clearly regards it as impossible to return home without her husband's support. There is no one else with whom she can stay. Discharging her to a state-supported nursing home might be possible, but the psychiatric as well as other care there is substandard and she, herself, rejects this option. Should the staff proceed and give her ECT, as she is requesting?

Our view is that her consent should be viewed as valid. The physicians were not only not doing the coercing, but they had no control over the coercing party, her husband. We regard Mrs. R's husband's coercion as a fact-about-her-life with which she must contend, much as a victim of appendicitis must contend with her abdominal pain in deciding whether to consent to an appendectomy. In each case, the patient's decision is significantly determined by a strong negative stimulus for which the physician bears no responsibility and over which the physician has little or no control. Both the appendicitis patient and Mrs. R may acknowledge that their decisions are being largely determined by a coercive stimulus but, on balance, wish to consent. Though the staff may believe that Mr. R's paternalistic behavior toward his wife is morally unjustified, they do not have Mrs. R's permission to intervene. We do not believe her consent is invalid, and we believe it is morally justified for her physicians to proceed with ECT. To refuse to treat would put the staff in the paradoxical position of refusing to give the one treatment that they themselves believe is most highly indicated.

It may seem paradoxical to regard coercion from the physician as invalidating consent but coercion from the family as not doing so. But to see that different moral considerations apply in the two cases, consider again the example of appendicitis. When a patient's intense appendiceal pain causes her to consent to surgery, that does not invalidate her consent and it is morally justified for the surgeon to operate. The same is true when the coercive cause of consent is from a family member. However the surgeon is acting immorally if he himself intentionally caused the painful condition which made the patient consent to surgery. Even though it might now be necessary for him to operate, he would be subject to severe penalties because he himself is the cause of the harm. The same is true if the surgeon initiates the coercive cause of consent from a family member.[25]

Obtaining an Ideal Consent

If a physician gives adequate information to a patient who is competent to make a rational decision, and does not coerce the patient into choosing some particular treatment option, then the physician has satisfied the moral requirements for obtaining a *valid consent,* and has fulfilled her professional duty. If the patient subsequently consents to a rational treatment option, the physician is morally justified in providing the treatment, even if it involves violating a moral rule, for example, "Do not cause pain." If the patient refuses all suggested treatments, then the physician is morally justified in not treating.

However, we have noted in this chapter several ways in which physicians can go beyond the minimal requirements of obtaining a valid consent. Since these additional steps all involve following moral ideals, rather than avoiding the breaking of moral rules, we call this additional process the obtaining of an *ideal consent.*

It is an ideal outcome of the consent process for patients to make treatment decisions which are based solely on their own stable ranking of the harms and benefits involved, as these rankings are applied to the treatment choices at hand. There are circumstances which sometimes make it difficult for even adequately informed and competent patients to do so. The overall *ideal* the physician should follow is to *try to prevent the patient from making an unreasonable or irrational decision.*[26] This means not only not making a decision it would be irrational for any patient to make in this situation, but a decision that, given the patient's own particular ranking of the harms involved, would be unreasonable for the patient to make. The doctor is following a moral ideal if she tries, insofar as justifiable, to prevent a patient from making an irrational or unreasonable decision.

There are several circumstances that can influence a patient to make an unreasonable decision, even when the required elements of a valid consent have been satisfied. These circumstances can be described in terms of the valid consent elements to which they are most closely related.

(1) Valid consent requires that the patient be given full information of the kind discussed above so that no misleading or deceptive withholding occurs. Ideal consent requires more. It requires that when there is more than one way of presenting information, and it is true that different ways commonly lead persons to have different impressions, that all applicable ways be presented and explained to the patient. Concepts like the NNTT can be particularly helpful in giving information about the possible efficacy of different treatments.

(2) Valid consent requires that the patient not be coerced into consenting by any member of the health care team. Ideal consent requires that the physician assure herself that the patient is not being coerced by anyone; if some third party is coercing the patient to consent, the physician should make every effort to remove that coercion or, at least, to assure the patient that she will support the patient in whatever decision the patient unilaterally makes. Similarly, even if the pressure being put on the patient to consent falls short of coercion and would be better described as manipulation, ideal consent requires that the physician help the patient understand and resist the manipulative attempt if the patient desires that the physician do so.[27]

(3) Valid consent requires that the physician determine that the patient is competent to make the kind of rational treatment decision confronting him.

Ideal consent requires that the physician try to determine whether the patient's decision, even if rational, is also reasonable, that is, is maximally consonant with the patient's own ranking of the harms involved in the different treatment options. For example, a physician can strongly recommend to an agitated patient who has quickly agreed to a treatment that he take a few days to consider his decision carefully. The physician is following the ideal of helping the patient make a decision in a "cool moment," so that the patient will make that decision most consistent with his own stable values.

Although pursuing the goals of ideal consent puts great emphasis on encouraging patients to express their own values in ranking the harms of alternative treatment options, we do not advocate that the physician always adopt a strict nondirective stance. In fact, trying to obtain an ideal consent may require the physician to make clear and forceful statements, sometimes even to challenge a patient's decision. Such statements may be "directive," but directive only in the sense that they direct the patient to consider pointedly a certain set of facts or they suggest to the patient that he seems to be making an unreasonable decision, based on the knowledge that the physician has about him.

Conclusion

The power of the concept of valid consent is significant and far-reaching. This chapter shows how the concept of consent, correctly understood and applied, has implications for topics as diverse as the proper way to convey statistical information to patients, and the regionalization of medical services. The topic of consent emerges repeatedly in chapters to come: for example, it plays a key role in determining the approach doctors should follow in managing private information about patients; the lack of appropriate consent is a defining feature of the concept of paternalistic behavior; and the obtaining of advance directives is best understood as a kind of anticipatory consent or refusal with regard to medical situations that may arise in the future.

Despite the power of the concept of valid consent, the moral requirements it imposes on the physician are neither ad hoc nor anything out of the ordinary. They are simply the everyday requirements of morality particularized in the consent situation. The elements of consent are all easily inferable from a knowledge of ordinary morality and a knowledge of the nature of the doctor-patient relationship. The elements could scarcely be anything other than what they are.

Notes

1. There are three situations which occur with respect to patients' making decisions about treatment. Patients may request a treatment themselves, as discussed in Chapter 12, "Euthanasia." Patients may refuse a treatment, as discussed in Chapters 9 and 10,

"Paternalism" and "Justification." Or patients may consent to a suggested treatment, the subject of this chapter.

2. We will talk throughout of doctors suggesting "treatments"; we use that term broadly, to include diagnostic tests, regimens, drugs, operations, psychotherapies, and so forth.

3. Including the moral rule "Do your duty," which, as explained above, may include actions that would generally represent following moral ideals, but which have been explicitly turned into duties by the members of a particular profession.

4. See, for example, "American College of Physicians Ethics Manual," *Annals of Internal Medicine,* 117 (1992), pp. 947–960, especially pp. 949–950.

5. See Chapter 2 for a discussion of the concept of an "unreasonable" choice.

6. See Teri A. Manolio, Jeffrey A. Cutler, Curt D. Furberg, Bruce M. Psaty, Paul K. Whelton, and William B. Applegate, "Trends in Pharmacologic Management of Hypertension in the United States," *Archives of Internal Medicine,* 155 (1995), pp. 829–837. The authors point out that between 1982 and 1993 there has been a dramatic shift away from the use of the traditional antihypertensive agents (diuretics and beta-blocking drugs) and toward such newer agents as calcium antagonists and ACE inhibitors. This has occurred despite the lack of evidence that the newer drugs are more beneficial than the older, and despite the greatly increased cost of the newer drugs. The average estimated monthly cost of beta-blockers (app. $24.00) is about three times that of diuretics (app. $8.00); ACE inhibitors (app. $36.00) are more than four times as expensive, and calcium antagonists (app. $48.00) are almost six times as expensive. Every patient for whom the newer drugs is prescribed should be aware of these data.

7. This is especially important now when doctors are often working for HMOs. Apropos of HMOs, "gag rules," which prohibit HMO physicians from disclosing information about alternative treatments to patients, are clearly morally unacceptable.

8. See Gina Kolata, "Diagnosis: Treatment Pending," *The New York Times,* Feb. 12, 1995, sec. 4, p. 1. One physician is quoted as saying, "I would like proof beyond a reasonable doubt that there is more benefit than harm." Another, however, states, "I don't think we should say that until all these questions are answered about the value of treatment that we should not try to detect cancer." A third physician takes a position closer to ours; he recommends that patients should be told about the disputes among experts. He asks: "Are patients getting accurate and evenhanded information, or are physicians playing on their fears to push them in a certain way when the data are inadequate?"

9. For a good example of needless apprehension, see Natalie Angier, "Ultrasound and Fury: One Mother's Ordeal." *The New York Times,* November 26, 1996. Two separate ultrasound tests indicated that this reporter's first baby had a clubfoot, but the baby was perfectly normal at delivery. The article concludes that "women should be entitled to have ultrasound and other prenatal tests, but . . . the process of informed consent must be taken far more seriously than it currently is."

10. For an excellent early description of this phenomenon, an exemplification of Bayes rule, see Paul E. Meehl and Albert Rosen, "Antecedent Probability and the Efficiency of Psychometric Signs, Patterns, and Cutting Scores," *Psychological Bulletin,* 52 (1955), pp. 194–216. For an application of Bayes rule to an issue in bioethics, see Charles M. Culver, "Commitment to Mental Institutions," in Warren T. Reich (Ed.), *Encyclopedia of Bioethics* (New York: Macmillan, 1995), pp. 418–423. For a discussion of Bayes rule and medical diagnosis, see K. Danner Clouser, "Approaching the Logic of Diagnosis" in Kenneth Schaffner (Ed.), *Logic of Discovery and Diagnosis in Medicine* (Berkeley: University of California Press, 1985), pp. 35–55.

11. August Piper Jr., "Truce on the Battlefield: A Proposal for a Different Approach to Medical Informed Consent," *Journal of Law, Medicine and Ethics,* 22 (1994), pp. 301–313.

12. See note 7.

13. Toby A. Gordon, Gregg P. Burleyson, James M. Tielsch, and John L. Cameron, "The Effects of Regionalization on Cost and Outcome for One General High-Risk Surgical Procedure," *Annals of Surgery,* 221 (1995), pp. 43–49.

14. Evidence of this kind has been accumulating for many years. For an early summary, see Harold S. Luft, John P. Bunker, and Alain C. Enthoven, "Should Operations Be Regionalized? The Empirical Relation between Surgical Volume and Mortality," *New England Journal of Medicine,* 301 (1979), pp. 1364–1369. For one response to this article, emphasizing the importance of communicating volume-outcome data to patients, see Charles M. Culver and Bernard Gert, "Regionalization of Surgical Services" (letter to the editor), *New England Journal of Medicine,* 302 (1980), pp. 1034–1035.

15. This may not be true for patients who have health insurance that covers the complete cost of all treatments, but even such patients may be concerned about the overall cost of medical care.

16. We think this is a plausible threshold number, but we know of no consensus about what the exact magnitude of this number should be. Most persons would probably agree that a risk of death of 1 in 1,000,000 need not be told and that 1 in 1,000 should be, but there could be disagreement where to put the threshold between these extremes.

17. Amos Tversky and Daniel Kahneman, "The Framing of Decisions and the Psychology of Choice," *Science,* 211 (1981), pp. 453–458.

18. Ibid.

19. See Andreas Laupacis, David L. Sackett, and Robin S. Roberts, "An Assessment of Clinically Useful Measures of the Consequences of Treatment," *New England Journal of Medicine,* 318 (1988), pp. 1728–1733. For a good general discussion of the use of the NNTT and other quantitative measures in evaluating treatment outcomes, see David L. Sackett, R. Brian Haynes, Gordon H. Guyatt, and Peter Tugwell, *Clinical Epidemiology: A Basic Science for Clinical Medicine,* 2d ed. (Boston: Little, Brown, 1991), especially Chapter 7: "Deciding on the Best Therapy."

20. Laupacis, et al., "An Assessment of Clinically Useful Measures of the Consequences of Treatment."

21. For additional examples related to the treatment of mild hypertension, see Lachlan Forrow, Steven A. Wartman, and Dan W. Brock, "Science, Ethics, and the Making of Clinical Decisions: Implications for Risk Factor Intervention," *JAMA,* 259 (1988), pp. 3161–3167.

22. For an excellent summary and discussion of the evidence mentioned here that challenges these assumptions, see David M. Eddy, *Clinical Decision Making: From Theory to Practice,* Sudbury, MA: Jones and Bartlett, 1996.

23. William Strull, Bernard Lo, and Gerald Charles, "Do Patients Want to Participate in Medical Decision Making?" *JAMA,* 252 (1984), pp. 2990–2994.

24. Bernard Gert, "Coercion and Freedom," in J. Roland Pennock and John W. Chapman, *Coercion (Nomos* XIV), p. 34 (Chicago: Aldine, 1972).

25. See Steven D. Mallary, Bernard Gert, and Charles M. Culver, "Family Coercion and Valid Consent," *Theoretical Medicine,* 7 (1986), pp. 123–126, for a more extensive discussion of this case.

26. We think that this is what is meant by those who talk of "promoting autonomy." On this interpretation, promoting autonomy is clearly a moral ideal, and should be distin-

guished from "respecting autonomy," which is morally required. We think that talking about autonomy is more liable to confusion and abuse than this way of describing the consent process.

27. For a definition and discussion of interpersonal manipulation, see Michael Kligman, and Charles M. Culver, "An Analysis of Interpersonal Manipulation," *The Journal of Medicine and Philosophy,* 17 (1992), pp. 173–197.

8

Confidentiality

In this chapter we analyze and define the concepts of privacy and confidentiality and discuss the ethical justification of disseminating private information in different situations. We argue that physicians should make clear to their patients what kinds of information and activities they believe they have a duty to regard as private and under what conditions they would engage in a breach of confidentiality. We show how our approach clarifies the understanding of privacy and can help reduce moral conflicts about confidentiality. We propose three guidelines that should govern physicians' conduct with regard to confidentiality.[1]

The Concept of Privacy

It is important to be clear about the concept of privacy in order to understand and attempt to solve problems of medical confidentiality. Discussions of privacy can be frustrating, because people hold divergent views not only about what should be private but about how the concept should be defined. Moreover, the concept of privacy has been evolving over the last two centuries. At least three different conceptions of privacy, or at least perspectives on the concept of privacy, can be found in the literature. We begin by untangling these different views of privacy, and then we integrate the various approaches into a common framework. Arriving at a clear understanding of the concept is crucial if one wishes to formulate coherent policy in this area.

A classic conception of privacy is *nonintrusion*. People in the United States regard themselves as private citizens and in most respects they believe the government should not intrude into their lives. A central purpose of the Bill of Rights of the United States Constitution is to express the limits of government's power to intrude into the lives of its citizens. Although the Constitution does not mention "privacy" explicitly, many, including members of the United States Supreme Court, believe that the "right to privacy" is implicit in several amendments that limit the government's right to intrude. For example, the Fourth Amendment states, "The right of the people to be secure in their persons, houses, papers, and effects, against unreasonable searches and seizures, shall not be violated." Other explicit prohibitions against specific forms of government intrusion are mentioned in the First, Fifth, and Fourteenth Amendments.

The conception of privacy as nonintrusion has been expanded over the years to include the right to be protected from the intrusions of other citizens. In a classic 1890 *Harvard Law Review* article Samuel Warren and Louis Brandeis argued for a broad concept of privacy. They believed that people have the right to be let alone not only by the government but by other persons as well. Warren and Brandeis were particularly concerned about intrusions by the press armed with a new technology—the camera. As they put it, "Instantaneous photographs and newspaper enterprise have invaded the sacred precincts of private domestic life; and numerous mechanical devices threaten to make good the prediction that 'what is whispered in the closet shall be proclaimed from the house-tops.'"[2] Warren and Brandeis regarded violations of privacy to be significant, because, as they argued, the resulting mental pain and distress could be even greater than that inflicted by bodily injury.

A second, related conception of privacy is the *freedom to act in personal matters*. This view of privacy has played an important role in matters of medical practice. Consider the situation of Dr. Buxton, who was the medical director at the Planned Parenthood League of Connecticut in New Haven, and Mr. Griswold, who was the executive director of the League. The doctor and his staff at the center gave medical examinations and also dispensed information about contraception. At that time this activity conflicted with Connecticut law which forbade even counseling on the topic of contraception. A challenge was brought against the center, and eventually the case went to the U.S. Supreme Court. In 1965, in *Griswold v Connecticut,* the Supreme Court, citing the Fourteenth Amendment and others, overturned those Connecticut statutes which forbade selling and counseling about contraceptive devices.[3] The court maintained that these statutes violated a married couple's right to privacy. The *Griswold v Connecticut* decision influenced another well-known U.S. Supreme Court decision, *Roe v Wade,* in which a woman's right to choose an abortion was predicated largely on the basis of the right to privacy.[4]

A third, popular, contemporary view of privacy is the *protection of personal information.* In American society, in which computers and electronic communicating devices are commonplace, there is a prevalent fear that personal information, such as medical records or financial records, can be used against individuals. As Charles Fried explains, "Privacy is not simply an absence of information about us in the minds of others, rather it is the control we have over information about ourselves."[5] Unfortunately, people rarely have much control or even awareness of the flow of information about themselves. For example, an unauthorized examination of computer medical records can be done so that patients remain unaware of the invasion of their privacy. As a practical matter, it is impossible for people personally to control all of the extant information about themselves, but they can insist that safeguards be used so that the flow of personal information is under the protection of responsible management.

Although no one of the three views of privacy, *nonintrusion, freedom to act,* and *protection of personal information,* is, taken individually, adequate to explain the full concept, these views can be organized into a single coherent framework for explicating the notion of privacy.[6] All of these aspects of privacy involve the restricted access of the government or of individuals either to some activities of other individuals or to some information about other individuals. Thus, we define privacy as follows: *An individual or group has privacy in a situation with regard to others if and only if in that situation the individual or group is normatively protected from intrusion, interference, and information access by others.* The notion of a "situation," which is central to the definition, is left deliberately vague so that it can range over the kinds of states of affairs which people normally regard as private. A situation may be an activity in a location, such as living in one's home, or a situation may be a relationship, such as the doctor-patient relationship, or a situation may be the storage and access of information, such as that stored in a filing cabinet or in a computer.[7]

The boundaries of private situations are defined normatively through law or through custom. The force of custom can be strong, even absent an associated law. In American culture if someone opens and reads someone else's personal diary, the intruder has seriously invaded the diary writer's privacy although, except in extraordinary circumstances, the diary writer has no legal reprisal.

To a large extent the nature and kinds of situations which are private are culturally determined: there are situations in a culture where rules, legal or conventional, explicit or implicit, exist about who may and may not have access to the activities of persons or information about persons. This does not mean that privacy is completely relative or totally arbitrary. It does mean that the articulation of normatively private situations varies from country to country and from time to time. As a result, cultures vary, at least to some degree, about which situations are considered normatively private and which are not.

In the United States, for example, there is a general rule, albeit one often violated in practice, that information about a competent patient's medical condition should be given primarily to the patient. To give it instead, without asking the patient, to the patient's family is regarded by many patients as an invasion of their privacy. To do the same in Argentina and many other Latin American countries is generally not so regarded. In both cultures, however, to give the information to a patient's neighbor is considered a breach of privacy. Both cultures define a normatively private situation about medical information, but they draw the boundaries of the situation somewhat differently. And, cultures can change over time in how they define a particular normatively private situation. It is probably true, for example, that the definition of medically private information, with respect to access by a patient's family, was at one time in the United States similar to what it is today in Argentina.

Why have normatively private situations? Why not let everyone intrude on and observe everyone else at any time? It seems clear that from an individual point of view private situations foster personal goods and prevent harms. Freedom, enjoyment, and personal development are often enhanced by the existence of private situations and embarrassment as well other social, political, and economic losses are frequently avoided.[8] Privacy in medical situations encourages trust and honesty, which in turn supports better medical care. Normally, privacy has a distinct payoff so that when privacy is invaded real harm can be done. As Warren and Brandeis suggested, the loss of privacy may be even more harmful than physical injury. Invading a person's privacy not only violates a moral rule with respect to that person, either violating a law or neglecting a duty, it increases the chances of futher harm. These violations often result in significant mental suffering and deprivation of freedom.

But privacy is not an unalloyed social good; it has costs as well.[9] Privacy sometimes makes social institutions less efficient and effective, which in turn may be detrimental to individuals. For example, treating medical records as totally private protects patients but also impedes the search for medical information by epidemiological researchers who often need to use medical record information to search for the causes of diseases.[10] This tension is manifested in the distinction between traditional medicine that addresses personal health and the allied discipline of public health that addresses the health of the community. Privacy may promote personal health while retarding public health.

Medical practice has many private situations. Some are legally defined but many are matters of convention. A physician's office, the doctor-patient relationship, medical records, financial records, a patient's room, and the adjoining bathroom are all examples of private situations. Within private situations different people are permitted to enter or share information. The hospital laboratory gathers information about a patient in a private situation: it is expected to share the information with the attending physician and referring physician but not with just any physician. These patterns of sanctioned behavior in a private situation can be shaped and adjusted to improve the beneficial outcomes of having the private situation. For example, the general rule in the United States that information about a patient may not be shared, without permission, with the patient's family is modified if the patient becomes seriously ill or mentally incompetent and some significant treatment decisions must be made. Then some aspects of the previously private situation may be revealed to certain family members.

We have explicated privacy in terms of situations and not in terms of specific information. Privacy is better tracked by the customary duties involved in the situation than it is by specific information. Suppose a male gynecologist has performed a routine pelvic examination on a patient. The situation in which the information has been gathered is private and proper. The gynecologist has detailed and intimate information about the patient. Now suppose the gynecologist later surreptitiously and voyeuristically peeks at the same patient through the examining room door. Although the gynecologist may gain no new information about the patient, he still is guilty of invading the patient's privacy because the situation is different—it is no longer a situation for the purposes of medical examination and treatment.

Although in this analysis of privacy we stress private situations as opposed to private information per se, it is plausible to talk in terms of private information as long as such talk is understood to be an elliptical way of claiming there is or ought to be a normative situation protecting the information. Some information is clearly private in this sense. The contents of a psychiatric interview, at least when not in the context of a forensic or disability evaluation, are presumed private. Patients would not feel free to divulge information that is crucial for their treatment to the therapist unless they believed that information would be kept private. However, information that a particular person is a practicing physician is not private. It is private that a patient is a patient of a particular doctor, but it is not private that that doctor is practicing medicine.

At times it is unclear whether to regard some information as private, that is, whether or how to define a restricted access situation to protect it. This is often true of information generated by new technology. Consider caller ID, a telephone device that displays the phone numbers of incoming calls. Does caller ID invade the privacy of the caller? Currently, the answer is unclear because there are few rules, legal or conventional, that define whether displaying caller phone numbers is private. Technology gives people access to previously unavailable information. Pizza parlors may like caller ID; those who call telephone hot lines to discuss sensitive issues often do not. Usually good guidelines, the norms for a new private situation, can be generated effectively and fairly through public debate and decision making. Then, of course, people need to know what the rules are. Pizza parlors should make it clear that they record callers' numbers; hot lines should make it clear they do not. The application of new technologies and the social conventions regarding privacy should interact and modify each other.

There are medical examples of new situations with uncertain privacy status as well. Technology can create new kinds of information and, therefore, new privacy concerns. Today lost hair is not regarded as a matter of privacy. But hair contains a wealth of genetic information about an individual. Perhaps in the near future this information will be readily analyzable. Should such information be protected? Should employers be forbidden to collect hair samples? Or, should submitting a hair sample be regarded as analogous to taking a psychological test given by an employer? In deciding whether to create a private situation of this kind the harms avoided and the goods gained by creating the private situation must be weighed against the harms avoided and the goods gained by not creating it.[11] The decision will depend largely on the facts of the situation. What kinds of information will be available from hair samples and what effects will knowledge of this information have on the parties involved? Thus the nature and kinds of situations that ought to be private are not merely a matter of habit or taste but are matters open to rational argument and criticism. Fully informed, impartial, rational persons do not always agree on what is best.

Privacy and Confidentiality

Confidentiality is part of the concept of privacy. We have defined privacy by saying, "An individual or group has privacy in a situation with regard to others if and only if in that situation the individual or group is normatively protected from intrusion, interference, and information access by others." Confidentiality is related to the information-access part of the concept of privacy. People hold information in confidence because the rules of a private situation require them not to reveal that information.

Confidentiality thus refers to a duty within a private situation.[12] Some party—a doctor, nurse, or physician assistant—has the trust and responsibility not to divulge information to inappropriate parties. Privacy is *invaded;* but confidentiality is *violated*—that is, the duty of confidentiality is violated (or broken, or breached). If confidentiality is violated, then privacy has been invaded and is lost. Confidentiality is a view from within a private situation looking out. It is the duty of some party to keep some information secret even if nobody on the outside is trying to invade the private situation. It is the duty of the physician, the lawyer, the nurse, or the physician assistant to limit access to information in that private situation.

Because confidentiality entails a duty to limit access to information, it is not surprising that confidentiality plays an important role in the professions. For professionals to do their work effectively, it is often essential that their patients and clients regard their mutual interactions as taking place in a private situation.

The success of a professional (and of the profession) often depends on the professional's ability to protect information. Therefore, in medicine and other professional fields discussions often center on the concept of confidentiality, which is the duty from the professional's perspective, and not on the more general concept of privacy.

Public Aspects of Confidentiality

One advantage of understanding confidentiality in terms of a duty to restrict access to a private situation is that it allows the normative details of the privacy situation to be tailored so that different people are allowed different kinds of access. A laboratory has information about a patient which it shares with a physician but the physician does not share all of his information about the patient with the laboratory. A lawyer's receptionist knows that someone is a client but does not know the details of the client's problems. A physician knows the patient's medical record and knows his charges to the patient but the physician is not given access to the patient's full financial transactions with the hospital. A psychiatrist knows in detail about a patient's psychiatric problems, while the patient's referring primary care physician need not in some cases. The restrictions on access must be worked out carefully to balance the needs for protection against the needs for doing efficient and competent work.

Because the different kinds of access in a private situation can be complex, it is useful to describe them as carefully as possible to all of those involved. Real situations frequently have residual vagueness and uncertainties, but the more these can be clarified, the more effective the privacy protections will be. Indeed, the parameters of confidentiality should be completely public. This means the conditions and rules of a private situation, and the procedures and the duties of those involved, should be spelled out publicly and explicitly so that all participants are clear in advance about what is expected. This is particularly important for patients and clients, who may not have any sense of what privacy protections they do and do not have. In some cases a patient may have a choice about how to proceed, and information about privacy or the lack of it may influence the patient's choice.

Private situations are not static. Circumstances change. Technology improves. Unexpected complications occur. From time to time the details of a private situation must be adjusted to accommodate a new reality. When private situations are redefined, altering who has what kind of access to what, the adjustments should be made public and clear to all relevant parties, so that people can plan their actions according to this new arrangement. In particular, if new circumstances would justify invasions of privacy, then the possibility of such invasions should be included in a redefinition of the private situation so that to the greatest extent possible everyone is informed ahead of time.

Informed Consent and Confidentiality

The notion of valid or informed consent (see Chapter 7) is widely accepted in medical ethics and is explicitly contained in many codes of medical ethics. It is also enshrined in legislation and common law. The doctor-patient relationship is fiduciary in nature. The doctor has vastly more information about illnesses and treatments than does the patient. The patient, however, can consent to or refuse any suggestions the doctor makes about treatments, regimens, diagnostic tests, and so forth. In order for patients to be able to make those choices which are most in accord with their own goals and values, doctors have a duty to supply patients with the relevant information required to make informed decisions. Of course, in addition to possessing sufficient information, if consent is to be valid, patients must be competent to make a rational decision of the relevant kind, and must not be coerced by the physician.

Thus, physicians should warn patients in advance whenever any treatment, regimen, or diagnostic test suggested to the patient carries with it some risk of loss of privacy. The disclosure of private information about a patient often carries some risk of harm to the patient. Doctors should make sure that their patients are informed about what kinds of information they do and do not regard as private and under what conditions and to whom they will or will not disclose information. Simply put, a physician's policies about confidentiality should not be kept private from her patients.

It may seem that our recommendation to divulge information about the rules governing confidentiality places a large burden on physicians, because most physicians encounter private situations routinely. We take the model of informed consent seriously and believe that the burden should be no less or greater than the normal burden on physicians to inform patients about risks of harms. Patients have a right to know about how information will be shared, just as much as they have a right to know other consequences of medical procedures. Of course, not all patients need to be informed about all possible situations, and some information can be included in pamphlets or presented on videotapes rather than explained in person to every patient. Also, physicians can make reasonable assumptions about what people know and do not know about standards of confidentiality. However, these caveats do not diminish a physician's responsibility to be proactive in informing patients about the nature and amount of privacy in relevant medical situations.

It is not always possible to define the parameters of confidentiality to patients in advance. Psychiatrists, for example, sometimes involuntarily hospitalize dangerously suicidal patients they see in emergency rooms and must, in the process, disclose information about the patient to the personnel in the psychiatric ward to which they send the patient, whether the patient wants the information disclosed or not. But such cases are the exception and not the rule. For most patients in most cases, there is plenty of time and opportunity to provide full disclosure about the nature of the rules governing confidentiality.

Disclosing Prima Facie Private Information

Physicians have a duty to keep confidential almost all information they obtain about a patient. This duty is explicitly stated in medical codes of ethics and is one of the oldest duties of the physician. It is derived from the intimate character of medical information and the therapeutic need for a trusting doctor-patient relationship. It is also true that states have laws safeguarding the privacy of medical information, and unwarranted disclosure may be a punishable criminal offense or give rise to civil liability or professional discipline.

Nonetheless the duty of confidentiality, though universal and strong, is not absolute and there are widely recognized exceptions to it. Most of the exceptions concern situations where it is necessary to divulge otherwise private information to prevent harm to the patient himself or to third parties, for example: the fact that a patient has certain communicable diseases, or the strong likelihood that the patient may carry out future actions which are dangerous to himself or to third parties.

When is it justified to reveal private information? In the particular situation, there must be a great likelihood that the harm caused by the disclosure is significantly less than the harm prevented. In calculating the harm caused by the disclosure one must take into account not only the harm likely to be caused to the particular patient but also to the therapeutic relationship. One must, as with all violations of moral rules, take into account all of the morally relevant features of the situation. Finally, one must consider the consequences of everyone knowing that information disclosure is allowed in all cases with the same morally relevant features. If one believes that the harms that will result from everyone knowing that information disclosure is allowed in these kinds of cases is less than the harms that will result from information disclosure not being allowed, it is justified to reveal that information.[13]

To whom is it justified to reveal confidential information? The goal, consistent with the above justification scheme, is to keep the harm or potential harm done by the disclosure, if there is any, as small as possible. This is usually done by revealing as little information as possible to as few persons as possible while still attaining the goal which justifies the breach in the first place. And it is not just the number of persons that is important but, if there is a choice, those persons should be selected who may be expected to keep the disclosure as limited as possible.

Consider a case in which revealing information against the wishes of the patient seems morally justified to most persons. A male patient, unbeknownst to his acquaintances, has homosexual relationships. Even his wife does not know he has frequently picked up male lovers when he has been out of town on business trips. He asks his doctor to order an HIV test; after hearing the distressing news that it is positive, the patient decides he does not want his wife to know.

The patient tells the doctor that the couple have unprotected vaginal intercourse about twice a week. His wife has no way of knowing that she is at risk of contracting AIDS from her husband. Her risk of becoming infected is probably about 20% per year (the best estimate is that the male-to-female transmission risk is about 1 in 500 with each act of unprotected vaginal intercourse).[14] Of course she may be infected already, although the chances are reasonably high that she is not.

Most persons believe that if the husband refuses to tell his wife, then the physician should tell the man that he believes the woman must know, and that if the man refuses to do so, the physician will tell her himself. If one balances the harms caused—the distress to the man on this occasion, the damage to the marriage, and the general weakening of trust that occurs when it becomes known that in this kind of case doctors will reveal private information—against the harm prevented (the 20% chance per year of saving the woman from contracting a fatal disease), rational persons can disagree on whether or not to advocate that disclosure be publicly allowed. Thus this violation is what we call weakly justified. It is an interesting feature of this case that rational persons can disagree on whether the doctor should inform the wife, even though the statistics about the likelihood of harm occurring with and without divulging the information are more precisely known than is true in many cases of privacy disclosures.

Certain plausible changes in the factual circumstances of the case affect one's moral intuitions. For example, if the doctor knew, with a virtual certainty, that the man was heterosexually impotent and that neither the man nor his wife had the slightest current or future interest in having sexual relations, the doctor might clearly feel that it is not morally justified to tell the patient's wife.

Reducing the Frequency of Moral Conflicts about Confidentiality

We believe that not only do professionals have a duty to disclose explicitly their policies about confidentiality, but that by so doing the frequency of ethical dilemmas in the area of confidentiality will be lessened. Making the rules clear ahead of time should lead to fewer anguishing situations later.

The case of the secretly homosexual HIV+ married man provides an illustrative example. If the doctor believes, before the testing is done, that the patient's wife must be informed if the results are positive, then we believe the patient should be given that information before he consents to testing. In fact this is the practice followed in many hospitals where HIV testing cannot be carried out without the patient's written consent, and the consent form explicitly informs the patient that if the results are positive, then any regular sexual partner of the patient must be informed of that fact. The patient is then free to decide whether to proceed, knowing that such seemingly confidential information will in fact be revealed even if he does not desire it to be, or whether to go to one of the laboratories that perform anonymous testing.

Explicitly informing patients ahead of time will not eliminate all problems concerning confidentiality. There is always the threshold problem of determining whether the particular facts of a situation justify breaching someone's right to privacy. Borderline cases are bound to occur, some with strong attendant disagreements among the involved parties. In addition, some patients will understandably object to the revelation of information about themselves, even if they do acknowledge that they knew of this possibility ahead of time.

One advantage of informing patients at the beginning about the parameters of confidentiality is that the physician is not violating a duty by disclosing information which is not protected. If the HIV + man knows his wife will be told if he is positive, then the doctor has not breached any duty of confidentiality toward the patient if he is later forced to tell her. The doctor has stipulated that he does not have the duty to keep that information private from the patient's wife.

Another advantage of physicians' making public their rules about confidentiality is the reduction in the number of clients who experience a good-faith surprise by such a disclosure. By a good-faith surprise we mean that the client neither knew nor reasonably should have known that what was disclosed would not be kept confidential. This sort of surprise is surely, for both patient and doctor, one of the most unpleasant aspects of disclosing personal information. Indeed, many good-faith surprises indicate a failure on the part of the doctor to inform the patient adequately about confidentiality rules ahead of time. Physicians who do breach confidentiality by disclosing private information without having warned their patients that they would do so should have the dual burden of justifying the breach and justifying the lack of warning.

Conclusion

The essence of our approach to privacy and confidentiality can be summed up with a definition and three normative guidelines.

Definition of Privacy

An individual or group has privacy in a situation with regard to others if and only if in that situation the individual or group is normatively protected from intrusion, interference, and information access by others.

Guidelines Concerning Confidentiality

1. *Publicity:* Rules and conditions governing confidential situations should be clear and known to the persons affected by them.
2. *Justification:* A breach of a confidential situation is justified if and only if there is a great likelihood that the harm caused by the disclosure will be so much less than the harm prevented by the disclosure that impartial rational persons can publicly allow such breaches in all situations with the same morally relevant features.
3. *Adjustment:* If special circumstances justify a change in the parameters of a confidential situation, then the alteration should become an explicit and public part of the rules and conditions governing the private situation.

We believe our approach helps to clarify and resolve some general issues concerning privacy and confidentiality and, in particular, some issues in medical practice. However, we do not suggest that all dilemmas surrounding confidentiality will suddenly disappear. Understanding actual private situations is sometimes neither easy nor clear, and decision making about when it is morally justified to breach confidentiality is often neither simple nor mechanical. Rather, our claim is that the concept of a private situation and the related duty of confidentiality, though not without residual vagueness, is frequently helpful when applied to particular cases. We believe that our guidelines concerning confidentiality, if applied in medical situations, will reduce misunderstandings and lead to greater protections and benefits for all patients.

Notes

1. This chapter is adapted from Charles Culver, James Moor, William Duerfeldt, Marshall Kapp, and Mark Sullivan, "Privacy," *Professional Ethics*, 3 (1994), pp. 3–25. We thank Arthur Zucker and Ohio University for sponsorship of the 1991 Conference on Privacy and the Professions which facilitated this collaborative work.
2. Samuel D. Warren and Louis D. Brandeis, "The Right to Privacy," *Harvard Law Review*, Vol. 4, No. 5 (1890), p. 195.
3. *Griswold v Connecticut*, 381 US 479 (1965).
4. *Roe v Wade*, 410 US 113 (1973).
5. Charles Fried, "Privacy," *Yale Law Journal*, 77 (1968), pp. 475–493.
6. James Moor, "The Ethics of Privacy Protection," *Library Trends*, 39 (1990), pp. 69–82.
7. There is a distinction between a naturally private situation and a normatively private situation. In a naturally private situation people and information are protected by natural means from intrusion and observation by others. Thus, a physician walking alone through a connecting tunnel to his office might be in a naturally private situation because the tunnel is otherwise empty and nobody can see into it from the outside. If someone else should appear in the tunnel, natural privacy is lost but there is no invasion of privacy. The other person may have every right to be there. In a normatively private

situation the protection is based upon ethical, legal, and conventional norms. Of course, normatively private situations are frequently naturally private as well. Filing cabinets have locks. But, when an unauthorized person enters a normatively private situation, privacy has been more than lost—it has been breached or invaded. In this chapter we are concerned with normatively private situations.

8. James Rachels, "Why Is Privacy Important?" *Philosophy and Public Affairs,* 6 (1975), pp. 323–333.

9. See Sissela Bok, *Secrets: On the Ethics of Concealment and Revelation* (New York: Pantheon, 1982).

10. James Moor, "How to Invade and Protect Privacy with Computers," in C. C. Gould, ed., *The Information Web* (Boulder, Colorado: Westview Press 1989), pp. 57–70.

11. This specific example of interpretation is discussed in detail in Chapter 3.

12. See Chapter 3 for a discussion of how duties arise in professions and why a violation of a professional duty represents a moral rule violation.

13. See Chapter 2 for a fuller discusion of justifying violations of moral rules.

14. N. Hearst and S. B. Hulley, "Preventing the Heterosexual Spread of AIDS: Are We Giving Our Patients the Best Advice?" *JAMA,* 259 (1988), pp. 2428–2432.

9

Paternalism

Paternalism may be the most pervasive moral problem in medicine. It is involved in many discussions of euthanasia, and often accounts for the failure of physicians to supply full information when attempting to obtain consent for a procedure they believe to be important. At one time doctors thought that they were supposed to act paternalistically toward their patients, now many of them think that they should never act paternalistically. Not only is there confusion concerning whether acting paternalistically is ever justified, there is even confusion about what counts as paternalism. In this chapter we shall be concerned primarily with the definition of paternalism; in the next chapter we shall be concerned with its justification.

Paternalism has an unusual combination of features; it is intended to benefit another person and yet everyone agrees that it needs moral justification. These seemingly conflicting features indicate the difficulty of understanding paternalism and may explain why it is discussed so often. We believe that a discussion of paternalism is valuable for several reasons. First, it illustrates clearly that having a good motive is not sufficient for the act to be morally acceptable. This is extremely important since many people think that meaning well is all that is needed for acting morally. An examination of paternalism shows clearly that morality requires more than good intentions. Paternalism is not always morally unacceptable; on the contrary, not only is it often justified, it is sometimes even morally required. However, it is also often unjustified, and unjustified paternalism involves good intentions as much as justified paternalism does.

Any adequate definition of paternalism must take into account both that all paternalistic behavior is done with good intentions and that it needs to be justified in order to be morally acceptable. An adequate definition must also allow for both justified and unjustified paternalism. Since the point of providing a definition of paternalism is to enable a more useful discussion of what is commonly regarded as paternalistic behavior, the definition must include all of the clear cases, and exclude behavior which is commonly not regarded as paternalistic. It is a misuse of philosophy to offer a definition of paternalism that has the provocative result that some kind of behavior that no one considers to be paternalistic, for example, buying one's child an educational toy, turns out to be so, or that behavior that is taken as a clear case of paternalism, for example, committing a suicidal patient to a mental hospital, turns out not to be so. An adequate definition can make the term somewhat more precise, so that it decides at least some cases about which there is dispute, but it should not result in a fundamental change in the way the term is used. Otherwise it cannot serve the point of defining it, which is to facilitate discussion of those cases to which the term is normally taken to refer.

The Definition of Paternalistic Behavior

We offer the following definition of paternalistic behavior: P is acting paternalistically toward S if and only if:[1]

1. P intends his action to benefit S;
2. P recognizes (or should recognize) that his action toward S is a kind of action that needs moral justification;
3. P does not believe that his action has S's past, present, or immediately forthcoming consent; and
4. P regards S as believing he can make his own decision on this matter.

From this definition, it is easy to derive accounts of paternalistic attitudes, persons, and so on. A paternalistic attitude is an attitude that indicates a willingness to act paternalistically, and a paternalistic person is one who is more inclined than most to act paternalistically. A paternalistic law is a law that is intended to benefit the person whom it deprives of freedom.

Paternalistic laws differ from paternalistic actions in that paternalistic laws almost always violate the moral rule against depriving people of freedom, whereas paternalistic actions commonly involve the violation of many of the moral rules, such as those prohibiting deceiving or causing pain, as well as the rule prohibiting depriving of freedom. A paternalistic law, for example a seat belt law, is one whose legislative intent is to benefit those who are being deprived of freedom by that law. Taking paternalistic laws as the paradigm for paternalistic action has led some people to define paternalism as if it necessarily involved the deprivation of freedom.[2]

We shall discuss each of the four features of our definition in a separate section.

The Action Benefits S

There is no dispute about Feature 1; P's action toward S is paternalistic because P intends to benefit S; P's benefiting himself or some third party is irrelevant to classifying his action as paternalistic. Of course, P's actions can be partially paternalistic; they can be intended for the benefit of others, including P himself, in addition to S. But what makes P's actions toward S paternalistic is never the intended benefit to anyone other than S. Although P may be involved in self-deception, he must at least intend to benefit S. For instance, a physician may believe that she is deceiving her patient about his prognosis in order to prevent him from feeling bad, whereas the physician is actually more concerned with avoiding the unpleasantness of telling the truth to the patient. In all standard cases of paternalism, P's belief that S will benefit from her action must provide a sufficient motive for P's acting in this way.

Although doing something to S is paternalistic only if it is intended to benefit S, it need not benefit S directly. The intended benefit to S may be the intended result of benefits to those who are taking care of S. For example, those taking care of S may find it very difficult to do so and therefore not treat S well. Giving S some drug, which makes it easier for them to take care of S, may make them less upset with S. If a physician gives S a drug to make it easier for the caregivers to provide S with better care in order to benefit S, giving S that drug can count as paternalistic. Making things easier for caregivers can benefit those in their care, but what is in the best interests of the caregivers is not always in the best interests of the patient.

Restraining a patient in a wheelchair may be paternalistic if done to prevent him from trying to stand and, as a result, falling. If the caregivers cannot provide the constant supervision needed, then they may regard it as in the best interests of the patient to be so restrained, and such an action can count as paternalistic. Whether this kind of paternalistic action is justified depends on the situation. However, if it is clear that the restraints are used in order to provide even less supervision with no net benefit to the patient from the restraints, but only to maximize the profit of the institution, then the action does not even count as paternalistic. If the reduction in supervision clearly results in greater harm to the patient than the small probability that he will try to stand, and so will fall and hurt himself, such restraint is not only not a case of justified paternalism, it is not paternalistic at all, but only a sham paternalism.

When one person benefits another who is not suffering any loss, by increasing her ability, freedom, or pleasure, that is, by providing some good for her, we call this acting on a utilitarian ideal.[3] If, however, the person is suffering from a disability, or is deprived of freedom or pleasure, then increasing her ability, freedom, or pleasure may count as relieving an evil or harm. Unless one has a duty to do so, preventing or relieving a harm such as pain or disability for a person is acting on a moral ideal. Paternalistic acts can involve acting on either utilitarian or moral ideals. Paternalistically acting on a utilitarian ideal is justified only if done by parents or others in a similar role. Although medical paternalism involves acting toward patients as if they were one's children, almost all paternalistic actions that occur in medicine involve acting so as to prevent or relieve harms, which is acting on a moral ideal.

When talking about paternalism, benefiting a person does not mean doing what that person wants you to do. A physician who is acting in accord with the expressed desires of a patient is not acting paternalistically at all. Acting paternalistically often involves acting to benefit a person by doing what you regard as providing a net benefit for her when you do not know whether she would regard this as a net benefit. However, even if a physician does know that a patient would regard the result of the act as a net benefit to her, if he does not know if she is willing to undergo the harm involved in order to gain the benefit, he is acting paternalistically. Normally, paternalism involves acting on one's own ranking of harms and benefits rather than that of the person toward whom one is acting paternalistically. However, even if the patient would prefer the outcome that would result from the paternalistic action, he may not want to be treated in a paternalistic way, for example, lied to for his own benefit. Some people do not want others to do anything to them without their explicit consent. Unless one knows that the person wants to be deceived, caused pain, and so on, doing so for his benefit is acting paternalistically.

P's Action toward S Is a Kind of Action That Needs Moral Justification

Feature 2, that the person recognizes (or should recognize) that his action toward S is a kind of action that needs moral justification, is a key element of paternalistic behavior. If the person does not recognize that his action is of a kind that needs moral justification, and if it is not the kind of action that he should recognize as needing justification, it is not paternalistic, even if it has the other three features of paternalistic behavior. This kind of behavior is paternal or parental behavior, and it includes many of the beneficial things that parents do for their children, like buying them a computer or an encyclopedia. In Chapter 2, we attempt to show that the only kinds of actions that need moral justification are violations of moral rules. Our arguments in that chapter show that only violations of moral rules with regard to S can be paternalistic actions.

Everyone agrees that killing, causing pain or disability, depriving of freedom or pleasure, deceiving, breaking a promise, cheating, violating the law, or neglecting a duty are kinds of acts that need justification in order to be morally acceptable. The only dispute is whether there are any other kinds of acts which need moral justification.

On our account of morality in Chapter 2, any general kind of action that needs moral justification is prohibited by a general moral rule. As we pointed out in Chapter 3, there are particular moral rules which prohibit doing less general kinds of actions; acting paternalistically can involve violating one of these rules. However, as we showed in Chapter 3, all violations of particular moral rules also involve violations of the general moral rules, so no paternalistic act is excluded by limiting paternalistic actions to violations of the general moral rules. We have, of course, not proved that there are no other general moral rules, but we believe that our rules do cover all actions needing justification.

To have a justification for acting paternalistically is to have a justification for violating a moral rule. What counts as an adequate justification for violating a moral rule is discussed in detail in Chapter 2 and we will use this account in providing the justification of paternalism. Someone who has a different account of justification, however, can still accept our account of paternalism, although they may differ from us in the way in which they decide which paternalistic acts are justifiable. We recommend comparing our account of moral reasoning with that provided by others, such as consequentialists, deontologists, contractarians, virtue theorists, principlists, or casuists, to see which provides the most help in deciding what action morally ought to be done or in explaining one's moral judgments.

We have already pointed out that those who take paternalistic laws as the paradigm of paternalism commonly say that paternalism always involves a deprivation of freedom of the person who is being treated paternalistically. Paternalism, however, need not involve violating the moral rule prohibiting the deprivation of freedom, but can involve violating any of the moral rules discussed in Chapter 2. Paternalism involving breaking a promise is even discussed by Plato, who advocates not keeping one's promise to return a weapon to someone who has gone mad and may hurt himself. A promise to discharge a patient on a given day may be broken when the physician thinks it would not be in the patient's best interests to go home on that day, even though the patient wants to go home. In medicine, many acts of paternalism involve deception, and are often not related, except in a very indirect way, to the patient's actions at all. Rather they are done in order to prevent the patient, at least for some time, from feeling bad because of receiving unpleasant news about her medical condition.

One can even imagine cases of paternalism that involve violating the rule against killing. Indeed, one of the arguments against legalizing voluntary active euthanasia is that it may lead to paternalistic nonvoluntary killing of patients, that is, killing a patient who has not explicitly requested to be killed. This argument against legalizing voluntary active euthanasia is that some doctors who are reluctant to talk to a patient about dying, may conclude that the patient would be better off dead. If the doctor acts on that belief and kills the patient, he would be acting paternalistically. Of course, many are against legalizing voluntary active euthanasia because they believe that doctors may be led to practice nonvoluntary active euthanasia for economic reasons; they may act against what they take to be the best interests of their patients in what they take to be the best interest of their hospital, or health care system, or society. But many also hold that legalizing voluntary active euthanasia is dangerous because some doctors may act with the best interests of their patients in mind, but do so paternalistically. This may not be a good argument, but it shows that the notion of paternalistic killing is a fairly straightforward notion.

It is easy to imagine cases of causing pain, disabling, or depriving of pleasure that would count as paternalistic. P can act toward S in any of these kinds of ways in order to prevent S from doing something that P considers dangerous. It may be more difficult to imagine paternalistic examples of cheating, violating the law, or neglecting one's duty, because acting in these kinds of ways is not usually directed toward particular persons. Although unusual, cheating a particular person in a card game can be paternalistic, if, for example, one believes that the person being cheated is too cocky and will benefit from losing the game.

It is now generally accepted that paternalism is not limited to depriving of freedom, but that there can be paternalistic deception, paternalistic causing of pain, and so forth. Paternalism requires only that P recognizes (or should recognize) that he is performing a kind of a action, such as deceiving, that requires moral justification. It does not require P to think that his particular action needs justification. P may recognize that deceiving needs justification, and he may know that he is deceiving a patient, but not think of his action in that way, but rather as comforting a patient. All that is necessary for an act to count as paternalistic is that the person acting recognize that he is performing a kind of action, such as deceiving, and that deceiving is the kind of action that needs justification. He need not, and usually does not, think that he is doing anything wrong, and may not even regard his particular act as needing justification. All paternalistic acts can be correctly described as violations of moral rules, but it is extremely unlikely that a person acting paternalistically will be thinking of moral rules, or of whether he is violating any of them.[4]

Some philosophers hold that some actions that are not violations of moral rules may still be paternalistic. Dworkin gives the following example: "we play tennis together and I realize that you are getting upset about the frequency with which you lose to me. So, for your own good and against your wishes I refuse to play with you."[5] Dworkin regards this as a case of paternalism, whereas we regard it only as showing a paternalistic attitude. On our account, refusing to play tennis is not paternalistic, because it does not need moral justification; there is no moral rule violation. Dworkin then says, "It begins to look as if the only condition that will work is one that depends on the fact that the person who is being treated paternalistically does not wish to be treated that way." However, Dworkin realizes that this definition does not work and says that paternalism requires "a violation of a person's autonomy." He thus seems committed to the view that refusing to play tennis with someone in the situation described above is a violation of that person's autonomy.[6] He seems to take a violation of a person's autonomy to be equivalent to "an attempt to substitute one person's judgment for another's" and regards that as paternalistic when it is done "to promote the latter's benefit."[7] Dworkin clearly regards paternalistic actions as needing moral justification, but not all actions that he counts as "an attempt to substitute one person's judgment for another's" do need moral justification. Even if he regards the example of refusing to play tennis as an attempt to substitute one person's judgment for another's, it does not violate a moral rule and so does not need moral justification.

Dan Brock provides a similar account of paternalism. He says, "Paternalism is action by one person for another's good, but contrary to their present wishes or desires, and not justified by the other's past or present consent."[8] He explicitly states, however, that it is not intended to be a precise definition. James Childress, on the other hand, puts forward without any qualification the following definition of paternalism. "Paternalistic action is non-acquiescence in a person's wishes, choices, and actions for that person's own benefit."[9] Childress distinguishes between active and passive paternalism. "In active paternalism an agent refuses to accept a person's wish or request that he not intervene, whereas, in passive paternalism, an agent refuses to carry out a person's wishes or choices."[10] Childress holds that active paternalism is harder to justify than passive paternalism, but seems to hold that passive paternalism still needs to be justified. Thus Childress agrees that it is a necessary feature of paternalism, that it needs to be justified. Since Dworkin and Brock also agree that paternalism needs to be justified, they disagree only with our claim that the only actions that need moral justification are violations of moral rules. They claim that some actions which are not violations of moral rules need to be justified.

Brock, Childress, and Dworkin all hold that paternalism involves acting contrary to the wishes of the person toward whom one is acting. We agree that these are among the paradigm cases of paternalism, but we think, as do Brock and Dworkin, that this is not an adequate way to characterize paternalism. It is possible to act paternalistically toward someone about whom you do not know whether your action is contrary to his wishes. That is why we phrase Feature 3, "P does not believe that his action has S's past, present, or immediately forthcoming consent." However, the point we wish to stress now is that not all actions that are contrary to the wishes of someone need to be justified. Although Childress recognizes that there is a difference between refusing to accept a person's wish or request not to intervene and refusing to carry out a person's wishes or choices, he holds that both need to be justified. We claim that only when refusing to acquiesce to a person's wishes involves violating a moral rule does that action count as paternalistic. Normally this involves intervening, but it can also involve not carrying out a person's wishes, when one has a duty to carry out those wishes.

Dworkin offers the following example to show that acting paternalistically does not require violating a moral rule. "A husband who knows that his wife is suicidal hides his sleeping pills. He violates no moral rule. They are his pills and he can put them wherever he wishes."[11] Dworkin regards the husband's action as paternalistic because it interferes with the wife's self-determination and it is a violation of her autonomy. Since "self-determination" and "autonomy" are technical terms with no clear or settled meaning, no one can say whether or not the husband's action does interfere with his wife's self-determination or violates her autonomy. It is clear that his action does not violate a moral rule with regard to her and so, unlike Dworkin, we would not regard such an action as paternalistic. Dworkin may be misled because he realizes that the husband certainly shows a paternalistic attitude, that is, a willingness to act paternalistically, for there seems no doubt that he would have hidden the sleeping pills even if they were his wife's and not his own.[12] However, in the circumstances it was not necessary to violate a moral rule in order to accomplish his end, preventing his wife from committing suicide. Thus, he did not act paternalistically toward her and his action needs no justification.

We think it is important to distinguish between performing the kind of action that needs justification in order to be morally acceptable (violating a moral rule) and failing to act in a way which is morally encouraged, but whose omission does not require justification (not following a moral ideal). We do not count it as paternalistic behavior if one refuses to give money to a beggar because one believes he will only buy whiskey with it, which will be harmful to him. Such behavior may reveal a paternalistic attitude, a willingness to act paternalistically toward the beggar if the situation arose, but it is not itself a paternalistic act. Only when one's action requires moral justification is it appropriate to call it paternalistic. There may be some disagreement concerning which acts need moral justification, but there is no disagreement that all of the clear cases involve violations of moral rules. Relieving pain is normally following a moral ideal, but a nurse sometimes has a duty to relieve the pain of her patients. If a nurse fails to act so as to relieve the pain of her patient, what needs justification is her failure to do her duty, which is a violation of a moral rule, not her failure to follow a moral ideal.

Suppose a very distraught patient goes to a psychiatrist and says that he feels that he is likely to harm himself in some significant way and that he would like the psychiatrist's advice about whether to be hospitalized. The psychiatrist is not acting paternalistically if he urges the patient to enter the hospital. His urging is not paternalistic not only because he has the patient's consent to give him advice, but because he is not violating any moral rule in urging the patient to enter the hospital. Urging a patient to take some action does not count as coercion (see Chapter 6), and so does not count as a paternalistic act unless it involves deception, or in some other way involves the violation of a moral rule. Physicians who have come to realize that paternalistic behavior needs justification may mistakenly believe that strongly supporting a treatment, even giving asked-for advice, is paternalistic. This prevents them from acting in ways that are completely appropriate, and do not need justification at all. We suspect that often when paternalism is defended as an appropriate behavior for physicians, it is not really paternalism that is being defended. Rather, it is what we call paternal or parental behavior, behavior which is done for the patient's benefit but without violating any moral rule, such as strongly advising or urging the patient to consent to treatment.[13] When this urging or advising is neither coercive nor deceptive, and is done in the appropriate manner, it does not require justification. On the contrary, it may be part of the duty of a doctor to advise and urge her patients to, say, take their medication.

The Action Does Not Have S's Consent

Feature 3 points out that P believes that his action with regard to S does not have S's past, present, or immediately forthcoming consent. If P has S's consent, or if P expects S's immediately forthcoming consent for his action, then an action which might otherwise be paternalistic is not so. Suppose I pull someone from the path of an oncoming car which I believe he does not see. This action needs justification, because it involves unconsented touching, which is a violation of a person's freedom. If, however, I do so because I think that he would have consented to my action if I had asked him, and that he will confirm this immediately after the action, my action is not paternalistic even though it may satisfy all the other conditions of paternalistic behavior. On the other hand, if I think that he is trying to commit suicide because of a temporary depression, then even if I think that he will thank me later when he recovers, my act is paternalistic, although it may be justified. It is only in situations where I cannot ask for consent prior to acting that immediately forthcoming consent prevents the act from being counted as paternalistic. Usually these are emergency situations.

It might be claimed that deceiving someone about a surprise party is not paternalistic, for one cannot ask for consent to give a surprise party. Indeed, the surprise party is a very useful case for distinguishing paternalistic behavior from behavior that is not paternalistic. If one believes that the person he is deceiving loves surprise parties and will be immediately delighted when she is surprised at her party, then his deceiving her about the party is not paternalistic. Suppose, however, he does not believe, but in fact doubts, that the person he is deceiving loves surprise parties, but he is certain that she would benefit from having one, because it would make her realize how many people care about her. He further believes that even if she is initially upset, by the end of the party she will be delighted. In this case, his deceiving her is paternalistic. No claims are being made here about whether either or both of these cases of deception are justified, only that the first should not be regarded as paternalistic, and the second should be.

The discussion of deceiving in order to give a surprise party makes clear that the expectation of receiving future consent, even when a virtual certainty, does not make an action nonpaternalistic. Consider a psychiatrist who has been treating a depressed patient for many years. Suppose, against the patient's wishes, he hospitalizes him because he is suicidal, but because the doctor has done this several times before in the same circumstances, he knows that the patient will be effusively thankful within two or three days. He is taking away the patient's freedom and even if the patient would be thankful almost immediately, that would not be sufficient to make the action nonpaternalistic. Immediately forthcoming consent does not make an action nonpaternalistic unless one believes one would have received consent beforehand if one had been able to ask for it.

Without this limitation on future consent, a clearly paternalistic injection of a fast-acting mind-altering drug would not count as paternalistic. If a physician could have asked for consent to inject the drug, but did not do so, then, given the other conditions of paternalism are satisfied, injecting the drug is paternalistic even if he expects immediately forthcoming consent. Since it is known that some drugs change one's mood and attitude, it would be a perversion of the concept of valid consent to say that the patient's immediately forthcoming consent after taking the drug counts as the kind of consent that make the physician's action nonpaternalistic. We will discuss the "thank you" theory of justifying paternalism in the next chapter; here we are merely claiming that a belief, even a justified belief, that the patient will immediately thank the physician, does not by itself prevent an action from being paternalistic.

Almost all nonemergency medical interventions would be paternalistic if one did not have the patient's valid consent. That is why obtaining a valid consent from a patient is so important morally. Medical interventions often involve causing pain, depriving of freedom, and so on, and these need justification. When such actions are done for the benefit of the patient and with his valid consent, all medically appropriate treatments are strongly justified. The very same intervention with the same benefit but without the patient's consent may not be. One serious problem with utilitarianism, or any form of consequentialism, as a moral guide is that it may not distinguish between these two situations. If the outcome of the treatment is the same (including the patient's attitude toward the treatment after it has been done), but in one case valid consent was obtained, in the other not, then the first is not paternalistic and the second is. Those utilitarians who hold that only actual consequences count must hold that, morally speaking, it is not important whether one obtains valid consent and whether an act is paternalistic.

We have already pointed out that belief in immediately forthcoming consent does not always make an action nonpaternalistic, but there are also medical situations in which past consent does not remove P's act from the class of paternalistic acts. Consider a patient who has considerable anxiety about undergoing an operation which the doctor believes to be important for him. After considerable persuasion, the patient consents to the operation which is to be done the next morning. However, the next morning his anxiety is such that, immediately after taking the preoperative medication, he refuses to go through with it. It would clearly be paternalistic for the physician to wait for the medication to take effect and to take advantage of the patient's condition and proceed with the operation. Past consent makes an action nonpaternalistic only if it is not rescinded.

Although we say that in order for an action to be paternalistic, P must believe that his action does not have S's past, present, or immediately forthcoming consent, it is clearly present consent that is primary. Past and immediately forthcoming consent prevent an action from being paternalistic only when they are believed to be signs that one has or would have had the patient's present consent to act toward him as one did. When it is clear that the past consent does not continue into the present, or that the immediately forthcoming consent would not have been given prior to the action, then neither past consent nor immediately forthcoming consent are sufficient to make an action nonpaternalistic.

S Believes He Can Make His Own Decision on This Matter

Feature 4, P regards S as believing he can make his own decision on this matter, is presupposed in many accounts of paternalism, but rarely is made explicit. One cannot act paternalistically toward infants because they do not believe that they can make their own decision on any matters, indeed they do not believe anything about themselves.[14] The same is true of comatose persons whose views could not be known beforehand, and for whom some action must be taken before they cease to be comatose. If S does not believe anything at all about himself, then it is inappropriate to regard any action with regard to him as paternalistic. P can be paternalistic toward S only if S is regarded as believing he can make his own decision on this matter.[15] This normally involves S holding that he understands at least something about what might happen to him and to have some desire about whether it is done. To say that P is acting paternalistically when he does not have S's consent, presupposes that P regards S as at least believing that he can make his own decision on this matter.

A physician should regard S as believing he can make his own decision about treatment if S understands enough to know that the physicians want to benefit him and that this involves their doing something to him which may have some risk of harm to him. A physician need not regard S as competent to give consent, or even think that S believes that he understands enough to make his consent valid. For example, both the physician and S may realize that S does not understand the important future consequences of his decision, only the immediate consequences of it. Nonetheless, if the physician regards S as believing he understands enough to make his own decision about treatment, then if she acts on S without his consent, her action is paternalistic. When S is not competent to give valid consent, whether he believes he can make his own decision on this matter or not, paternalism is often justified. But even in this kind of case, it should be the patient's guardian, not the physician, who acts paternalistically.

A patient who is incompetent to make a rational decision may be regarded as deficient in two different ways. First, he may be regarded as not having sufficient *cognitive competence,* for example, he cannot understand enough about the benefits and/or the risks to be able to make a rational decision. Or he does not have sufficient information about future consequences to make a rational decision. Or he may not understand probabilities at all, thinking that a 5% probability of serious injury is the same as a 95% probability, both being equivalent to a 50% probability, because either it will happen or it will not. Children between the ages of five and nine are often cognitively competent to make rational decisions on simple matters, but incompetent to make rational decisions on complex matters, and the same is true of some who are mentally retarded.

A patient can be sufficiently intelligent to understand all of the information necessary to make a rational decision concerning a certain kind of treatment, yet still be cognitively incompetent to make that decision, if he cannot appreciate that this information applies to him. This lack of appreciation may be due to a mental disorder which involves delusions (for instance, he believes that his physicians are trying to kill him), so that although he understands what is said about the benefits and risks of treatment, he does not believe it applies to his case. A delusion which prevents a person from making a rational decision in a certain kind of case is sufficient to make that person cognitively incompetent to make that kind of decision, no matter how intelligent he is and how well he understands the information presented to him.

Second, a patient may be regarded as not having sufficient *volitional competence.* However, it is inappropriate to regard anyone as volitionally incompetent unless he is suffering from some relevant mental disorder. Addictions, phobias, and compulsions may render a person volitionally incompetent; a person with a phobia of needles may irrationally refuse a lifesaving injection that has no significant side effects, or a person with an irrational fear of ECT may irrationally refuse that treatment (see Chapter 6, Case 6.7). People who are addicted often cannot make rational decisions concerning their addiction, even when they seem as if they are doing exactly what they want to do. Mood disorders like depression can also make a person volitionally incompetent, if they are sufficiently severe. However, there are degrees of depression, from relatively mild to very severe, and even if severe depression can make one volitionally incompetent, mild depression usually does not do so.

Often, whether a person is regarded as volitionally incompetent depends on the degree of irrationality of his decision to refuse treatment. If a patient makes what is regarded as a mildly irrational decision—for example, without an adequate reason he does not take his medication or otherwise treat his moderately high blood pressure—he is not normally regarded as volitionally incompetent. However, if the irrational decision making persists, or if the irrational decision is more serious—for example a person on the edge of hepatic failure refuses to stop drinking—he is more likely to be regarded as volitionally incompetent. If the irrational decision will soon lead to death or severe permanent injury—for example a severely depressed person refuses to eat or drink—he would be regarded as volitionally incompetent by almost everyone.

Violating a moral rule without their consent, with regard to those who are only volitionally incompetent, is always acting paternalistically. Similarly, violating a moral rule without their consent, with regard to those who are incompetent to give valid consent, but believe that they can make their own decisions, is also acting paternalistically. Paternalistic behavior toward both of these kinds of patients is often justified, but not always. In the next chapter we will discuss in more detail how one determines when it is justified to act paternalistically in a given case. Only violating a moral rule without their consent, with regard to those who are so cognitively incompetent that they do not even believe that they can make their own decision concerning treatment, does not satisfy Feature 4 and so is not paternalistic.

As discussed in Chapter 7, someone who is cognitively incompetent because of lack of understanding to make a rational decision about a certain kind of treatment is incompetent both to validly consent to and to validly refuse that treatment. It is his lack of understanding of the relevant information that renders him unable to make a rational decision, and so no decision that he makes, either to consent or to refuse, can be taken as valid. However, if someone is cognitively incompetent to make a rational decision about a certain kind of treatment because of a delusion, or is volitionally incompetent to do so, there may be an asymmetry between consent and refusal. If the person irrationally refuses treatment because of a mental disorder, such as an addiction or a phobia, then his irrational refusal shows that he is volitionally incompetent to make a rational decision in this kind of situation. However, were he to consent to treatment, this would show that, at least on this occasion, his mental disorder did not cause him to make an irrational decision and so his consent would count as valid.

Making a distinction between cognitive incompetence and volitional incompetence helps resolve the dispute we have had with those who claimed that one could be competent to consent to a treatment, but incompetent to refuse the very same treatment.[16] If cognitive competence is the kind of competence at issue, which is what we assumed in our previous criticism of the legal definition of competence, then people who are competent to consent to a treatment are also competent to refuse the very same treatment. However, if volitional competence is the kind of competence at issue, which now seems to be included in the legal interpretation of competence, then competence to consent does not imply competence to refuse, when the former is rational and the latter is not.[17] When a person irrationally refuses treatment because of a volitional disability, that refusal is not valid, although this does not necessarily justify overruling that refusal. However, even though the person still has the associated volitional disability, if he changes his mind so that he makes a rational decision, his consent can count as valid. On this occasion he is regarded as having overcome his associated volitional disability.

It is crucial not to confuse irrational decisions with unusual or unpopular ones; irrational decisions harm the decision maker without a rational belief about a corresponding benefit for anyone. Normally, only serious or persistent irrational decisions raise the question of the competence of the person to make the decision.[18] Since irrational decisions harm the decision maker without a corresponding benefit for anyone, it is not surprising that it is implausible that anyone knowingly and voluntarily makes an irrational decision, especially one that is seriously irrational. In all cases where a patient persistently and irrationally refuses treatment, it is appropriate to consider whether he is cognitively competent (whether he knows what he is doing) or whether he is volitionally competent (whether his decision on this matter is voluntary). That a patient is incompetent in either of these ways does not automatically justify acting paternalistically with regard to him, but requires further consideration.

Cognitive incompetence requires a guardian to be appointed to approve both consent and refusal, whether rational or not. This guardian must consider whether it is justified to overrule both refusals and consents to treatment by considering what the patient would do if he were cognitively competent, that is, if he understood the benefits and harms involved. Unless the patient's decision is irrational, the guardian should overrule the patient's present decision only because she believes that if the patient understood the benefits and harms involved, he would have decided differently; that given his values his decision was unreasonable. Such paternalism, if based on genuine knowledge of the patient's preferences and rankings of harms and benefits, is usually justified.

Volitional incompetence presents more difficulties. In these cases the patient does understand the benefits and harms involved, but still makes an irrational or unreasonable decision. Thus, the person acting paternalistically cannot say that she is overruling the patient's decision because she believes that if the patient understood the benefits and harms involved, he would have decided differently. However, especially if the decision is seriously irrational, that is, if it involves a high risk of death or significant permanent disabilities, then it may be justifiable to act paternalistically. Involuntary commitment involves this kind of paternalism and is explicitly allowed by law in nearly all states, even though the person is not cognitively incompetent. However, it requires a finding of mental disorder, so as to guarantee volitional incompetence. In cases of involuntary commitment, serious irrational actions constitute prima facie evidence of such a mental disorder.[19]

Those who hold that paternalism is never justified must both (1) define paternalism in terms of interfering with a patient's "autonomous" choices, and (2) claim that the choices of those who are cognitively or volitionally incompetent are not autonomous choices. We hold that some paternalism is justified for we think it is incorrect not to regard overruling a volitionally incompetent patient's irrational decision as paternalistic. Such overruling is for the benefit of the patient, it needs justification, it does not have the consent of the patient, and he believes he can make his own decision on this matter. Thus, such overruling satisfies all four features of the definition. The recognition that overruling even incompetent patients' decisions is paternalistic forces physicians to consider whether overruling is justified. We think that this may lead to less unjustified paternalism. A metaphysical discussion about whether a decision is "autonomous" may be more interesting to philosophers than a moral discussion about whether a doctor is justified in overruling an incompetent patient's decision, but it is less likely to have a beneficial effect.[20]

Examination of Cases of Paternalism

We shall now examine some cases of paternalism in order to show how our account of paternalism applies to them.

CASE 9.1

Mr. N, a member of a religious sect that does not believe in blood transfusions, is injured in a serious automobile accident and loses a large amount of blood. On arriving at the hospital, he is still conscious and informs the doctor of his views on blood transfusion. Immediately thereafter he faints from loss of blood. The doctor believes that if Mr. N is not given a transfusion he will die. Thereupon, while Mr. N is still unconscious, the doctor arranges for and carries out the blood transfusion.

<h2 style="text-align:center">Case 9.2</h2>

Miss X is a 22-year-old single woman brought to the emergency room by her roommate, who accidentally came home and discovered her soon after Miss X ingested what appears (and later proves) to be a quantity of barbiturate capsules sufficient to kill her. Miss X did this because her fiancée was killed the day before in an automobile accident and she feels she does not want to live without him.

Dr. W tells Miss X that it will be necessary to insert a naso-gastric tube in order to evacuate the contents of her stomach. She refuses permission, saying that she wishes to die. Dr. W nonetheless inserts the tube, despite Miss X's angry objections, and recovers a large quantity of the capsules.

Both doctors' actions seem to be clearly paternalistic and do, in fact, satisfy the proposed definition of paternalism. Their actions are clearly done for the patients' benefit; they need moral justification for they are violations of the rule against depriving of freedom; not only do the doctors not have the patients' consent, the patients have clearly refused the suggested treatment; and the doctors regard the patients as believing they can make their own decisions on these matters.

In our previous discussion of the blood transfusion case in *Philosophy in Medicine,* we did not realize that the doctor violated the patient's freedom, for we limited depriving of freedom to attempting to control behavior.[21] We now realize that someone can deprive another of freedom by taking away control of what touches or goes into his body. In the blood transfusion case there is no behavior to control, but there is still a deprivation of freedom, namely, a deprivation of the freedom to control what touches or goes into one's body. Thus, even though there is no attempt to interfere with action and no coercion, the doctor's action is still a violation of the moral rule against depriving of freedom. The second case involves a deprivation of freedom in both senses, deprivation of freedom of action and deprivation of freedom to control what touches one's body.

That paternalism does not always involve attempting to control behavior is also shown by an example of paternalistic deception which is intended to affect feelings rather than behavior. A doctor lies to a mother on her deathbed when she asks about her son. The doctor tells her that her son is doing well, although he knows that the son has just been killed trying to escape from prison after having been convicted of multiple rape and murder. The doctor behaved paternalistically but did not attempt to control behavior or to apply coercion. Even in political rather than personal situations, paternalism may involve deception in order to affect the body rather than behavior, as when officials surreptitiously introduce fluorides into a city's water supply in order to reduce tooth decay in the inhabitants.

Of course, many paternalistic acts do involve attempts to control behavior by depriving a person of freedom, as illustrated in the following case.

CASE 9.3

Mr. K is pacing back and forth on the roof of his five-story tenement and appears to be on the verge of jumping off. An observant neighbor calls the police. When questioned by the police, Mr. K sounds confused so they take him to the emergency room. When interviewed by Dr. T in the emergency room, Mr. K admits to being afraid that he might jump off the roof and says that he fears he is losing his mind. However, he adamantly refuses hospitalization. Dr. T decides that for his own protection, Mr. K must be committed to the hospital for a period of 48 hours.

This is a classic example of paternalistic behavior on the part of the physician. He is acting for the best interest of the patient; he is depriving the patient of freedom; he does not have the patient's consent; and he regards the patient as thinking he can make his own decision on this matter. The only point that is at all controversial about regarding this case as one of paternalism is the last feature. It may not seem clear that the patient thinks he can make his own decision concerning hospitalization, so that the doctor may not regard him as thinking this. However, we think that a doctor should regard any patient who responds to a request for consent in a way that shows that he knows what he is being asked to consent to, as thinking that he can make his own decision on the matter being considered. Only if the patient is so cognitively incompetent that he does not regard himself as understanding what is being requested is it not paternalistic to treat without his consent.

CASE 9.4

Mrs. B will undergo a radical mastecomy in two or three days for a malignant tumor of her right breast. She has obviously understood her situation intellectually, but her mood has been rather blasé and she appears to be inappropriately minimizing the emotional gravity of her situation. Dr. C's experience is that women in Mrs. B's situation who before mastectomy do not experience some grief and at least moderate concern about the physical and cosmetic implications of their operation often have an unusually severe and depressive postoperative course. Mrs. B insists that she does not wish to talk about the effects of the surgery. Nonetheless, before surgery Dr. C tells her about such effects in order to facilitate her emotional preparation for her impending loss.

This example shows that a physician can act paternalistically by causing mental suffering, when he does this in order to prevent what he believes will be even greater pain or suffering. This case not only shows that paternalism need not be concerned with how a patient will act, but only with how she will feel, it also goes against another common view of medical paternalism. If presented with the question of which doctor is acting paternalistically, one who confronts a patient with a painful truth, or one who withholds the truth in order to avoid the pain it will cause the patient, many people would choose the latter. However, as this example makes clear, this need not be the case. Which doctor is acting paternalistically, if either one is, depends upon whether he will proceed with what he thinks is best for the patient regardless of the patient's expressed wishes. If the patient wants to be told the truth, then to withhold it simply to prevent her suffering the effects of being told is paternalistic. If the patient says that she does not want to be told the truth about the effects of her mastectomy, however, then it is paternalistic of the doctor to cause suffering by forcing the truth on the patient on the grounds that it is better for her to face the painful truth now.

CASE 9.5

> Mrs. P, on her first visit as an outpatient, is insistent during the last few minutes of her session that Dr. Z give her some medicine for her nerves and for the vague, diffuse pains which she describes. He feels there is no medical reason for her to have medication but judges that if he refuses her request outright, a useful and productive initial interview will end on a very sour note. However, he believes strongly in not administering active drugs when there is no medical reason for doing so; therefore, he writes a prescription for a week's supply of a placebo and makes a note on her chart to discuss the issue of medication with her in detail at their next appointment.

Dr. Z has given Mrs. P. a placebo for what he believes is her benefit; he knows he is deceiving her and that he does not have her consent (in this case, even her knowledge); and further, he regards her as someone who not only believes she can make her own decision on this matter, but is, in fact, competent to give valid consent. Dr. Z is attempting to affect both actions and feelings; he wants Mrs. P. to return and he wants her to feel better. Someone might claim that Dr. Z's action is not really paternalistic because he planned to discuss the issue of medication at the next meeting. However, although this may show that his paternalism is limited, he recognizes that his writing a prescription for a placebo is clearly deceptive and thus is the kind of action that need justification. Whether he is, in fact, justified in this time-limited deception is a separate question, but it is quite clear that his act is of a kind that needs justification and it also satisfies all of the others features of paternalism.

CASE 9.6

> Dr. Q is leading a new therapy group during its second session. The group consists of patients who have all claimed to have difficulty in relating to other people. One

patient, Mr. G, is a single professional man in his early thirties who has complained of an inability to maintain lasting friendships with either men or women. It has become apparent to Dr. Q through watching the group interaction that Mr. G, while not totally unlikeable, is self-centered, critical of others, and smugly certain about his own opinions. It has also become apparent that Mr. G has little insight into these characteristics and the way they irritate other members of the group. Dr. Q believes it would be useful for Mr. G to acquire insight into the effect his personal style has on others. Of course, whether Mr. G will then try to change his style will be his own decision. Accordingly, midway through the session, Dr. Q begins to encourage other group members to confront Mr. G with their feelings about him, despite Mr. G's obvious anger and great discomfort when they begin to do so.

This satisfies three of the four elements of the definition. Dr. Q believes that this confrontation is for Mr. G's benefit, recognizes that his causing Mr. G mental suffering needs justification, and regards Mr. G as someone who believes he can make his own decision about being confronted by others in the group. What is not clear from the example as given is whether Dr. Q believes he has Mr. G's consent to have others confront him. This is not clear because nothing is specified about the nature of the prior agreement between Dr. Q and Mr. G. In particular, nothing is said about whether Mr. G has or has not consented to confrontational activities like being exposed to (confronted by) the painful judgments of others. Thus, on the information given, it is not known whether Dr. Q's actions are paternalistic. Dr. Q might claim that Mr. G's presence in group therapy demonstrates implicit consent to being confronted in an emotionally painful way, but that claim would be weak unless Dr. Q had evidence that essentially *all* patients had such expectations, which seems unlikely.

This example is similar to the dilemma posed by many psychiatric interventions; whether or not they are paternalistic (and thus require justification) turns heavily on the nature and quality of the consent given by the patient and the degree to which the psychiatrist acts independently of that consent for what he believes is the patient's good. In this case, if Dr. Q has obtained Mr. G's consent to be exposed to emotionally painful experiences, then Dr. Q's actions are not paternalistic. If this consent has not been obtained, then he is acting paternalistically.

In the above examples the harms, if any, perpetrated by the physician and (possibly) prevented for the patient vary considerably in their intensity. Health professionals in particular should be sensitive to the pervasiveness of paternalistic actions that are concerned with relatively minor harms. Not allowing a patient to nap during the daytime so that he sleeps better at night can be a thoroughly paternalistic action and in as much need of justification as depriving someone of more extensive freedom. Thus, it would probably be best to explain the situation to the patient and obtain his consent. We are aware that legally one does not need to obtain consent for many minor interventions; however, from the moral point of view, it is always preferable to get consent. This point will be discussed in more detail in the next chapter.

This account of paternalism clarifies many of its features. It explains why doctors, nurses, and other health professionals who act to benefit their patients usually resist the charge of paternalism; people generally do not want to be in a position of having to justify their actions. However, our account does not allow paternalism to degenerate into a term of abuse, for not only is paternalism sometimes justified, it is sometimes morally required. Nonetheless, it is clear that paternalism requires justification because it involves doing, without consent, a kind of action which needs justification, that is, a kind of action which is a violation of a moral rule. Our account also explains why the absence of valid consent is so closely tied to the concept of paternalism. Insofar as it is not clear whether and to what extent the patient has given valid consent to the doctor, it is not clear whether and to what extent the doctor is acting paternalistically. The example of the patient in group therapy illustrates this close connection between paternalism and lack of consent.

In addition to clarifying the concept of paternalism, we think that our account of paternalism provides the conceptual framework for interesting empirical research. For example, what factors, if any, in medical training lead some doctors to act paternalistically? To what extent does awareness that acting in a given way is paternalistic (as defined in this chapter) decrease (or increase) a doctor's tendency to do so? Is there a significant difference in belief concerning the ability of patients to make correct decisions affecting their own welfare between doctors who often act paternalistically, and those who do so infrequently? Perhaps the most important questions concern whether medical training can be developed that leads a doctor to act paternalistically only when this is justified, and whether there are factors in medical training that lead a doctor to act paternalistically when it is not justified.

Notes

1. Throughout our analysis we assume that P's beliefs are at least rational, though they need not be true. If P's beliefs are irrational, if he thinks for instance that flowers are competent to give consent, it is implausible to maintain that he is acting paternalistically toward the flowers when he waters them though he believes that they would prefer to remain dry. We are indebted to Timothy Duggan for calling our attention to this latter point.

2. Gerald Dworkin, in an important article, "Paternalism," *Monist,* No. 1 (1972), pp. 64–84 (reprinted in *Paternalism,* ed. Rolf Sartorius [Minneapolis: University of Minnesota Press, 1983], pp. 19–34—all page references are to this volume), seems to make this mistake. "By paternalism I shall understand roughly the interference with a person's liberty of action justified by reasons referring exclusively to the welfare, good, happiness, needs, interests, or values of the person being coerced" (p. 20). Dworkin's view that paternalism always involves the restriction of liberty used to be the standard one.

See, for example, Michael D. Bayles, "Criminal Paternalism" (pp. 174–188) and Donald
H. Regan, "Justifications for Paternalism" (pp. 189–210), both in J. Roland Pennock and
John W. Chapman (eds.) *The Limits of Law–Nomos XV* (New York: Lieber-Atherton,
1974). However, partly in response to criticisms that we made, Dworkin had second
thoughts, and in a 1983 article titled "Paternalism: Some Second Thoughts" (*Paternalism*, pp. 105–111) he admits that a broader definition is needed. Indeed, he now holds
that "the attempt to broaden the notion [of paternalistic behavior] by including any violation of a moral rule is too restrictive" (p. 106). He now thinks, "There must be a violation of the person's autonomy, (which I conceive as distinct from that of liberty) for one
to treat another paternalistically. There must be usurpation of decision-making, either by
preventing people from doing what they have decided or by interfering with the way in
which they arrive at their decisions" (p. 107). However, Dworkin seems to agree that
something like our Feature 2, that A recognizes that his action toward S is a kind of
action that needs moral justification, is a feature of paternalism. Thus our only disagreement with Dworkin seems to be on what kinds of actions need moral justification. However, this will result in our classifying some cases in different ways. See discussion later
in this chapter.

3. See Chapter 2.

4. They can also be described as violations of rights. Those who prefer the language
of rights to that of moral rules might plausibly hold that all paternalistic behavior involves the violation of a person's rights. The close connection between rights and liberties may then partly explain the widely held but mistaken view that paternalism always
involves the restriction of liberty of action. For example, paternalistic behavior involving
deception may sometimes be taken as violating the person's right to know when it cannot
be taken as restricting his liberty of action. There may be no substantive difference
between violating a moral rule with regard to someone independently of his past, present, or immediately forthcoming consent and violating his rights. However, since we find
the terminology of moral rules to be clearer than that of rights, we have presented our
analysis of paternalism solely in terms of violating a moral rule. See Gert, *Morality*, pp.
113–116.

5. Dworkin, "Paternalism: Some Second Thoughts," p. 106

6. This is another example of why "autonomy" is a term that is best avoided.

7. Ibid., p. 107

8. Dan Brock, "Paternalism and Promoting the Good," in Sartorius, *Paternalism*, p.
238.

9. James F. Childress, *Who Should Decide? Paternalism in Health Care* (New York:
Oxford University Press, 1982), p. 241.

10. Ibid., p. 115.

11. Dworkin, "Paternalism: Some Second Thoughts," p. 106. This example is a very
slightly revised version of a case that we provide in *Philosophy in Medicine (PIM)*, p.
128. However, the slight revision is quite significant, for in that case, the husband removes all of the sleeping pills, and it is not clear whether he is removing only his own
pills, or also those of his wife. See *PIM*, note 5 on p. 140 for further discussion of the
implication of this unclarity. Dworkin's example makes clear that it is only his own pills
that he hid.

12. The issue here is whether by hiding the pills he is depriving his wife of the
opportunity to take the pills, hence breaking a moral rule. Since they were his own pills,
we would say that he was not depriving his wife of opportunity. For further discussion of
what counts as depriving, see Gert, *Morality*, pp. 111–112.

13. We do not intend this statement to be taken as a complete account of paternal or parental behavior. We recognize that the term "paternalistic" is often used to describe behavior that we think is more appropriately described as parental, but we do not think this significantly affects our analysis. (In a similar way, an analysis of jealousy is not significantly affected by the fact that "jealousy" is often used to refer to an emotion which is more appropriately referred to as "envy.")

14. Feature 4 seems to be suspended in one very unusual kind of case: killing a severely defective neonate in order to prevent it from the great suffering it will experience due to its severe defects. It does not seem paternalistic to take action to save the life of the neonate even if this involves causing considerable pain. Killing the neonate to prevent his pain seems paternalistic, whereas causing him pain to prevent his death does not, because the former prevents the neonate from ever becoming a person, whereas the latter does not. Thus the only time one can be paternalistic toward someone who does not even believe he is competent to give consent is when one's act prevents that being from developing into a person who would believe himself competent to give consent. It may be paternalistic even if it is known that he would never develop into such a person. These are very special cases, and we shall not consider them further here.

15. Thus, acting for the mildly retarded without their consent, if it meets the other elements of the definition, is clearly paternalistic. See Daniel Wikler, "Paternalism and the Mildly Retarded," *Philosophy and Public Affairs,* 8 (1979), pp. 377–392, reprinted in Sartorius, *Paternalism.*

16. See particularly A. E. Buchanan and D. Brock, "Deciding for Others," *Milbank Quarterly* 64 (1986), pp. 17–94, and *Deciding for Others: The Ethics of Surrogate Decision-Making* (New York: Cambridge University Press, 1989), and J. Drane, "The Many Faces of Competency," *Hastings Center Report* 15 (1985), pp. 17–21.

17. See Charles M. Culver and Bernard Gert, "The Inadequacy of Incompetence," *Milbank Quarterly,* 68 (1990), pp. 619–643.

18. An unreasonable action, that is, one that is rationally allowed but conflicts with the rankings of harms and benefits of the person acting, can also raise the question of competence. In these cases it must be clear that the rankings of harms and benefits are not merely those that the patient had in the past, but are those that he continues to have at present, even though his decision conflicts with those rankings. Most of these cases are those in which the patient is regarded as incompetent because of his inability to understand or to appreciate the information provided, but they can also be the result of a volitional disability which the patient, himself, regards as unreasonable. Sometimes these can be serious enough that the patient can be regarded as incompetent.

19. See *DSM-IV* definition of mental disorder and Chapter 5, "Malady."

20. Cf. discussion of autonomy in Tom L. Beauchamp and James F. Childress, *The Principles of Biomedical Ethics,* 4th ed. (New York: Oxford University Press, 1994).

21. This was pointed out by James Childress in his critique of our previous account of paternalism.

10

Justification

The justification of paternalism is an interesting and important topic because it provides such a clear and discriminating test of the various accounts of morality. It tests both those accounts of moral reasoning that have some special appeal to those in bioethics—principlism, casuistry, and virtue theory, as well as the two dominant general accounts of morality: consequentialism and deontology. There are, of course, many variations of consequentialism and of deontology, and it is impossible to examine all of them. We confine our examination to the clearest variation of each of these two types of theories, act consequentialism and absolutist deontology. We restrict our examination to these extreme versions because we believe that as the versions become more qualified they turn into variations of the account of morality that we have outlined in Chapter 2. As consequentialism comes to acknowledge the necessity of moral rules, it needs more than consequences to justify the violation of a rule; as absolutist deontology comes to acknowledge that some violations of moral rules are justified, it needs to determine how violations are justified. We think that our account of morality explains how to justify violations of moral rules in a way that incorporates the insights of both consequentialism and deontology.

Since paternalism is an extremely common kind of behavior in medical contexts, the justification of paternalism has special relevance for those accounts of morality that are most widely used in bioethics, namely, principlism, casuistry, and virtue theory. We have already pointed out the inadequacies of principlism in Chapter 4, so here we limit our comments to casuistry and virtue theory.

217

After principlism, these two kinds of accounts of moral reasoning are the most widely discussed. One problem with both of these accounts is that they do not explain why paternalism needs any justification. We show that this is the result of neither of them having any concept that corresponds to what we call a moral rule, that is, they have no general concept of a kind of behavior that needs justification but that, in particular circumstances, may turn out to be justified.

An adequate account of morality has value not merely, perhaps not even primarily, because it enables one to resolve a moral problem. One of the most valuable features of an adequate account of morality is that it alerts one to the presence of a moral problem. This is the primary value of the moral rules. Acknowledging these rules does not enable one to resolve a moral problem, but it does enable one to know when one has a moral problem, for example, when one's behavior is paternalistic. Knowing that violating a moral rule needs justification enables one to plan one's behavior so as to avoid, as far as possible, breaking any moral rules. Of course, that is not always desirable or even possible, but sometimes it will be, and so our account of morality, unlike either casuistry or virtue theory, can be helpful by alerting one to when there is or will be a moral problem.

Casuistry

Casuistry involves concentrating on a particular case and comparing it to other cases so as to determine what rules are most applicable to it, and how these rules should be interpreted when dealing with this case.[1] Casuistry, when it is not explicitly a part of the kind of public system that was described in Chapter 2, may help to resolve problems, but it can do nothing to help avoid them, because casuistry, considered by itself, has no concept comparable to that of a moral rule. Of course, casuistry, properly understood, is part of the kind of moral system that we present; it is a useful method for interpreting and applying the moral system. As we pointed out in Chapter 2, it is not always clear what kind of behavior counts as killing, deceiving, and so on; casuistry helps with such interpretation. Casuistry is also helpful in determining whether the case under consideration should be viewed as a justified exception to the rule. Concentrating on the particular case and comparing it to other cases may make more salient the morally relevant features of the case. Further, this comparison of cases can also help one to see whether one would want everyone to know that this kind of violation is allowed. Divorced from the moral system, however, casuistry is of little value and simply promotes ad hoc solutions to problems.

Of course, to use casuistry successfully, one need not explicitly adopt a moral system; one need only employ it implicitly, as most of us do, in interpreting that moral system. Casuistry, for example, can help in deciding whether a particular case of not telling a patient some information counts as withholding that information and thus as deception, or whether, on the other hand, there is no moral requirement to provide that information. Indeed, it is not even clear what it would be to use casuistry without using the moral system, at least implicitly. Without the moral system, casuistry seems to be nothing more than ad hoc reasoning about moral matters. It contains no way to resolve disputes if people choose different cases as models that they claim should be used to resolve the case under consideration. More importantly, it does not make clear what is even causing the dispute, nor why people are using different cases as models. Most importantly, casuistry, independent of a moral system, does not even identify what counts as a moral matter.

Although it seems to be against moral systems, casuistry has the appeal that it does because everyone implicitly uses some moral system; we think it is the moral system we have described. We do not consider casuistry as an alternative account of moral reasoning, rather we regard it as emphasizing that morality is not a deductive system in which one simply applies absolutely clear rules to absolutely clear cases in order to determine the correct course of action. Although there are many cases in which everyone agrees what the correct course of action is, these are not the cases that anyone discusses. The cases that present problems are those that, for example, involve differing interpretations of the rules or different rankings of the evils. That our account of morality is intended to provide a clear framework for moral reasoning, may explain why some have mistakenly taken us to be advocating a deductivist model of moral reasoning.[2] But our view of morality as an informal public system which allows for unresolvable moral disagreement is incompatible with a deductivist model.

Casuistry makes clear that the moral rules need interpretation, and that such interpretation is often essential before one can apply a rule to a particular case. Casuistry also emphasizes the need to look for all of the morally relevant features of the case, although it does not provide a list of such features. Casuistry realizes that a particular detail, such as the relationship between the parties involved, may change the act from one that is morally unacceptable to one that is morally acceptable, but it provides no explanation of when or why this is so. Since casuistry requires a moral system, it is not an alternative to our account of morality, rather it has the subsidiary but important role of helping to apply the moral system to particular cases.

Virtue Theory

Those who take virtues to be fundamental to morality we call virtue theorists. A significant problem with many virtue theorists is that they do not distinguish the moral virtues, such as honesty and kindness, from the personal virtues, such as courage and temperance. The moral virtues are those virtues which all rational persons want other people to have. The personal virtues are those virtues that all rational persons want to have themselves. The moral virtues are directly related to the interests of others, and only indirectly related to one's own interests, while the opposite is true for the personal virtues. Understanding the personal virtues does not require understanding morality, whereas understanding the moral virtues does. We are concerned with virtue theory only insofar as it purports to provide an account of morality that takes moral virtues as more fundamental to morality than moral rules and moral ideals.

Virtue theory, like casuistry, is closely related to the moral system which we have described. However, unlike casuistry, it is not a method of applying morality to a particular case, but an alternative and incomplete way of formulating the moral system. A complete account of morality must, of course, include an account of the moral virtues and vices.[3] Such an account lists the moral virtues and vices and relates them to particular moral rules and ideals. It describes them so that one can not only identify those who have the virtues, but also describes the way a virtuous person would act in a particular situation. Of course, this is an idealized scenario, because even those who have the virtues do not always exemplify them. As Hobbes pointed out, a person is not virtuous simply because he acts morally, nor does he cease to be a virtuous person simply because he performs one morally unacceptable act.

Some virtue theorists claim to provide a useful guide to conduct by enabling virtuous persons to be identified and then used as role models. This account of virtue raises several critical questions, such as how does one pick out a virtuous person? and how does the virtuous person decide how to act? Further, it is not only possible, but common, for a person to have some of the virtues, but not others. For virtue theorists who advocate the use of role models as basic guides, these are serious problems. If no particular person can serve as a role model for all situations, and there is general agreement that few if any can, there needs to be some way to determine what virtue is called for in a particular situation so that a role model with the relevant virtue can be selected. Even more serious, no virtuous person can be depended upon to act virtuously 100% of the time, so there has to be some independent way of determining when he is acting virtuously and when not. These are not new problems that we have just discovered, indeed, in a different context, Kant explicitly raised these same points.[4]

Unless it is possible to provide a description of the virtues such that one can tell in every situation what counts as a virtuous act in that situation, virtue theory is of no use to people without completely reliable role models. We have already pointed out that such role models are usually not available. An even more serious objection is that the notion of a completely reliable role model strongly suggests that there is complete agreement among all fully informed impartial rational persons on the best way to act in any moral situation. This false view plagues almost all moral theories and can lead to intolerance of differing views on particular topics, such that, for example, people on one side of the abortion issue must view those on the other side as lacking a particular virtue. However, fully informed impartial rational persons can sometimes disagree on what is the best way to act in a particular situation. This means they can also sometimes disagree on what is the virtuous way to act in that situation. On those occasions when they do disagree, two completely reliable role models provide different models of how to act, creating a quandary for anyone who depends solely on role models to determine the morally best way of acting.

Since reliable role models are in short supply, and sometimes even disagree with each other, for virtue theory to be of practical use there must be some other way to determine what counts as acting virtuously in a particular situation. Common morality does provide a way to make that determination. Having a moral virtue is being disposed to obey the moral rules or follow the moral ideals in a given situation in the way that at least some fully informed impartial rational person would do. Although fully informed impartial rational persons do not always agree, there are always limits to their disagreement. The moral theory presented in Chapter 2, by providing clear accounts of the concepts of impartiality and rationality and by providing a clear account of the moral system, including the moral rules and ideals, does provide a way of determining what counts as a virtuous way of acting in any particular situation.

The virtue of truthfulness is not exemplified by telling the truth when one should have remained silent. Telling the truth in such circumstances exemplifies the vice of tactlessness. Kindness is not exemplified by withholding the truth to avoid causing unpleasant feelings when one should have told the truth. Virtue, as Aristotle points out, consists in following the rule or ideal appropriately or, as we put it, as a fully informed impartial rational person would. Knowing when one should obey a rule or follow an ideal and when one should not requires judgment. That is why it is so misleading to regard any of the virtues simply as dispositions to obey the moral rules or follow the moral ideals. Having those virtues that are connected to the moral rules, such as truthfulness, and the moral ideals, such as kindness, involves knowing when it is appropriate to act on them and when it is not. Of course, having the virtue involves more than knowing how to act, it also involves regularly acting in that way. Neglect of the question of how one knows what the virtuous way to act is, may lead to the false claim that acting virtuously is acting because it is the virtuous way to act, that is, it is sufficient for acting virtuously that one's intention in acting is virtuous.

If the moral virtues are understood primarily as possessing the appropriate motivation for one's actions, then serious problems arise, particularly with regard to paternalistic behavior. All cases of genuine paternalism with regard to patients involve the health care worker being motivated to act for the benefit of the patient. On the motive-reading of virtue theory, the doctor who acts paternalistically is necessarily a virtuous person. He is disposed to act benevolently, to try and help others and so exemplifies the virtue of beneficence. Unfortunately, his beneficence may obscure the fact that he is also violating a moral rule, for instance the rule prohibiting deception, and so it may not even be recognized that there is a moral problem. Virtue theory not only makes one less likely to consider whether a particular paternalistic act is justified, it also provides no method for determining whether it is justified. A proper account of the moral virtues must explain not only when but why an impartial rational person should violate a moral rule or follow a moral ideal in specific kinds of circumstances.

Just as with casuistry, virtue theory is valuable if it is not taken as the fundamental feature of morality. It emphasizes a dimension of moral behavior that we do not, that morality is usually concerned with a consistent pattern of behavior, and does not call for special decisions in every particular case. The virtues also provide the most powerful way to show that it is rational to be moral, for though it may be beneficial to act immorally on a particular occasion, one is far more likely to live a satisfactory life if one has the moral virtues than if one does not. Thus it is perfectly appropriate for parents to present morality to children as the acquiring of the moral virtues and to teach them by example. However, as a theoretical guide to behavior the virtues are dependent on the guide provided by the moral system. Parents can teach morality by the virtues only if they appreciate the connection of the virtues to the moral system. It may be valuable to select a role model, but some way of selecting the right role model is needed, and also some way of determining if the role model is acting in the right way in a particular situation. All of this requires a clear understanding of the moral system and of how to apply it. Virtue theory is not an alternative to our account of the moral system or its foundation, rather it is an important and practical supplement to it.

Why the Justification of Paternalism Is Interesting

Paternalistic behavior requires justification because it involves violating a moral rule. Since the violation is done in order to benefit the person toward whom the rule is violated, the consent of that person would make it a justified violation but, of course, with consent the violation is no longer paternalistic. All impartial rational persons would publicly allow violating a moral rule with regard to a person if that person gives rational and valid consent to the violation and the violation benefits her.[5] What makes justifying paternalism interesting is that although a paternalistic act is done to benefit a person, it involves breaking a moral rule with regard to that person without her consent, when she believes she is able make her own decision. Two of the traditional philosophical accounts of morality give incompatible answers to the question of how paternalistic behavior is justified: act consequentialism says that only the consequences of one's actions are morally relevant, and strict deontology says that, without consent, only the conformity or nonconformity of one's action with a moral rule is morally relevant.

For the purpose of using paternalism as a test of various moral theories, it is convenient that all of the positions that can be maintained with respect to the justifiability of a common kind of paternalistic behavior can be put into three categories: (1) it is always justified, (2) it is never justified, and (3) it is sometimes justified. It is even more convenient that in the kind of paternalism in which the action provides a net benefit to the person and no other person is harmed, act consequentialism says that paternalism is always justified, strict deontology says that it is never justified, and we say that is sometimes justified. This is what makes the discussion of the justification of paternalism so important philosophically; it provides a real test of the various accounts of morality. Since the opportunity and temptation to act paternalistically is ubiquitous in the field of health care, it is of great practical value to show which theory best determines when acting paternalistically is justified.

Act Consequentialism: Always Justified

Act consequentialism is a very simple guide to conduct. It claims that an act should be done if it results in the best overall consequences. There are many sophisticated variations of this view, but in its simple form it is held by many who do not regard themselves as holding any philosophical view at all. People who hold this view often state that all that really matters is that things turn out for the best, or that as long as no one gets hurt, you can do anything you want. As noted above, ignoring alternative actions, the ethical theory of act consequentialism implies that all paternalistic behavior which provides a net benefit to the person toward whom one acted paternalistically (and no other person is harmed) is justified. Of course, in many cases of paternalism it is not clear if the person gains a net benefit, for the physician may rank the harms differently than the patient does, and both rankings are rational. Further, even accepting the physician's rankings there is so much self-deception as well as so many mistakes about the outcomes of paternalistic intervention, that paternalism often does not yield any net benefit for the person who is being treated paternalistically.

Some act consequentialists claim that what determines the moral rightness of an act are its *actual* consequences. This view is probably the result of failing to realize that "morally right" is not a redundant phrase. Sometimes "the right act" means the same as "the act which produces the best consequences," but this is never the case when talking about what is morally right. *Actual* consequences are not even relevant when considering whether an act is *morally right,* it is the *foreseeable* consequences at the time of acting that are relevant. Those who claim that actual consequences are the relevant kind of consequences probably are contrasting them with intended consequences. They are right that consequences of actions that are not intended are often relevant to our moral judgments. This is shown by our making an adverse moral judgment of someone by saying that "he should have known that would happen." What this shows, however, is not that unforeseeable actual consequences are relevant to moral judgments, but that foreseeable consequences are as relevant as, or even more relevant than, intended consequences.

Unforeseeable actual consequences cannot be used by anyone in deciding how to act in any moral situation, nor should they be used by anyone in making a moral judgment on the act that was performed. On the most plausible interpretation, act consequentialism holds that in any situation, a person does what is morally right by choosing that action which, given the foreseeable consequences, will produce at least as favorable a balance of benefits over harms as any other. This is the type of ethical theory that underlies what is sometimes called "situation ethics." Since this theory denies that there are any kinds of acts which need justification, that is, it denies the significance of moral rules, it denies that violations of moral rules need justification. According to act consequentialism, if the foreseeable consequences of the particular paternalistic act provide at least as favorable a balance of benefits over harms as any other act, then the act is morally right, and if the foreseeable consequences are not as favorable, then the act is not only morally wrong, there is no justification for it.

The implicit holding of this false ethical theory is probably responsible for some unjustified paternalistic behavior, especially in those cases in which the foreseen consequences are beneficial. But since the paternalistic cases may be controversial, it is best to start with a self-interested violation of a moral rule. That the theory is false is seen most clearly when considering a case of cheating on an exam in a course taken on an honor system that is not graded on a curve. If the foreseeable consequences are that no one will be hurt by the cheating and the cheater will benefit by passing, act consequentialism not only says that cheating is justifiable, but that it is unjustifiable not to cheat. Common morality, however, correctly judges cheating in this kind of situation as morally unacceptable, for no impartial rational person would publicly allow such a violation. Act consequentialists, however, are unconcerned with the consequences of this kind of act being publicly allowed, and consider only the foreseeable consequences of the particular act. Thus they must make up facts about human nature, saying, for example, that given human nature, the foreseeable consequences of cheating in this kind of situation will never result in as favorable a balance of benefits over harms as not cheating. But this is playing around with hypothetical facts in order to prevent the theory from conflicting with the moral judgments that everyone would actually make.

Act consequentialism is not an accurate description of the common moral system. Although act consequentialism is sometimes presented as if it were a description of the moral system that is actually used by people in deciding how to act in moral situations or in making moral judgments, it is really an alternative guide to conduct. Although the common moral system recognizes that foreseeable consequences are morally relevant, unlike act consequentialism, it does not hold that only consequences are morally relevant. Common morality recognizes the moral significance of the moral rules and does not allow a rule, such as the one against cheating, to be broken, whenever doing so has a more favorable balance of foreseeable consequences. More than the balance of benefits over harms is relevant to determining the justifiability of violating a moral rule. Further, insofar as consequences are the decisive factor in justifying the violation of a moral rule, they are not the consequences of the particular act, but the consequences of everyone knowing that this kind of violation is allowed. Many factors besides the consequences of the particular act determine the kind of violation. (See Chapter 2 for a fuller discussion of justifying the violation of a moral rule.)

Strict Deontology: Never Justified

According to the strict deontological view, it is never justified to break a moral rule without the valid consent of the person toward whom you are breaking it.[6] Some hold that even valid consent does not justify violating some moral rules, against disabling for instance, so that it is immoral to violate these moral rules even with regard to oneself. This extreme position usually has a religious foundation, holding, for example, that the moral rules were ordained by God to govern the behavior of human beings. However, this position can also have a metaphysical basis, as in Kant, where reason takes the place of God as the author of the moral rules. Without such a religious or metaphysical foundation, the view that it is never justifiable to violate a moral rule with regard to a competent person who has rationally consented to your violating the rule toward her, including oneself, has no support.

Further, almost everyone who holds a deontological view holds that it is justified to violate a moral rule, sometimes even the rule prohibiting killing, with regard to someone who has himself violated a moral rule. Punishment, even capital punishment, is accepted as justified by most deontological thinkers including Kant and most religious philosophers. It is only with regard to the innocent, that they hold that it is never justified to violate a moral rule without consent. It is quite common for strict deontologists to hold that only consent can justify violating a moral rule with regard to an innocent person and even on this less radical account, no paternalistic behavior is justified.

Some strict deontologists, like some act consequentialists, claim that they are presenting a description of the common moral system. However, like act consequentialism, strict deontology does not provide an accurate account of common morality. Common morality sometimes justifies deception if necessary to save an innocent person's life. If the only way to prevent very serious harms is by breaking a moral rule and the violation prevents so much greater harms than it causes that one could publicly allow such a violation, common morality holds that such a violation is at least weakly justified. Common morality does not hold that in order for a violation to be justified an impartial rational person must will that everyone act in that way; all that is necessary for justification is that an impartial rational person can publicly allow such a violation.

Similarly, common morality may hold that paternalistic behavior, paternalistic deception, say, is justified if it is the only way one can prevent very serious harm to the patient. Paternalistic deprivation of freedom, in the form of involuntary commitment, is even sanctioned by law if there is a high enough probability of the person seriously harming herself. Common morality thus sometimes sanctions an individual violating a moral rule with regard to an innocent person who has not given consent for such a violation. To support their views, some strict deontologists, like some act consequentialists, have put forward accounts of human nature which make their views seem more plausible. They have claimed that any violation of a moral rule with regard to an innocent person without his consent inevitably results in wholesale violations of moral rules with disastrous consequences. It is interesting that this defense of strict deontology seems to depend upon consequences, but closer inspection shows that it presupposes the view that we have put forward, that the decisive factor in determining the morality of an act is the consequences of everyone knowing that the violation is allowed.

One attempt to maintain the strict deontological position with regard to paternalism has been to claim that it is never justified to violate a moral rule with regard to a *competent* innocent person. The addition of the term "competent" is supposed to eliminate those cases of paternalism which are generally regarded as justified. Indeed, strict deontology tries to define paternalism so that one cannot act paternalistically toward someone who is not competent to make a rational decision in this kind of situation. Those who want to hold that paternalism is never justified in effect substitute "S is competent to make a rational decision" for our Feature 4 from Chapter 9, "P regards S as believing he can make his own decision on this matter"). This does eliminate many cases of what we regard as justified paternalism, but not all. It often still is justified to lie to a patient with a serious heart condition if telling the truth has a high enough probability of killing him.

A more serious problem is that this way of characterizing paternalism may sometimes sanction morally unacceptable behavior toward those who are not competent to make a rational decision. Just because people are not competent to make a rational decision does not mean that it is justified to violate any moral rule with regard to them as long as they benefit from that violation. If the benefit is small, it generally is not justified to deceive or deprive of freedom. By making competence of the patient a necessary feature of paternalism, strict deontology seems to justify treating large numbers of patients in a way that would be paternalistic if they were regarded as competent. Just as extreme views of the political left and right often seem to justify violence when more moderate views do not, so act consequentialist and strict deontological views seem to justify what would be viewed by common morality as unjustified paternalistic behavior. The act consequentialist would claim that his act is justified because there is a net benefit to the patient, while the strict deontologist would claim that his behavior is not even paternalistic because the patient is not really competent. Someone who simply concentrated on the relevant behavior, however, might not be able to distinguish the strict deontologist from the act consequentialist when dealing with those patients toward whom physicians are most tempted to act paternalistically.

Another serious problem with making it true by definition that no behavior toward any incompetent person is paternalistic, is that it transforms a genuine moral problem of justifying paternalism into a question of whether the action is really paternalistic. This may sound like a merely verbal dispute. It is a dispute about the proper use of a word, but it can have significant practical consequences. On our broad definition of paternalism, *any* violation of a moral rule, toward a person who believes himself able to make his own decision, and done for his benefit but without his consent, counts as paternalistic. Anyone who acts in this way must seriously consider whether her act is justified. Defining paternalism in a narrow way, so that one can only act paternalistically toward those who are competent to make a rational decision, may lead physicians not to be concerned with justifying their violation of a moral rule with regard to someone they view as incompetent. Since many cases of medical paternalism are with regard to patients whom the physician regards as not competent, this is a serious problem.

The strict deontological proposal shifts the emphasis from the genuine moral problem of justifying violating a moral rule for a patient's benefit without his consent, to the problem of determining if the person is competent. If he is not, the interference is not paternalistic and need not be justified. On our account, even if the patient is incompetent, if he believes he can make his own decision, it still may not be justified to intervene. The harm prevented by interfering may not be great enough to justify the violation of a moral rule with regard to the patient. On the strict deontological proposal there is an absolute dichotomy between the way the two classes of patients may be treated. No matter how great the harm prevented and how minor the violation of the moral rule, competent patients can never be interfered with for their own benefit without their consent. With regard to incompetent patients, interference is justified by determining that even a little more harm is prevented than caused. There is not such a sharp line separating competence from incompetence and, even if there were, it has not yet been reliably enough determined to allow it to play such an important role in determining whether it is justified to break a moral rule toward someone without consent.

The strict deontologist, who holds that genuine paternalism (paternalism toward the competent) is never justified, like the act consequentialist, who holds that genuine paternalism (paternalism that has a net benefit for the patient) is always justified, has a serious problem. Neither presents us with a practical way of deciding whether or not particular patients should be deceived or deprived of freedom, when the foreseeable consequences are that they would benefit from this violation of moral rules with regard to them. Both of these views present overly simple accounts of how physicians do and should go about determining whether it is justified to act paternalistically. Of course it is just their simplicity which makes them so attractive, for if physicians accept either of these views, they have a simple way of dealing with troublesome cases. However, those physicians who are serious about the matter have to be prepared to look at the morally relevant features of each case and only then decide whether paternalistic behavior is justified.

Common Morality: Sometimes Justified

Many writers maintain, as we do, that some paternalistic behavior is justified and some is not. However, we know of none who use an explicit account of morality to determine when paternalism is justified. Showing that common morality applies to cases of medical paternalism provides strong reasons for thinking that there is no need for a special ethics for medicine. This is very important, for holding that common morality does not apply in medical situations may lead some physicians to think that they are not subject to the same moral constraints that all other people are. This may be one explanation for the many instances of unjustified paternalism in medicine.

Most philosophical discussions of the justification of paternalism oversimplify. The act consequentialist considers morally relevant only the consequences of the particular act, and the strict deontologist considers morally relevant only whether a moral rule is being broken with regard to an innocent person who has not given consent for the violation. All of these features are morally relevant, but there are also many other morally relevant features. Failure to take into account all of these features often leads to a failure to distinguish between cases that might differ in only one crucial respect, such as whether that situation is an emergency. Casuistry is helpful in distinguishing between these cases, although it does not even try to provide a list of those features of a situation that are morally relevant.

For ease of reference, we repeat below the questions, the answers to which are the morally relevant features. These were listed and discussed in Chapter 2.

1. What moral rules would be violated?
2. What harms would be (a) avoided (not caused), (b) prevented, and (c) caused? (This means foreseeable harms and includes probabilities as well as kind and extent.)
3. What are the relevant beliefs and desires of the people toward whom the rule is being violated? (This explains why physicians must provide adequate information about treatment and obtain their patients' consent before treating.)
4. Does one have a relationship with the person(s) toward whom the rule is being violated such that one has a duty to violate moral rules with regard to the person(s) without their consent? (This explains why a parent or guardian may be morally allowed to make a decision about treatment that the health care team is not morally allowed to make.)
5. What benefits are being caused? (This means foreseeable benefits and also includes probabilities, as well as kind and extent.)
6. Is an unjustified or weakly justified violation of a moral rule being prevented?
7. Is an unjustified or weakly justified violation of a moral rule being punished?
8. Are there any alternative actions that would be preferable?
9. Is the violation being done intentionally or only knowingly?
10. Is it an emergency situation that no person is likely to plan to be in?

It may be worthwhile to make explicit that in cases of medical paternalism some of the questions on this list have obvious answers, for instance the answer to Question 7 is clearly no. In medical paternalism, the moral rule violation is being done to benefit the person, not to punish him. In some cases of involuntary commitment, however, there may be nonpaternalistic reasons as well as paternalistic ones for justifying commitment, to prevent the patient from harming another person, say, so that the answer to Question 6 might occasionally be yes. In this kind of case, an act which may not be justified on paternalistic grounds may nonetheless be justified. The answer to Question 9 is almost always that the violation is being done intentionally. The answer to Question 10 also is usually no, for paternalism normally occurs in a situation where the physician or other health care worker has time to ask consent. Actions done in emergency situations are usually not considered paternalistic for, as discussed in the previous chapter, when one cannot ask for consent prior to acting, immediately forthcoming consent usually prevents the act from being counted as paternalistic.

The answer given to Question 4, about the duties of physicians, distinguishes our view from many others. We claim that physicians do not have a duty to violate moral rules with regard to their patients without their consent unless they are in an emergency situation, that is, unless the patient will suffer very serious harms if action is not taken immediately. Act consequentialism claims that all persons, including physicians, have a duty to do that act which has the most favorable balance of benefits and harms. Strict deontology defends paternalistic actions toward incompetent patients by claiming that physicians have a duty to act so as to benefit their incompetent patients, even if that involves violating moral rules with regard to them. We do not accept these claims. Except in emergency situations, a physician has no duty to achieve the best consequences for her competent patients, especially when this involves violating moral rules with regard to them without their consent. Physicians do have a duty to consult with the guardians of incompetent patients or, if an incompetent patient has no guardian, to apply to the court to obtain a guardian for the patient. Physicians also must not act against the best interests of incompetent patients.

All of the other questions, 1, 2, 3, 5, and 8, are ones that need to be answered in each particular case in order to determine whether or not that paternalistic action is justified. These questions help one know what facts one should seek to discover. Everyone says, quite correctly, that finding all the relevant facts is crucial in making any moral decision. However, often no guidance is given in determining which facts are relevant. This lack can sometimes be serious, as shown by the following example: A physician wanted to perform blood tests on a 50-year-old woman who refused to have them performed. The physician regarded these tests as necessary in order to have any chance of discovering the woman's problem and treating it appropriately. He consulted the Ethics Committee of his hospital to ask for advice about whether it was morally acceptable to perform these tests without the woman's consent. He described the woman as sometimes delirious, so that there was some serious question about her competence. Accepting his claim that the tests were not dangerous in any way and only slightly unpleasant, the Ethics Committee concluded that it was morally acceptable for him to proceed with the tests without the woman's consent.

It was later discovered that he had neglected to tell the Ethics Committee that the woman was a devout Christian Scientist who had refused the tests because of her religious beliefs. Further, although she was sometimes delirious, her refusal was consistent and did not change when she was not delirious. She had no immediate family, but other members of her family made it clear that she had never accepted any medical treatments even in serious situations. Thus there was no doubt that her refusal was not due to her delirium and that even if she were fully competent she would have refused the tests. If the physician had been aware that it was morally required to consider the answers to Question 3, about the patient's relevant beliefs and desires, both his presentation to the Ethics Committee and their advice to him would have been different.

Perhaps the most overlooked question, but one which is often the most important, is Question 8, concerning alternatives. If there is a nonpaternalistic alternative that does not involve any unconsented to violation of a moral rule and does not differ significantly in the harms and benefits to the patient, then paternalistic behavior cannot be justified. This is a very significant matter, for often there is an alternative to paternalistic behavior, namely, long conversations with the patient trying to explain the benefits of accepting a treatment. Often it is lack of time to spend with the patient rather than lack of alternatives that leads to paternalistic behavior.

If lack of time does tempt some physicians into acting paternalistically, then someone else who has the time can be assigned to do what the physician does not have time to do. Allowing nurses more of a role in talking to patients about proposed treatments, even in obtaining valid consent for treatment, is a plausible option when the physician does not have the time. As discussed in Chapter 7, nurses could be encouraged to answer patients' questions about proposed treatments and to make them feel more comfortable about accepting the treatment. They can do this in conjunction with brochures, videotapes, interactive discs, and the like. Once the moral problems with paternalism are taken seriously, it is likely that physicians will discover some innovative nonpaternalistic methods of dealing with patients. Of course, often there is no alternative that will benefit the patient as much as acting paternalistically, and so deciding whether or not it is justified to act paternalistically will remain a problem.

Act consequentialists claim that the answers to Questions 2, 5, and 8, about harms, benefits, and alternatives, are the only morally relevant features that need to be considered in determining what morally ought to be done. This claim is incorrect. Not only are there other morally relevant features that are necessary to determine the kind of moral rule violation, but determining the kind of moral rule violation is only the first step. The next step requires considering whether one could advocate publicly allowing that kind of violation (a violation of that rule in those kinds of circumstances). Failure to move to the next step puts one back into a kind of act consequentialism, considering only the consequences of the particular act. The function of the morally relevant features, including the foreseeable consequences, is to determine the kind of violation, which, although absolutely crucial, is only the first step of a two-step procedure.

The second step is answering the morally decisive question, which is: would the foreseeable consequences of that kind of violation being publicly allowed, that is, of everyone knowing that they are allowed to violate the moral rule in these circumstances, be better or worse than the foreseeable consequences of that kind of violation not being publicly allowed? Consequences are crucial, but it is not the consequences of the particular act, rather it is the consequences of that kind of act being publicly allowed that are decisive. This account of common moral reasoning incorporates the insights of both Kant and Mill. Previous philosophers oversimplified common morality. We not only recognize the diverse nature of the morally relevant features, we realize that moral reasoning involves a two step procedure: (1) using the morally relevant features to determine the kind of violation, and (2) estimating the foreseeable consequences of that kind of violation being publicly allowed.

Disagreement about moral decisions and judgments can occur in either step. People can disagree about the kind of act, or they can disagree about whether they favor that kind of act being publicly allowed. Of course, one cannot even begin to decide whether one favors a kind of act being publicly allowed until the kind of act has been determined. This explains why discovering all the relevant facts is so important. It also explains why it is important for all of the morally relevant features to be recognized, for they tell one what facts to look for. Only after determining the kind of violation, by finding all the facts indicated by the morally relevant features, can the morally decisive question be asked: does the harm avoided or prevented by this kind of violation being publicly allowed outweigh the harm that would be caused by it being publicly allowed? If all rational persons would agree that the harm prevented by the violation being publicly allowed would be greater than the harm caused by it being publicly allowed, the violation is strongly justified; if none would, it is unjustified. If there is disagreement, we call it a weakly justified violation, and whether it should be allowed is a matter for decision.[7]

Our goal is not to provide a solution to every case, but rather to provide a framework that enables fruitful moral discussion of paternalistic (and other) behavior. We think that this framework always limits the range of morally acceptable answers. Further, we believe that using this explicit account of moral reasoning makes it less likely for mistakes to be made, such as failing to consider a patient's religious beliefs. Perhaps most important, it enables people to disagree without any party to the dispute concluding that the other party must be ill informed, partial, or acting irrationally or immorally. Providing limits to legitimate moral disagreement and at the same time getting people to acknowledge that, within these limits, moral disagreements are legitimate and to be expected, provides the kind of atmosphere which is most conducive to fruitful moral discussion.

Justifying Paternalistic Behavior: Cases

In most if not all cases, in order to justify paternalistic behavior it is necessary, but not sufficient, that the harm prevented for S by the moral rule violation be so much greater than the harm, if any, caused to S by it, that it would be irrational for S not to choose having the rule violated with regard to himself.[8] When this is not the case, then the behavior cannot be justified on paternalistic grounds. If it is not irrational for S to choose suffering the harm rather than having the moral rule violated with regard to himself, then no rational person can publicly allow the violation of the rule in the same circumstances. For that is the same as publicly allowing someone to force their own rational ranking of harms on someone else who has a different rational ranking. No rational person wants this kind of violation to be publicly allowed.

We now consider situations in which there are different combinations of morally relevant features. One of the most interesting set of cases is where the violation of different moral rules is involved (so that there are different answers to Question 1), but the amount of harm caused, avoided (not caused), and prevented, and the benefits caused (the answers to Questions 2 and 5) are very similar. This set of cases enables one to test whether our two-step procedure of justification does provide a more adequate account of moral reasoning than act consequentialism in those unusual but difficult cases where the two accounts give different answers. We begin by applying this moral framework (the morally relevant features and the two step justification procedure) to two cases of paternalistic behavior, one justified and one not.[9]

Case 10.1

Mr. K was brought to the emergency room by his wife and a police officer. Mrs. K had confessed to her husband earlier that evening that she was having an affair with one of his colleagues. He became acutely agitated and depressed and, after several hours of mounting tension, told her he was going to kill himself so "you'll have the freedom to have all the lovers you want." She became frightened and called the police because there were loaded guns in the house and she knew her husband was an impulsive man.

In the emergency room Mr. K would do little more than glower at Dr. T, his wife, and the officer. He seemed extremely tense and agitated. Dr. T decided that for Mr. K's own protection he should be hospitalized, but Mr. K refused. Dr. T therefore committed Mr. K to the hospital for a 72-hour emergency detention.

Using the above moral framework, Dr. T could attempt to justify his paternalistic commitment of Mr. K by claiming that by depriving Mr. K of his freedom for a very limited time, there was a great likelihood that he was preventing the occurrence of a much greater harm, Mr. K's death or serious injury. Dr. T need not claim that self-inflicted death is a harm of such magnitude that paternalistic intervention to prevent it is always justified. Rather, he could claim that it is justified in Mr. K's case on several counts. First, Mr. K's desire to kill himself seems irrational for he appears to have no reason at all, let alone an adequate one, for killing himself. An adequate reason would be a belief on his part that his death would result in the avoiding of great harm(s) or the attaining of great goods for himself or others. His statement to his wife, "You'll have the freedom to have all the lovers you want," is not intended as an altruistic reason, but is merely a sarcastic expression which, even if taken literally, would not be an adequate reason for his suicide.

Second, there is evidence that Mr. K suffers from a condition that is well known to be transient. Dr. T can support this conclusion by citing his professional experience that the majority of persons in Mr. K's condition who were hospitalized subsequently recovered from their state of agitated depression within 72 hours and then acknowledged the irrational character of their former suicidal desires. Third, the deprivation of freedom which Dr. T has imposed on Mr. K is a much lesser harm than the harm (death) which Mr. K may perpetrate on himself, even when one takes into account that the former is certain and the latter is only somewhat probable. Of course, Dr. T must have a justified belief that the probability of suicide is high enough, say, more than 15%, that it would be irrational to choose the risk of death over the loss of three days of freedom, and the psychological suffering involved.

It is, however, not sufficient justification for Dr. T merely to show that the harms prevented for Mr. K by his paternalistic action outweigh the harms caused to Mr. K; he must also be willing to publicly allow the deprivation of freedom of anyone in these circumstances, that is, he must be willing for everyone to know that in these circumstances everyone may be deprived of his freedom for a limited period of time. In this case, since Dr. T actually supports the law allowing exactly this kind of action, it is clear that he does advocate publicly allowing it. If the case is filled out such that all of Dr. T's beliefs are well supported, Dr. T's action could be regarded as strongly justified. However, if there is some disagreement about the facts, and the probability of Mr. K harming himself is taken to be lower, say, less than 5%, then Dr. T's behavior might be regarded as only weakly justified or not justified at all.[10]

CASE 10.2

Mrs. R, a 29-year-old mother, is hospitalized with symptoms of abdominal pain, weight loss, weakness, and swelling of the ankles. An extensive medical workup is inconclusive, and exploratory abdominal surgery is carried out, which reveals a primary ovarian cancer with extensive spread to other abdominal organs. Her condition is judged to be too far advanced for surgical relief, and her life expectancy is estimated to be at most a few months. Despite her oft-repeated request to be told "exactly where I stand and what I face," Dr. E tells both the patient and her husband that the diagnosis is still unclear but that he will see her weekly as an outpatient. At the time of discharge she is feeling somewhat better than at admission, and Dr. E hopes that the family will have a few happy days or weeks together before her condition worsens and they must be told the truth.

Dr. E could attempt to justify his paternalistic deception by claiming that the harm, namely, the psychological suffering, he hoped to prevent by his deception is significantly greater than the harm, if any, he caused by lying. While this might be true in the short run in this particular case, it is by no means certain. By his deception, Dr. E is depriving Mrs. R and her family of the opportunity to make those plans that would enable her and her family to deal more adequately with her death. In the circumstances of this case as described, Mrs. R's desire to know the truth is a rational one; in fact, there is no evidence of any irrational behavior or desires on her part. This contrasts sharply with Mr. K's desire to kill himself, which is clearly irrational.

In this case, Dr. E is violating the rule against deception in circumstances in which there is a high probability that he is preventing psychological suffering for several days or weeks and at least an equally high probability that he is depriving the patient and her family of the opportunity to make the most appropriate plans for her future. The person affected by the deception has a rational desire to know the truth about her condition. Given this description of the kind of violation, would a rational person publicly allow it, that is, be willing that everyone know that they are allowed to deceive in the circumstances described? The following discussion shows that no rational person would publicly allow such a violation.

Suppose someone ranks one harm, like unpleasant feelings for several weeks, as greater than another, such as the loss of some opportunity to plan for the future, but another person ranks them differently.[11] If both rankings are rational, should the first person be allowed to deceive the second, if his deception results in the second person suffering what the deceiver regards as the lesser harm? Would any rational person hold that such deception be publicly allowed, that everyone know that they are allowed to deceive in these circumstances? Since publicly allowing this amounts to allowing deception in order to impose one's own ranking of harms on others who have an alternative rational ranking, we think no rational person would publicly allow such a violation. Publicly allowing deception in such circumstances would clearly have the most disastrous consequences on one's trust in the words of others. Thus, this kind of violation being publicly allowed would have far worse consequences than it not being publicly allowed. This analysis shows Dr. E's deception, though clearly done with benevolent motives, is an unjustified paternalistic act.

CASE 10.3A

Mrs. V is in extremely critical condition after an automobile accident which has taken the life of one of her four children and severely injured another. Mrs. V is about to go into surgery and Dr. H believes that her very tenuous hold on life might be weakened by the shock of hearing about her children's conditions, so he decides not to give her that information until she has had the operation and recovered sufficiently.

CASE 10.3B

Mrs. V is in extremely critical condition after an automobile accident which has taken the life of one of her four children and severely injured another. Mrs. V is about to go into surgery and asks Dr. H how her children are. He believes that her very tenuous hold on life might be weakened by the shock of hearing of her children's conditions, so he decides to deceive her by simply telling her that they are concerned about her. He plans to tell her after she has had the operation and recovered sufficiently.

In Case 10.3A, Dr. H is not deceiving by withholding information, so he is not acting paternalistically. A physician's withholding information is deceiving when he has a duty to provide that information, as in Case 10.2. A physician has a duty to provide the diagnosis and prognosis to a patient unless he can justify not doing so. A physician has no duty to provide information that is irrelevant to the treatment that he is providing, so that not telling the mother about her children is not even withholding information, it is simply not providing it. Dr. H may be demonstrating a paternalistic attitude by not telling her that information, that is, he may be demonstrating that he would act paternalistically if deception were required to keep the information from Mrs. V. This is the situation in Case 10.3B, where Dr. H's answer to Mrs. V's question is deceptive, even if it is not clearly a lie.

Dr. H is acting paternalistically in Case 10.3B. This is, however, an example of justified paternalism. This assessment depends upon accepting that telling Mrs. V that one of her children died would increase her own chances of dying significantly, say, by more than 1%. It also depends upon Mrs. V not being in a situation where she is being deprived of any significant opportunity to make appropriate plans or decisions. She is going to be operated on immediately and so is not able to make any plans, even if plans need to be made.

Anyone acting rationally who had to choose between a loved one (1) being deceived for a short period of time, when this would have (almost) no effect on her planning for the future, and (2) being fully informed but thereby significantly increasing her chance of dying, would choose the former. If, in this situation, Mrs. V said that she wanted to know now, it would be assumed that she did not realize that knowing the truth now might kill her. (We are assuming that she wants to live and there are no other morally relevant features, such as religious beliefs, that would make knowing now especially significant.) In these circumstances, deception significantly decreases the chance of death and causes no significant harm. Would a rational person publicly allow this kind of violation? What would be the effect of publicly allowing this kind of violation? There might be some loss of trust, but whatever loss might occur would seem to be more than balanced by the number of lives that would be saved. Thus we hold that deceiving in this case is at least weakly justified, and may even be strongly justified.

In discussing the justification of paternalism, it is very easy to fall into the error of supposing that all that needs to be done is to compare harms prevented with harms caused and always decide in favor of the action that results in lesser harms. This kind of view, a relatively straightforward negative utilitarianism, seems to be held by many doctors and may account for much of their paternalistic behavior. A physician who holds this view thinks that if she is preventing more harm for a patient than she is causing to him, that justifies her violation of a moral rule with regard to him. This straightforward negative utilitarian view may explain why paternalistic acts of deception done in order to prevent or postpone psychological suffering, as in the case of Mrs. R described above, are so common. Little if any harm seems to be caused, and mental suffering is prevented, at least for a time; thus it seems as if such acts are morally justified. Paternalistic acts in which someone is deprived of freedom, as in commitment to a mental institution, are seen as more difficult to justify, for it is certain that some significant harm, the loss of freedom, is caused, and there is only a degree of probability that the more serious harm is prevented.

As noted earlier, negative utilitarianism, however, is not an adequate ethical theory. As discussed above, the foreseeable consequences of a particular act are not the only morally relevant features. Such consequences are significant, for, as part of the morally relevant features, they help determine the kind of act involved. However, knowing all of the morally relevant features, such as the beliefs and desires of the person toward whom the rule is being violated, is only the first step. The next step is considering the consequences of everyone knowing that this kind of violation is allowed. In many cases, balancing the harm that would be caused against the harm that would be prevented by everyone knowing that this kind of moral rule violation is allowed, leads to the same moral judgment as if only the consequences of the particular act had been weighed. Since the simpler balancing often provides the correct answer, people may not realize that answer is correct only because it is the same answer that would result if one used all the morally relevant features and the two-step procedure.

Those cases in which the two-step procedure and act consequentialism yield the same answer, however, are those in which there is usually no question about how one should act. Many of the problem cases are those in which considering other morally relevant features in addition to the consequences and applying the two-step justification procedure yields a different answer than act consequentialism yields. These latter kinds of cases make the inadequacy of act consequentialism apparent. Part of the standard philosophical literature against act consequentialism consists of examples in which it is inadequate to consider only the foreseeable consequences of a particular act. Consider a particular example discussed earlier in this chapter. A medical student has always been in the middle of his class, but for fairly trivial reasons has not studied during the weeks preceding the state medical examinations he is now taking. He has good reason to believe himself to be qualified for the practice of medicine. He therefore cheats in order to increase his chance of qualifying for the practice of medicine now and thereby prevent the unpleasant feelings to himself and his parents which would accompany failure. His cheating has not caused harm to anyone (the exam is not graded on a curve) and on a simple negative act consequentialist view would therefore be morally justified, perhaps even morally required.

Now consider the consequences if everyone knows that they are allowed to cheat for the purpose of decreasing unpleasant feelings, if they have good reason to believe that no one will be hurt by their particular act. Included in their belief that no one will be hurt is their belief that they either have or do not need the qualifications that the test is designed to measure. People have limited knowledge and are fallible. If everyone knows that cheating is allowed in these circumstances, it is very likely that some individuals, who believe themselves qualified when they are not, will cheat and thereby pass. Further, if everyone knows that everyone is allowed to cheat in these circumstances, this destroys the value of these tests on which people rely to determine who is qualified for, say, medical practice. The consequences of everyone knowing that they are allowed to cheat will result in some people having positions, say as doctors, for which they are not qualified. This will result in an increased risk of the population's suffering greater harms, such as pain and disability. Counting the anxiety caused to everyone, especially patients, who know that cheating is allowed, it seems clear that this outweighs the occasional suffering caused to those who cannot qualify without cheating.[12] Using the two-step procedure yields the judgment that is intuitively obvious; cheating in these circumstances is morally unjustified. Act consequentialism tries to avoid the conclusion that cheating in these circumstances is justified, if not morally required, by invoking very implausible features of human nature, claiming for instance that anyone who cheats once will continue cheating forever and so will cause great harm eventually.

Paternalistic acts committed by physicians may involve the violation of many different moral rules, but the three most common violations seem to be depriving of freedom, deceiving, and causing pain or suffering. Each of these three kinds of violations can be either justified or unjustified paternalistic acts. The examples of depriving of freedom in Case 10.1 (Mr. K) and of deception in Case 10.3B (Mrs. V) are justified, and the example of deception in Case 10.2 (Mrs. R) is not. Agreement on the facts is crucial. In order to show how what may seem like minor changes in the facts can affect the final moral judgment reached, we present the following cases of medical paternalism.

CASE 10.4

Mr. L is a 26-year-old single male patient with a past history of intense participation in physical activities and sports, who has suffered severe third-degree burns over two-thirds of his body. Both of his eyes are blinded due to corneal damage. His body is badly disfigured, and he is almost completely unable to move. For the past nine months he has undergone multiple surgical procedures (skin grafting, removal of his right eyeball, and amputation of the distal parts of the fingers on both hands). He has also required very painful daily bathings and bandage changings in order to prevent skin infections from developing over the burned areas of his body. The future he now looks forward to includes months or years of further painful treatment, many additional operations, and an existence as an at least moderately crippled and mostly (or totally) blind person. From the day of his accident, he has persistently stated that he does not want to live. He has been interviewed by a medical center psychiatrist and found to be bright, articulate, logical, and coherent. He is firm in his insistence that treatment be discontinued and that he be allowed to die. Nonetheless his physicians are continuing to treat him.[13]

According to our definition, Mr. L's doctors are acting paternalistically: they believe that saving Mr. L's life benefits him; they know they are causing him great physical and psychological pain without his consent; and they know that Mr. L believes that he can make his own decision on this matter. Mr. L's physicians could claim that they are acting as they are because they believe that the pain they are causing him by continuing treatment is a lesser harm than the death that would occur should they stop. Most burn victims have the same ranking and consent to treatment. It is certainly a rational ranking on their part. If Mr. L agreed, then, although the physicians would still be violating the moral rule against causing pain, their having Mr. L's consent would make their actions strongly justified. Indeed, it would be morally unacceptable for them not to treat Mr. L. However, Mr. L ranks the harms differently: he prefers death to months of daily pain and months or years of multiple surgical procedures, all of which will still result in his being a severely disabled person. His ranking, like the opposing one of his physicians, is rational.

The kind of violation being engaged in by the physicians involves their causing a great amount of pain by imposing their rational ranking of harms on a person whose own rational ranking is different. No rational person would publicly allow this kind of violation because of the terrible consequences of living in a world where great pain could be inflicted on persons against their rational desires whenever some other person could do so by appealing to his own different rational ranking of harms. Thus consideration of the consequences of publicly allowing the kind of violation in which the physicians are engaged leads to the conclusion that their paternalistic act is unjustified. Note how similar the reasoning and conclusion of this analysis are to Case 10.2, the cancer patient who is deceived by her doctor. An advantage of using the moral framework we provide is that it facilitates seeing the similarity in superficially dissimilar cases.

We mentioned above that if Mr. L agreed with the ranking of his physicians, it would be morally unacceptable not to treat him. A change in moral judgment would also occur if the case were varied in another way. Suppose Mr. L had to undergo only one week of painful treatment and then had a high probability of resuming an essentially normal life, one in which he could resume all of his former activities. If he claimed to prefer death over one week of treatment, we would deny that his ranking of harms was rational, in fact, we would regard it as seriously irrational. We would now describe the kind of violation being engaged in by the physicians as involving their preventing death by causing a great amount of pain for a short time for a person whose contrary ranking of harms is irrational. A rational person could publicly allow this kind of violation. We believe that consideration of the consequences of publicly allowing this kind of violation yields the conclusion that the paternalistic intervention of the physicians in this kind of case would be at least weakly justified.

The following two psychiatric cases involve decisions by physicians about whether to administer ECT without the patients' consent. The first case shows that mildly irrational decisions usually do not justify significant paternalistic interventions.

CASE 10.5

Mrs. D, a rather frail 55-year-old woman, was admitted to a psychiatric inpatient service with a six-month history of a moderately severe depression. She was transferred from a community hospital where her local psychiatrist had tried two different antidepressant medications but had stopped both because of her marked drop in blood pressure when given even the usual low starting dosages.

When she came to the inpatient ward Mrs. D was severely depressed. She had lost a moderate amount of weight and was sleeping poorly but had maintained a fairly adequate intake of food and water. Her psychiatrist recommended ECT to her. However, she firmly and consistently refused. She had had a close friend who had received ECT; while her friend's depression had improved at the time, she had killed herself a year later. Mrs. D acknowledged that ECT "may not have been responsible" for her friend's suicide but said she was terrified of it.

Her psychiatrist therefore devised a drug regimen in which she was given a very small nighttime dosage (10 mg) of desipramine, a tricyclic antidepressant, which was later increased slowly in small (10 mg) steps. He also gave her small morning and noontime doses of methylphenidate, a stimulant. She suffered from significant lowering of blood pressure, but with close nursing care this problem proved manageable. After two to three weeks, her depression began to respond. In another two weeks she was feeling quite well and her low blood pressure had ceased to be a significant problem.

Mrs. D's physicians viewed her not only as believing herself competent to make her own decision, they also viewed her as cognitively competent: she fully understood and appreciated the facts of her illness, knew that she was refusing her physicians' suggested treatment, and understood what her physicians believed might be the possible consequences of her refusal. Her refusal of ECT seemed, on balance, clearly mistaken if not irrational to her physicians. This was because ECT seemed to offer a high probability of significant and rapid benefit with extremely little risk, while it was not clear that continued drug treatment would help, at least not very quickly. It also seemed that her fear of ECT was based in part on what she herself seemed to acknowledge as the mistaken belief that ECT may have caused her former friend's death. Nonetheless, the harm she risked by not choosing ECT was limited to a prolongation of her marked depression. She was eating adequately, maintaining good fluid intake, and was not suicidal, so that there appeared to be no immediate danger of her dying. Therefore, the harms that ECT might ameliorate did not seem great enough to justify the harms that would be caused by forcing her to take ECT, especially since the alternative, continued and meticulous drug therapy, had at least some chance of success. Although we regard Mrs. D's refusal of ECT as irrational, perhaps sufficient to regard her as incompetent to make a decision about ECT, we do not believe her psychiatrist would have been morally justified in paternalistically overriding her refusal.

CASE 10.6

Mrs. O, a 69-year-old woman, was admitted to the inpatient unit with a depressive illness of six months' duration. Approximately one year before admission she was discovered on a routine examination elsewhere to have an enlarged spleen. No further studies were carried out.

Approximately six months before her hospitalization, Mrs. O's husband suffered a heart attack and was subsequently confined to a nursing home. She stated in retrospect that her "world went to pieces" at that time. She gradually became depressed and experienced characteristic changes in appetite, weight, and sleep. She refused to seek medical attention. Eventually her husband called his lawyer, who summoned the police to her home where they found her in a state of neglect and brought her to the emergency room at her local hospital. She was admitted and noted to be depressed, but was alert, oriented, and cooperative. Positive physical findings included low red and white blood cell counts and a further increase in spleen size. She was seen by a consulting psychiatrist, who thought she was significantly depressed and recommended treatment with antidepressant medication. She agreed to take the medicine but did not improve. The patient's internist recommended a bone marrow examination and other laboratory studies. Mrs. O refused for reasons that she would not discuss, saying only that she did not "want to bother." She was transferred to a university medical center for a further attempt at evaluation and possible treatment.

This second evaluation confirmed the above impressions. She was seen by a neurologist and by a hematologist, who recommended a CT scan, an electroencephalogram, a spinal tap, and a bone marrow examination. The patient's clinical condition continued to deteriorate, and she began refusing most food and fluids. She refused to allow most of the recommended diagnostic tests to be performed. Repeated efforts by the staff and by her family to obtain her consent for these studies were unsuccessful and were now met by her saying, "I deserve to die."

Her doctors believed that she was indeed at risk of death through malnutrition and a body chemistry disturbance resulting from inadequate fluids and nutrition. Her husband and son were informed of the seriousness of the situation. Her son obtained an attorney, went to court, and on the basis of the clinical details provided, obtained temporary legal guardianship of his mother. He then authorized proceeding with the diagnostic procedures deemed necessary. These were done despite her objections. The hematology consultant concluded that the most likely diagnosis was myelofibrosis. Her long-term prognosis from this disorder was thought to be uncertain, but her prognosis for the next several years was quite good.

Her son authorized proceeding with ECT for her now severe melancholia. She was treated initially without her consent and over her stated objections.

After the second treatment, she gave verbal consent to further treatments; after the fourth treatment she became brighter in mood, began eating well, and was much more verbal. After a total of ten treatments, Mrs. O reported that she felt quite well. She exhibited a mild post-ECT confusion, which subsequently cleared. She was able to express appropriate feelings of sadness about her husband's illness. She said that she was very grateful she had been treated. At her last follow-up visit, several months after discharge, she was doing quite well.

Mrs. O not only believed herself competent to make her own decision, she was cognitively competent, she understood and appreciated what her physicians believed to be the facts concerning her condition, knew that she was refusing her physicians' suggested treatment, and understood what her physicians believed would be the consequence of her refusal, namely, her death. Since her refusal of ECT seemed seriously irrational to her physicians in that it seemed almost certain that she would die without ECT and there was little if any risk associated with it, they regarded her as incompetent to make a rational decision in this kind of situation. They believed that she was suffering from a volitional disability due to her depression. She offered no reason, let alone an adequate one, for wanting to die, and this desire seemed to be associated with her depression, a kind of mental malady which is usually quite responsive to treatment. Thus, we believe that paternalistically forcing treatment on her was morally justified. However, given that it was not an emergency, it would not have been justified for the physicians to act paternalistically (force treatment) toward the patient without court proceedings. It is also preferable that it was her son, who was appointed legal guardian, who authorized the paternalistic intervention. Since the authorization was made by the court specifically for this purpose, it is clear that at least some, if not all, rational persons would publicly allow such an intervention.

All of the above cases involve the balancing of great harms, such as dying, deception about terminal illness, and the infliction of severe pain. The paternalistic interventions described have been obvious and often dramatic: commitment to a mental hospital or lying to a mother about the death of her child. The health care professionals making the decisions were all physicians, and in most of the cases (though we have not mentioned this feature) the possibility of legal intervention was present, in the form of suits for negligence or battery or injunctions to stop treatment. However, the vast majority of paternalistic interventions in medicine take place on a smaller scale. The following case not only illustrates a much more common type of paternalism, it also provides an excellent example of the value of using all of the morally relevant features and the two-step procedure that are essential to moral reasoning.

CASE 10.7

Mr. J was a 50-year-old patient in a rehabilitation ward who was recovering from the effects of a stroke. A major part of his treatment consisted of daily visits to the physical therapy unit, where he was given repetitive exercises to increase the strength and mobility of his partially paralyzed left arm and leg. He was initially cooperative with Ms. Y, his physical therapist, but soon became bored with the monotony of the daily sessions and frustrated by his very slow progress in regaining his ability to move his partially paralyzed limbs adequately. He told Ms. Y that he did not wish to attend the remaining three weeks of daily sessions. Ms. Y knew that patients like Mr. J rarely regress, that is, become worse than they presently are, if they stop exercising. But her experience showed that if patients like Mr. J stopped the sessions early, they did not receive the full therapeutic benefit possible and might suffer for the remainder of their lives from a significantly more disabled arm and leg than would be the case if they exercised now in this critical, early post-stroke period. Accordingly, she first tried to persuade him to continue exercising. When that was not effective, she became rather stern and scolded and chastised him for two days. He then relented and began exercising again, but it was necessary for Ms. Y to chastise him sternly almost daily to obtain his continued participation over the ensuing three weeks.

Ms. Y's scolding and chastising was paternalistic behavior by our account: she caused Mr. J some psychological pain and discomfort without his consent for what she believed to be his benefit and she knew that Mr. J believed himself competent to make his own decision about physical therapy.

Ms. Y could have attempted to justify her action by claiming that the relatively minor amount of harm she inflicted by chastising him to exercise was so much less than the relatively greater harm Mr. J would suffer by being significantly more disabled than necessary for the rest of his life, that it would be irrational to rank harms in the opposite way. We agree that the kind of violation engaged in by Ms. Y was inflicting a mild degree of suffering on Mr. J (through her chastising and his resumed exercising) by imposing her rational ranking of harms on Mr. J, whose ranking was not rational. A rational person could advocate publicly allowing this kind of violation, and we conclude that Ms. Y's paternalistic behavior was at least weakly justified.

This case involves the balancing of harms which, while significant, are not of the intensity of our earlier cases. Refusing three weeks of exercising versus greater lifelong disability seems irrational, although it is quite likely that Mr. J did not believe the facts or, at least, did not appreciate that they applied to him. The amount of harm associated with the possibility of Mr. J's needlessly greater lifelong disability seems significant enough to at least weakly justify causing him a mild to moderate degree of transient suffering without his consent. However, there are some kinds of violations that would not have been justified in Mr. J's case. It would have been unjustified to inflict intense physical pain on him to force him to exercise. The amount of harm associated with the possibility of his increased disability was not great enough that a rational person could publicly allow that kind of violation.

Philosophically, the most interesting alternative to consider is Ms. Y's deceiving Mr. J. Suppose Ms. Y told him that if he continued to exercise not only might he improve, but more important, she could guarantee that he would not regress to the point that he might be unable to walk at all. She would thus be strongly suggesting that unless he continued to exercise for three more weeks he might regress and end up not being able to walk at all. Thus Ms. Y did not quite lie, but she clearly intended to deceive Mr. J. Suppose that deceiving in this way has the same probability of getting Mr. J to resume exercising as daily chastising. In addition, such deception causes Mr. J less total suffering than daily chastising, for he now is not bothered by his slow progress, but, on the contrary, is pleased by what he perceives as his successfully preventing any regression, especially a complete inability to walk. Two questions now seem to arise: Is this paternalistic deception justified? and Is this kind of deception morally preferable to daily chastising?

Using a simple negative act consequentialist method of calculation, it might seem that if chastisement were justifiable paternalism, this kind of deception would be even more strongly justifiable. This is not a case of deception in order to impose one person's rational ranking of the harms on another person's different rational ranking, but rather deceiving in order to substitute a rational ranking for an irrational one. It is deception that results in a temporary (three weeks) mild physical discomfort (of physical therapy) in order to prevent the possibility of a permanent (twenty or thirty years) moderate amount of disability. Mr. J does not want to be deceived and Ms. Y does not have a duty to deceive him, but she nonetheless intentionally does so. The situation is not an emergency situation, although that might be disputed by some, for some action must be taken now to prevent the increased level of disability.

Would a rational person publicly allow deceiving in these circumstances? Allowing deceiving in a situation where trust is extremely important, such as in medical situations, in order to prevent a harm significant enough that it is irrational not to avoid it (the high probability of permanent moderate disability) is an issue on which rational persons can disagree. The erosion of trust that would follow from everyone knowing that deceiving is allowed in these circumstances might have such harmful consequences (for instance, legitimate warnings might come to be disregarded) that it is not clear that even preventing a significant number of persons from suffering permanent moderate disability is enough to counterbalance these consequences. If deceiving were the only method whereby Ms. Y could get Mr. J to continue his treatment, and deceiving has a high probability of being successful in doing so, rational persons might disagree; some might publicly allow this kind of violation, some might not. However, if there is an alternative to deceiving, namely, the method of chastising and scolding, then deceiving would not be justified.

We believe that when presented with these alternative methods of getting Mr. J to continue treatment, rational people would regard chastising and scolding as morally preferable to deceiving, and that some would regard intentional deception as completely morally unacceptable. Simple negative utilitarianism cannot account for this result since in this particular case deceiving results in no more and probably less overall suffering than chastising and scolding. The method of justification that we have been presenting, however, accounts for these moral intuitions quite easily. The two alternatives differ *only* in two morally relevant features: (1) the moral rules violated: causing pain (the unpleasantness caused by the scolding) versus deception, and (2) the harms caused, for it seems that more harm is caused to Mr. J by the scolding than by deceiving. We have assumed that the harm prevented, including probabilities, seems the same: permanent moderate disability in both cases; and Mr. J has the same relevant beliefs and desires in both cases. Since it is clear that the two alternatives do not differ in any other morally relevant feature, the primary difference is which moral rule is violated. Taking the second step and determining the consequences of publicly allowing these two kinds of violations, shows that the consequences of publicly allowing deceiving has worse consequences than publicly allowing scolding and chastising. This result accounts for the moral intuitions that one actually finds.

The key morally relevant feature is the presence of the alternative of scolding and chastising, which by hypothesis has the same probability of getting Mr. J to continue his exercising as deceiving him does. Without this alternative, deceiving prevents a harm significant enough that it is irrational not to avoid it (the high probability of permanent moderate disability). With the alternative of chastising and scolding, deceiving only prevents three weeks of mental discomfort caused by chastising and scolding. When one considers the harmful consequences of everyone knowing that they are allowed to deceive in order to prevent the amount of harm caused by three weeks of chastising and scolding, it becomes clear that no rational person would advocate publicly allowing such deception. The amount of harm, that is, the suffering due to the scolding and chastising, that might be prevented by everyone knowing that deception is allowed seems far less than the amount of harm that would be caused by the loss of trust.[14]

Lying versus Other Forms of Deception

Suppose that instead of deceiving Mr. J in the way described, namely, guaranteeing Mr. J that if he continued exercising he would not fall below his present level of ability to function, and in particular would never become completely unable to walk, Ms. Y simply lied to him and said that unless he continues to exercise for three more weeks he would regress and might end up unable to walk at all. She knew that this was not true because stroke victims are at their worst right after the stroke and never get worse later even if they do not exercise at all. In both cases, the deception and the lying, she knew that Mr. J would think that it was the exercise that guaranteed that he would get no worse, and so believe that if he did not exercise he might get considerably worse. Would violation of the rule against deception by lying be publicly allowed? Is lying worse than the previously described intentional deception?

It is commonly believed that lying is a more serious form of deception than withholding or misleading in other ways. Insofar as intentionally breaking a moral rule is worse than doing so only knowingly (morally relevant Feature 9), intentionally deceiving is worse than only knowingly deceiving. Since lying is intentionally deceiving, whereas withholding information and misleadingly communicating may sometimes involve only knowingly deceiving, lying does seem worse than other forms of deception. However, since in this case, it is clear that the deception is intentional, it does not seem to make much difference if it is done by lying or in some other way. The loss of trust that would arise from everyone knowing that deception is allowed in these circumstances would have the same, or nearly the same, harmful consequences as publicly allowing lying. Theoretically the consequences may seem not quite so bad since patients presumably could ask questions which would prevent them from being deceived if they knew they would not be lied to, but we think the difference in loss of trust would be negligible at best.

The above case is typical of a multitude of everyday situations in medicine in which doctors, nurses, and other health care professionals act or are tempted to act paternalistically toward patients. For example, consider the problems presented by the patient with emphysema who continues to smoke, by the alcoholic with liver damage who refuses to enter any treatment program, or by the diabetic or hypertensive patient who exacerbates his disease by paying little heed to dietary precautions. Each of these patients is apt to stimulate paternalistic acts by a variety of health care professionals (as well as members of his own family). Before acting, it is crucial for health care professionals to determine all of the morally relevant features of the situation, including the feasibility of alternatives. A clear and full account of the kind of situation involved is essential for deciding which paternalistic acts are justifiable and which are not.

Another Theory of Justification

One approach to justification which physicians sometimes cite and use deserves brief discussion: the "thank you" test. According to this test, one may justifiably act paternalistically if one is certain that at some later time one will be thanked by the person (patient) toward whom one is acting. Alan Stone's "thank you theory of civil commitment" is a variation of this approach.[15] John Rawls has similarly written: "We must be able to argue that with the development or the recovery of his rational powers the individual in question will accept our decision on his behalf and agree with us that we did the best thing for him."[16] James F. Childress has labeled these approaches "ratification theories," though it is not clear whether he wholly agrees with them.[17]

The simplicity of these theories make them seem attractive. However, while the recipients of justified paternalistic acts are often subsequently grateful, thank you theories are inadequate accounts of the justification procedure. That obtaining future thanks or ratification is neither necessary nor sufficient to justify paternalistic acts, can be seen by imagining a case in which one is certain a patient will be thankful (and thus justifiable according to this test) and then imagine that the patient, a rather grudging person, is not thankful. No one would say that the action had turned out to be unjustified after all. It is never actual consequences, only foreseeable ones, that determine the morality of an act.

Moreover, receiving future thanks is not sufficient for justification either. It seems true that some patients are so obeisant toward physicians that they forgive them and even thank them for a variety of what appear to be unwarranted violations of the moral rules with regard to them. Patient obeisance does not justify paternalistic acts. Nor does unexpected gratitude from a previously unpleasant patient justify paternalistic intervention. What justifies is not the patient's actual thanks, rather the justification depends on factors known at the time of the decision to act paternalistically: the foreseeable consequences, not the actual ones.[18]

If a physician has paternalistically deceived her patient and it would be counterproductive to reveal the deception, the patient may never know that his physician has acted paternalistically toward him. The thank you theory seems inapplicable in such a case. It is tempting to say that the patient would thank the physician if it were possible to let the patient know what had actually happened. This shows that whether one will later be thanked is not important. It seems important because it is related to the morally relevant features of a given case at the time that one decides to act paternalistically. These features, which determine the kind of violation, and the consequences of publicly allowing that kind of violation are what count. Thank you theories have an illusory simplicity, but they do not allow one to avoid the task of isolating the actual criteria for justified paternalism. The plausibility of these theories comes from the fact that doctors usually judge whether a patient will say thank you, at least implicitly, by using the criteria we have developed in our account of the justification of paternalism. It is a mistake to think there is some special theory of moral justification for paternalistic interventions in medicine.

Notes

1. The most prominent defense of casuisty is *The Abuse of Casuistry* by Al Jonsen and Stephen Toulmin (Berkeley and Los Angeles: University of California Press, 1988), but as with principlism, we are primarily concerned with the general approach of casuistry, not any particular version of it.

2. Al Jonsen has a favorite analogy that he uses to contrast casuistry with a theoretical account of morality like ours. Casuistry is compared to a bicycle and a moral theory is compared to a hot-air balloon. Supposedly the person on a bicycle has a better view of what is going on at the ground level (real cases) than the person in the hot-air balloon. However, it is quite clear that both persons would do better if there were constant communication between them. The person in the hot-air ballon can provide better information about traffic patterns (much as helicopters are used to give traffic reports at rush hours), and the person on the bicycle can provide detailed information about particular problems.

3. That account is provided in Chapter 9 of *Morality,* but we do not discuss the virtues in Chapter 2 of this book because we do not consider them to be useful in helping to resolve the moral problems that arise in medicine.

4. See *The Grounding for the Metaphysics of Morals,* 408–409 trans. James W. Ellington (Indianapolis: Hackett, 1981), pp. 20–21.

5. Except for killing, where, because of the public nature of morality, there may be some disagreement. See Chapter 12, "Euthanasia," for fuller discussion.

6. The person must also be innocent, for strict deontologists usually do not think punishment of the guilty is unjustified. See the next paragraph in the text.

7. See Chapter 2 for a fuller discussion. Since some disagreement is unavoidable in many cases, having a public policy about who makes the decision is essential. Further, whenever possible, we think that in cases of bioethical disagreement, there should be a public policy that involves consulting some experienced advisory body, such as an ethics committee.

8. Throughout this chapter when we say that it would be "irrational" for S not to choose having the rule violated with regard to himself, we mean "irrational" if he knew all of the relevant information. Thus, we are not claiming that S's decision is actually irrational, only that it would be irrational if he knew all of the relevant information. Thus we use "irrational decisions" to refer to decisions that are seriously mistaken, as well as those that are irrational. Also, if S's rankings are reliably known, it might be justified to act paternalistically if S's decision is unreasonable rather than irrational, and in what follows this should be taken into account.

9. This framework is presented in Chapter 2 and more fully described in Gert, *Morality.*

10. See Charles M. Culver, "Commitment to Mental Institutions," *Encyclopedia of Bioethics* (New York: Macmillan, 1995), pp. 418–423.

11. The particular harms being ranked make no difference; completely different harms could be used, for example, prolonged severe pain versus an earlier death. See Chapter 12, "Euthanasia," for a fuller discussion of situations when these latter harms are involved.

12. It is this limited knowledge and fallibility of persons, their inability to know all the consequences of their actions, which explains not only why no rational person would publicly allow cheating simply on the grounds that no one would be hurt by it, but also why moral rules are even needed. The nature of a violation cannot be determined after it

is seen how things actually turn out, rather it must be determined when the violation is being contemplated; then the limited knowledge of persons and their fallibility will play their proper role. See Chapter 2.

13. This case is adapted from Case No. 228, "A Demand to Die," *Hastings Center Report,* 5, no. 3 (1975), p. 9, and refers to Dax's case, one of the most famous cases in the medical ethics literature. It is also available in two different videotape formats. A test of the adequacy of our description is whether one would find other morally relevant features in the more detailed descriptions and also whether these would affect the decision one would make. We realize that our description lacks detail, for we have provided only the morally relevant features. Real cases presented in full detail are often the best kinds of cases to present, because one has to search for the morally relevant features. Learning how to find the morally relevant features amid the complexities of real life is one of the most important skills in moral reasoning. It is indispensable in the process of ethics consultation. In making real-life decisions, often only limited precision and certainty is possible. These are factors that make coming to decisions in real cases sometimes so difficult. See Aristotle, *Nicomachean Ethics,* 1.3.1094b.

14. Considering the consequences of this kind of deception being publicly allowed alerts one to the far greater harm that is risked by deception even in the particular case, that is, the lost of trust, and not only by Mr. J. If Mr. J finds out about the deception he is extremely likely to tell other patients that they should not trust what their therapists say. Although there might be a very small chance of Mr. J finding out that he had been deceived, if he does find it out, the consequences could be very great. The chances of any particular house being burned down are very small, yet almost everyone regards it as imprudent not to spend their money in order to buy fire insurance.

15. See Alan A. Stone, *Mental Health and Law: A System in Transition* (Rockville, Md.: United States Department of Health, Education, and Welfare, 1975), p. 70.

16. John Rawls, *A Theory of Justice* (Cambridge, Mass.: Harvard University Press, 1971), p. 249.

17. James F. Childress, "Paternalism and Health Care," in Wade L. Robison and Michael S. Pritchard, eds., *Medical Responsibility* (Clifton, N.J.: Humana, 1979), pp. 15–27.

18. Childress acknowledges this point in a note (p. 26): "Since many individuals who are subject to paternalistic interventions in health care will never regain rational powers, the ratification theory often takes a hypothetical form: what individuals would consent to if they *could* consent. This version of the ratification theory, of course, appeals to some vision of what rational individuals do and should desire." Even in this form, ratification theories are still too simple.

11

Death

Definitions

Definitions of words are often not merely verbal matters. Some words are so closely related to a concept that is part of social and legal practices that whether or not that word is correctly applied determines whether or not it is appropriate to initiate or terminate those practices. The word "dead," with all of its close relatives ("die," "death"), is so closely related to the concept of death that when it is correct to refer to a person as dead, it is appropriate to terminate all medical care and to initiate funeral proceedings. Many other social and legal practices are initiated when a person is declared dead, for instance, if he is president of the country, someone else immediately takes over that office. Insurance policies, social security, and many other things are affected. Failure to recognize how many practices are dependent on the correct application of the term "dead" has led some physicians to think that the determination of the time of death affects only medical practices. The time at which a person is declared dead has many practical consequences and only a small number of them have anything to do with medical practice. For most of these practices, it is usually not important to determine the time of death with split-second accuracy, but it is often important to determine it within hours.

One new reason for trying to determine the time of death with some greater precision is due to advances in medical technology. It is often very expensive to keep someone on life-support systems; being able to determine the time of death more precisely may prevent a serious waste of medical resources. But for many, what now seems the most important reason for determining the time of death with greater precision concerns the transplantation of organs. The sooner after death that organs can be removed for transplantation, the greater the likelihood that the transplanted organ will function properly in a new body. Indeed, some physicians are so concerned about assuring that the organs to be transplanted are in the best possible condition, that they want to change the definition of death to further that end.[1] But changing the meaning of a word that plays such an significant role in so many important social and legal practices is a dangerous thing to do. This is especially true if one does not realize that one is changing that definition, but thinks that he is simply bringing new scientific information to bear on the question of how the word is best defined.

When it is very important that a word have a clear and precise meaning, ordinary use is often supplemented by law in order to eliminate any troubling vagueness. When a word is very widely used, as the word "death" is, it is important that any legal definition of it not result in any significant changes in the way that word is ordinarily used; otherwise there will be widespread confusion about the proper use of the term. If a term plays an important part in social and legal practices, as "death" does, then the greater the change in the meaning of the term the greater the likelihood that there will be significant social and legal problems. Any attempt to make a term clearer and more precise than it is in ordinary use necessarily results in some people being bothered by what they perceive to be a change in its use. This perception of change cannot always be avoided, but it is important that any change be a reduction in vagueness. There should be no cases where in ordinary use it is clear the term "dead" correctly applies, but according to the new definition it does not apply. Even more important, there should be no cases where in ordinary use it is clear the term "dead" does not correctly apply, but according to the new definition it does apply. When a precise definition is needed, an overriding goal should be to change ordinary use as little as possible.

As can easily be seen by looking at any dictionary, a definition of a word that refers to an object or a property, that is, a "referring term," such as "table" or "rectangular," consists of a description of the essential features of that which is referred to by the term. In defining a referring term like "dead," that plays a significant part in important social and legal practices and is very widely used, the features included in a description of what is referred to by that term normally cannot conflict with what people ordinarily think. The only time that it is necessary to conflict with what is ordinarily thought is when advances in knowledge, usually scientific or technical knowledge, show that mistakes are embedded in the ordinary use of the term. The meaning of the term "atom" had to be changed when it was shown that what was referred to by that term, contrary to earlier belief, could be split. Atoms ceased to be the ultimate building blocks of the universe. But the term "atom" played no significant role in any social or legal practice, so that changing its meaning had no disturbing practical effects.

In biology and medicine, the definitions of terms change not only when new knowledge shows that the ordinary use of the term depends on false assumptions, but also when new classification schemes are adopted. For example, whales ceased to be fish when a new scientific classification scheme was adopted. Insofar as this changed the meaning of the ordinary word "fish," and that word played a role in some social and legal practices, some adjustments had to be made. But most scientific terms do not play significant roles in social or legal practices, and most are not widely used by the general public. When a term is widely and appropriately used by the general public, and plays a significant role in social and legal practices, even strong practical reasons for changing one or two of those practices is not sufficient reason for defining the term in ways that conflict with ordinary use. It is, nevertheless, understandable that physicians, who are primarily concerned with medical practices, should think only of the benefits of changing those practices when proposing to change the meaning of a term like "death."

Changing the meaning of a term is likely to confuse people and to create general distrust of those proposing the change in meaning. Thus when a term plays a significant role in so many social and legal practices, as "death" does, then, rather than trying to bring about a change in some medical practice by changing the meaning of a key term involved in that practice, it is preferable to argue explicitly for changing that particular practice. It is almost impossible to conceive of a situation in which it is appropriate to redefine a term with widespread ordinary use in order to change any particular medical, or even social or legal practice, in which that term plays a significant role. George Orwell has shown the bad consequences of redefining ordinary words in order to serve the political purposes of those in power. But even when the purposes to be served are worthwhile, changing the meaning of ordinary words is not the appropriate way to bring about those changes.

Proposed Definitions of Death

Death as a Process or an Event

A prominent and influential example of a physician neglecting the ordinary use of the term "dead" is Robert Morison's claim that death is a process rather than an event (1971). He supports this claim by citing the following scientific description of dying. He correctly notes that a standard series of degenerative and destructive changes occurs in the tissues of an organism, usually following but sometimes preceding the irreversible cessation of spontaneous ventilation and circulation. These changes include: necrosis of brain cells, necrosis of other vital organ cells, cooling, rigor mortis, dependent lividity, and putrefaction. This process actually persists for years, even centuries, until the skeletal remains have disintegrated, and could even be viewed as beginning with the failure of certain organ systems during life. Because these changes occur in a fairly regular and ineluctable fashion, it is claimed by some that the stipulation of any particular point in this process as the moment of death is arbitrary.

We do not deny any of the biological facts cited in the previous paragraph, however we think that they are not relevant to determining the definition of death. The use of many terms, for example many of the common color words, is even more arbitrary, from a scientific point of view, than the use of the term "dead." But even though pink is related to red as pastel blue is related to blue, it is misguided to say that pink is really pastel red. The following considerations show some serious problems confronting any definition which makes death a process. If death is regarded as a process, then either (1) the process starts when the person is still living, which confuses the process of death with the process of dying, for everyone regards someone who is dying as not yet dead, or (2) the process of death starts when the person is no longer alive, which confuses the process of death with the process of disintegration. Although there is some inevitable vagueness in determining the precise instant of death, this vagueness is no greater than that involved in determining the precise instant of other important events, such as birth and marriage. In ordinary use the word "death" refers to not a process but the event that separates the process of dying from the process of disintegration.

A physician recently writing on this matter admitted, "The reigning view has assumed that life and death are nonoverlapping dichotomous states."[2] Unfortunately, she seems to think that this view reigns only among philosophers and physicians, that it is a technical view about the biological processes that accompany dying. However, as stated before, "death" is not a technical term, but one that is used by ordinary people. It is they, as well as almost all philosophers and physicians, who use "dead" as a term that cannot be correctly applied at the same instant to the same organism to whom the term "alive" is correctly applied. This is what makes life and death "nonoverlapping dichotomous states." In ordinary language, "dead" is used to describe persons only when it is appropriate to have a funeral for them, and to bury or cremate them.

As Wittgenstein pointed out, philosophical problems often arise from a misunderstanding of ordinary language. It is a failure to understand ordinary language that leads to the following kind of remark: "To say 'she is dead' is meaningless since 'she is' is not compatible with 'dead.'"[3] Consider a daughter concerned about her dying mother who asks the doctor how her mother is doing. The doctor replies, "She is dead." Only someone overcome by metaphysical arguments could regard the doctor's statement as meaningless. A decent respect for the ordinary use of language requires that a definition of death be provided that fits with its use in ordinary language.

It is very tempting, however, to give a technical sense to ordinary words without realizing what one is doing. When *Philosophy in Medicine* was translated into Japanese, the translators were physicians. In a note discussing our introduction of the term "malady" as a technical term, they denied our claim that there was no ordinary word in any language that included both diseases and injuries. They claimed there was a word in Japanese that did include both diseases and injuries.[4] Upon investigation it turned out that ordinary speakers of Japanese never apply that term to a broken arm or leg. The Japanese translators had done what American doctors sometimes do, they had taken an ordinary Japanese term, analogous to the English word "disease," and had not realized that they had enlarged it so that it no longer had its ordinary use (see Chapter 5). A similar process seems at work among those who propose new and more elaborate definitions of death, definitions that are "a more descriptively accurate model of life's progressive cessation."[5]

On a practical level, regarding death as a process makes it impossible to declare the time of death with the level of precision that already has been achieved. As mentioned earlier, this is not a trivial issue, for there are not only pressing medical reasons to declare the time of death with some precision, there are also serious legal, social, and religious reasons for doing so. These include not only decisions regarding the aggressiveness of medical support, but also burial times and procedures, mourning times, and the interpretation of wills. There are no countervailing practical or theoretical reasons for regarding death as a process rather than as an event in formulating a definition of death.

Nor are there adequate reasons to introduce several senses of the term "death," each of which is used in a different medical practice, for example, one for ceasing treatment and another for retrieving organs. Imagine a situation in which someone is told that a spouse has died, and then has to ask, in what sense, in the normal sense when it is appropriate to have funeral services, or only in one of the newer senses, when various medical procedures can be stopped and started, or organs removed. We agree that it may not always be appropriate to use the time of death, in the normal sense of that term, to determine the appropriateness of stopping or starting some particular medical procedures. However, it is not necessary to change the ordinary meaning of "death" or to introduce new senses of death, in order to change the timing of these procedures. It is both possible and preferable to use new precisely defined technical terms or phrases, like "in a persistent vegetative state," in order to devise a policy for when it is morally acceptable to discontinue any life support, retrieve organs, and so on.[6] To use the same term "death" for all of these different stages is to invite confusion, mistrust, and abuse.

Ordinary Features of Death

The definition of death must capture our ordinary use of the term, for "death" is a word used by everyone, and is not primarily a medical or legal term. In this ordinary and literal use, certain facts are assumed, such as that all and only living organisms can die, that the living can usually be distinguished from the dead with complete reliability, that the time when an organism leaves the former state and enters the latter can be determined with a fairly high degree of precision, and that death is permanent.[7] Recent advances in science have not called into question any of these assumptions, but they have made plausible some scenarios that were formerly regarded as limited to science fiction. It now seems that an animal can be kept alive for a significant time even when its head has been severed from its body, so that the organism is no longer functioning as a whole. To insist that the animal is dead, even though its head responds to sounds and sights, has little or no plausibility and is incompatible with our ordinary understanding of death.[8] Therefore it is important that our definition apply not only to all current situations, but also to some plausible science fiction speculations, for example, about brains continuing to function independently of the rest of the organism.[9]

Some who believe in what is called "life after death" believe that after the organism dies, the person who was that organism, or the soul that inhabited that organism, continues to be conscious. However, both those who believe in life after death and those who do not, agree in their ordinary application of the term "dead." Someone who believes in life after death does not believe that the organism which has permanently ceased to function is still conscious, but only that something that had been closely related to that biological organism is still conscious. We do not take any stand on the plausibility of a belief in life after death, but we think that this belief has no relevance to determining the meaning of the word "dead." We claim that regardless of what one believes concerning life after death, there is no dispute about the permanence of the death of the organism that used to be a living organism.

In the literal use of the term "die," which is also the medical use of that term, all and only living organisms can die. In this same literal sense, death is regarded as permanent. Some people may claim to have been dead for several minutes and then to have returned to life, but this is only a dramatic way of saying that both consciousness and (most) clinically observable functioning of the organism as a whole was temporarily lost (for example, because of a brief episode of cardiac arrest). But a temporary loss of consciousness and (even complete but temporary) clinically observable functioning of the organism as a whole is not sufficient for what is meant by "death." The loss must be permanent; when it is, even those with the relevant religious beliefs do not doubt that the organism has died. In fact, when the facts are not in dispute, there is almost no disagreement in ordinary life about whether and when someone has died.

In its basic sense, the terms "alive" and "dead" normally apply only to whole organisms such as a cat, a dog, a mosquito, or a tree. The tail of a cat or dog, or the wings of a mosquito, are not said to be either alive or dead. Nor is the fruit of a tree said to be either alive or dead. However, people do talk about dead branches of a tree, and some people talk about keeping parts of a body alive, so that they can be transplanted. If only part of the organism is kept alive, normally the organism is regarded as dead, but if the part of the organism that is alive is sufficiently important, the organism may be regarded as alive. If any part of a human organism retains consciousness, that organism is regarded as still being alive. Thus the presence of consciousness is sufficient to establish that the human organism is not dead. It was formerly assumed that consciousness depended on the functioning of the organism as a whole, but recent scientific studies have cast some doubt on this assumption.

In some moral, but not in legal, contexts, it is not important to distinguish between the death of an organism and the permanent loss of consciousness of the person who was that organism; for example, killing someone does not seem any worse than causing him to be permanently unconscious.[10] In other contexts, however, it may be important; for example, only after the death of the organism is burial or cremation appropriate. But purely from the point of view of the victim, and apart from some unusual religious or metaphysical beliefs, it does not seem to make any difference whether one has been killed or simply caused to be permanently unconscious. However, the use of the term "dead" is not determined from the point of view of the victim, rather "dead" is used by conscious living persons to describe someone who can be buried, whose will can be probated, and so forth. This use of "dead" plays a significant role in a wide variety of legal and social practices.

Definitions, Criteria, and Tests

Much of the confusion arising from the current brain death controversy is due to the failure to distinguish three distinct elements: (1) the definition of death, which should be determined so as to capture most accurately the ordinary use of the term "dead" and related terms; (2) the medical criterion for determining that death has occurred, which must stay current with changes in our scientific understanding of the organism; and (3) the tests to prove that the criterion has been satisfied, which often change with improvements in medical technology. We concentrate on defining death in a way which makes its ordinary meaning explicit. We use our present scientific understanding of the organism to provide a criterion of death. When there is any doubt about whether a person is dead, it is this criterion which is used to determine whether the definition of death has been satisfied. Since the tests to prove that the criterion is satisfied change as technology improves, we simply mention some past tests that have demonstrated perfect validity in determining that the criterion of death is satisfied.

It is a source of some confusion that both the "definitions" of death that appear in legal dictionaries and the new "statutory definitions" of death are not actually attempts to provide a definition of the term "death," that is, they are not attempts to describe what the term means in ordinary usage. Rather, these "definitions" are actually statements of the criteria by which physicians should legally determine when death has occurred. Since "death" is not a technical term but a common term in everyday use, a proper understanding of the ordinary meaning of this word or concept must be achieved before a medical criterion is chosen. A definition of death must make explicit what is ordinarily meant by death before physicians can decide how to medically determine death has occurred. Agreement on both the definition and medical criterion of death is literally a life-and-death matter.

Whether a spontaneously breathing patient in a persistent vegetative state is classified as dead or alive depends on whether one accepts a definition of death that makes explicit its ordinary meaning, or thinks that a new definition is required. The definition that we propose makes explicit the ordinary meaning of "death." However, more than a definition is needed. A definition, by itself, does not completely determine the status of a patient with a totally and permanently nonfunctioning brain who is being maintained on a ventilator. That determination depends on the criterion of death employed. Defining death is primarily a philosophical task. Providing the criterion of death is primarily a medical matter. But it must be recognized that the criterion of death is a criterion for the definition being satisfied, and so depends upon what that definition is. Choosing the tests to prove that the criterion is satisfied is solely a medical matter. In this chapter we concentrate our discussion on the definition of death, but we also say something about the criterion of death. We say very little about the tests which are used to determine whether the criterion has been satisfied.[11]

The Definition of Death

The definition of death that we provide is one that we believe describes and explains the ordinary use of "death" and related words. We do not claim that anyone explicitly uses this definition, only that, if explicitly used, the definition results in people, who are aware of all the relevant facts, describing as dead all and only those whom they ordinarily describe as dead. We are providing an ordinary dictionary definition, only slightly more detailed than most dictionary definitions, and perhaps one that makes the term slightly more precise. Its correctness is determined by seeing if there is any clear case where use of this definition is in conflict with the ordinary use of the term "death." The following is our definition: *Death is the permanent cessation of all clinically observable functioning of the organism as a whole and the permanent absence of consciousness in the organism as a whole and in any part of that organism.*

By "the organism as a whole," we do not mean the whole organism, that is, the sum of its tissue and organ parts, but rather the highly complex interaction of all or most of its organ subsystems. The organism need not be whole or complete—it may have lost a limb or an organ (such as the spleen)—but it still remains an organism. By "the clinically observable functioning of the organism as a whole," we mean a sufficient amount of spontaneous and innate activities of integration of most subsystems, and at least limited response to the environment, that results in clinically observable activity. It is not necessary that all of the subsystems be integrated with one another. Individual subsystems may be replaced (for example, by pacemakers, ventilators, or pressor drugs) without changing the status of the organism as a whole. There are science fiction examples in which almost all parts of the organism have been replaced by nonliving mechanisms, but even in these examples these mechanisms have been integrated into the organism which has clinically observable functioning.

It is possible for individual subsystems to function for a time after the organism as a whole has permanently ceased all clinically observable function. Spontaneous ventilation ceases either immediately after or just before the permanent cessation of functioning of the organism as a whole, but spontaneous circulation, with artificial ventilation, may persist for several months after the organism as a whole has ceased to function, and the same seems to be true for temperature regulation. The control of this complex process, which is important for normal maintenance of all cellular processes, is located in certain neuroendocrine cells in the hypothalamus. These neuroendocrine cells usually, but not always, cease functioning when the organism as a whole has permanently ceased all clinically observable function. However, even if they do not completely cease functioning, if the organism as a whole has permanently ceased all clinically observable functions, the patient is still dead.[12] As we discuss in more detail below, the only subsystem that is sufficient to establish life, even after the organism as a whole has permanently ceased all clinically observable functions, is that subsystem responsible for consciousness.

If science develops replacement parts for every part of the organism, including the brain, that may force a change in our concept of death. Such a scientific development would also force a change in our concept of personal identity. Indeed, it is hard to predict what it would be correct to say about the death of a person, or about who counts as the same person at two different points in time, if enough of our present beliefs about those organisms that are persons change.[13]

We are attempting to describe the present concept of death, one that is based on acceptance of present facts about those organisms that are persons. We are not making metaphysical claims about death, claims that hold in all possible worlds; our aim is to clarify our present concept, that which accounts for the ordinary use of the term "dead."

An important practical benefit of clearly defining the present concept of death is that it enables the evaluation of the various criteria of death that have been proposed. Including in the definition of death "the permanent absence of consciousness in the organism as a whole and in any part of that organism" does not entail that death does not mean the same for the members of all biological species. Although death is a biological phenomenon common to members of all species, criteria for the death of a plant are not as precise as the criteria for the death of a conscious animal. Further, since plants have no consciousness, it is only the permanent cessation of the function of the organism as a whole that is used to decide whether a plant has died. The death of a conscious animal, especially human beings, usually must be determined with some precision, whereas that of a plant need not be. It is relatively unimportant whether a plant is very sick or dead, whereas this is a crucial distinction for conscious animals, especially human beings. The importance of consciousness to a conscious organism has no counterpart in nonconscious animals or plants. Thus, it is not inappropriate for the definition to acknowledge the importance of consciousness in the life of conscious animals. Indeed, this seems especially true as technology advances and if, as now seems likely, it becomes possible for a part of the organism to remain conscious while the organism as a whole ceases to function.

Consciousness is not limited to human beings. All mammals are conscious to some degree and other animals and birds seem to be conscious as well.[14] Although consciousness is usually manifested only by an organism that is functioning as a whole, as noted before, it now seems possible to sever an animal's head from its body and for that severed head to manifest consciousness, that is, to respond appropriately to external stimuli. Given that death requires both a permanent cessation of the organism functioning as a whole and the permanent absence of consciousness in the organism as a whole and in any part of that organism, a dog, whose head has been separated from its body, does not count as dead if that head continues to manifest consciousness.[15] Even though there has been a permanent cessation of the functioning of the organism as a whole, an identifiable part of that organism continues to be conscious. Any criterion of death must take into account that consciousness of any part of the organism is sufficient for that organism to count as still living.[16]

Previously we had held that permanent cessation of the functioning of the organism as a whole was sufficient for death.[17] We did not realize that an identifiable part of an organism might continue to be conscious even when the organism as a whole has permanently ceased to function. This was simply a mistake on our part, and the new facts do not require a change in the concept of death. However, as previously unknown facts are discovered, our concept of death may have to change. Nonetheless, even if these new facts require a change in our concept of death, they do not allow the concept to be changed without significant constraints. The concept must accomodate the newly discovered facts, but it should be be changed as little as possible. Indeed, it may turn out, as it did before, that the new facts simply make it clear that our previous description of the concept was mistaken. This possibility explains why it is sometimes useful to consider science fiction examples. Contemplating the possibility that these examples might be facts can sometimes make clear the inadequacy of previous accounts.

We now recognize that our previous definition of the concept of death was inadequate. The chapter on death in *Philosophy in Medicine* contained the following paragraph:

We believe that the permanent cessation of the functioning of the organism as a whole is what has traditionally been meant by death. This definition retains death as a biological occurrence which is not unique to human beings; the same definition applies to other higher animals. We believe that death is a biological phenomenon and should apply equally to related species. When we talk of the death of a human being, we mean the same thing as we do when we talk of the death of a dog or a cat. This is supported by our ordinary use of the term *death*, and by law and tradition. It is also in accord with social and religious practices and is not likely to be affected by future changes in technology.[18]

Most of what we said in that paragraph remains correct. However, the first sentence needs to be modified so as to include the addition of the phrases "all clinically observable" and "the permanent absence of consciousness." We would now rewrite that first sentence as follows. "We believe that the permanent cessation of all clinically observable functioning of the organism as a whole and the permanent absence of consciousness in the organism as a whole and in any part of that organism, is what has traditionally been meant by death." It is both interesting and important to note that this change in the first sentence does not require any changes in the rest of the paragraph. Improvements in technology have made clear that there can be laboratory-determined functioning of some of the cells responsible for the function of the organism as a whole, even though there has been a permanent cessation of all clinically observable functioning of the organism as a whole. Also, developments in biology seem to have established that a part of the organism can remain conscious even though the organism as a whole has ceased to function. Consciousness, even of a part of the organism, is always sufficient to establish that the organism is alive.

In our previous account we recognized the importance of consciousness, claiming, "Consciousness and cognition are sufficient to show the functioning of the organism as a whole in higher animals, but they are not necessary."[19] If we had taken science fiction more seriously, we would have realized what recent research has demonstrated: that consciousness of a part of the organism was possible independent of the functioning of the organism as a whole. In these science fiction stories, it was quite clear that the only sense in which the organism as a whole continued to function, was that a part of the organism remained conscious. We realized that when consciousness is maintained even though the head, or the brain, has been separated from the rest of the organism, the organism has not died. However, we were so invested in our account of death as the permanent cessation of the functioning of the organism as a whole, that we made consciousness subordinate to it.

We erred in not recognizing consciousness as a sufficient condition for life, independent of the functioning of the organism as a whole. The opposite error was made by those who claimed that permanent loss of consciousness was a sufficient condition of death. Both of these errors arose from a desire to frame a simple definition of death. We defined death as the permanent cessation of functioning of the organism as a whole, whereas others defined it as the permanent loss of consciousness. Both of us were partly right; death does require the permanent cessation of functioning of the organism as a whole, and it does require the permanent absence of consciousness. Both of us were also partly wrong, holding that what was a necessary condition for death was also a sufficient condition. We both wanted one feature to be both a necessary and sufficient condition for death. Although it would be far more elegant if either of us had been correct, the concept of death, like many of the concepts in our ordinary language, is more complex than philosophers and others have usually portrayed it. Death requires both the permanent cessation of all clinically observable functioning of the organism as a whole and the permanent absence of consciousness in the organism as a whole and in any part of that organism. Attempts to eliminate either component result in a distortion of the concept.

Unlike those who maintain that consciousness, or the possibility of future consciousness, is necessary for an organism to be alive, we maintain only that it is sufficient. Even when higher organisms, including human beings, are comatose, evidence of any clinically observable functioning of the organism as a whole, especially when it does not depend on any artificial life support, is sufficient to show that the organism is still living. Both the permanent cessation of the organism functioning as a whole and the permanent absence of consciousness in the organism as a whole and in any part of that organism, such as the head, are necessary before that organism can correctly be said to have died.

A definition that took permanent absence of consciousness to be sufficient for death was proposed by Veatch (1976) and has attracted some support. This definition does not mention consciousness, but defines death as *the irreversible loss of that which is essentially significant to the nature of persons*. Although it may initially seem very attractive, it does not state what is ordinarily meant by death. It is not self-contradictory to say that a person has lost that which is essentially significant to the nature of a person, but is still alive. Many human beings have lost sufficient mental function so that they have lost that which is essentially significant to the nature of a person, but everyone acknowledges that they are not dead. Indeed, it is often regarded as a blessing for such persons if they were to die very quickly. Permanently comatose patients in persistent vegetative states (PVS) are extreme examples of this kind of human being, but they are still considered to be living.[20]

The patients described by the Multi-Society Task Force on PVS are in this category.[21] These patients have complete neocortical destruction with preservation of the brain stem and diencephalic (posterior brain) structures. They have isoelectric (flat) electroencephalograms (EEGs) and are permanently comatose (indicating neocortical death), although they have normal spontaneous breathing and brain stem reflexes. They retain many of the vital functions of the organism as a whole, including neuroendocrine control (that is, homeostatic interrelationships between the brain and various hormonal glands) and spontaneous circulation and breathing.

The definition of death as the irreversible loss of that which is essentially significant to the nature of a person, or as the permanent loss of consciousness, actually states what it means to cease to be a person rather than what it means for that person to be dead. *Person* is not a biological concept but rather a concept defined, not only in terms of certain kinds of abilities and qualities of awareness, but also in terms of the attitudes it is appropriate to take toward it. It is inherently vague. Since death is a biological concept, in a literal sense, death applies directly only to biological organisms and not to persons. Of course, it is perfectly ordinary to talk about the "death of a person," but this phrase in common usage actually means the death of the organism which was the person. For example, one might overhear in the hospital wards, "The person in room 612 died last night." In this common usage, the speaker is referring to the death of the organism that was a person. We think that Veatch and others have not appreciated that the phrase "death of a person" is normally applied to an organism which has died, not to an organism which has ceased to be a person but has not died.

A patient in a persistent vegetative state is usually regarded as living in only the most basic biological sense, but this basic biological sense is just what our definition of death makes explicit. The death of an organism which was a person must not be confused with an organism ceasing to be a person. The loss of personhood in persistent vegetative patients makes it inappropriate to continue treating them as if they were persons. Consciousness and cognition are essential human attributes. If they are lost, life has lost its meaning. Unless there are religious reasons to the contrary, we recommend that nothing be done to keep such patients alive. This alternative is preferable to considering these persistent vegetative patients as already dead. No one favors burying or cremating a patient who is still breathing spontaneously. Unless one favors "killing" such patients, it is still necessary to wait for the organism as a whole to permanently cease to function. In most cases there is no practical advantage to regarding such patients as dead rather than as ceasing to be persons.

The only cases in which there might be a practical advantage in regarding patients who have ceased to be persons as dead, is in the procurement of organs for transplantation. Waiting until the organism as a whole has ceased to function may sometimes reduce the chances of a successful transplant. However, changing the definition of death in order to gain some practical advantage in transplantation is exactly the kind of maneuver that concerns many people. If it is known that the definition of death has been changed to obtain better quality organs for transplantation, distrust of the medical profession is bound to increase. Changing the meaning of ordinary words for practical advantage is far too likely to be mistrusted and misused for it to confer any overall practical advantage.[22] It is better to explicitly argue in favor of removing organs from living but permanently unconscious patients, than to change the meaning of the word "death" in order to accomplish the same goal.

Apart from obtaining more viable organs, considering permanent loss of consciousness and cognition as what it means for an organism to be dead rather than for an organism to cease to be a person, has no practical advantages. It is far less troubling to argue for nonvoluntary cessation of life support for the permanently comatose, than to claim that the patient is already dead. The justification of nonvoluntary passive euthanasia, just as the justification of obtaining organs for transplantation, must be kept strictly separate from the definition of death. Most people would prefer to die when they cease to be persons, but few think that this should be accomplished simply by redefining "death" so that when they have ceased to be persons, they have died.

Organisms that are no longer persons have no claim to be treated as persons. However, just as human corpses are treated with respect, even more so, living organisms that were persons should be treated with respect. Treating these organisms with respect does not mean that one should strive to keep them alive. No one benefits by doing this; on the contrary, given the care needed to keep such organisms alive, it is an extravagant waste of both economic and human resources to attempt to do so. On the other hand, allowing, let alone requiring, anyone to kill them creates serious practical problems. Even though these organisms are no longer persons, they still look like persons, indeed, are almost indistinguishable from persons in deep sleep. Since these patients are not suffering in any way, there is no overwhelming reason for killing them. On the contrary, since killing them might weaken the prohibition against killing, there are strong reasons for not doing so.

It is important to note that since these patients have permanently lost all consciousness and cognition, they do not suffer from lack of care. Any patient who retains even the slightest capacity to suffer pain or discomfort of any kind remains a person and must be treated as such.[23] Of course, all patients should be encouraged to make out Advance Directives, in order to make clear whether or not they want to be allowed to die if they become permanently comatose. In the absence of any Advance Directive to the contrary, we propose that the legal guardian or next of kin be allowed to direct that all treatments, including food and fluids, be discontinued and the patient be allowed to die. Discontinuing all treatment, including food and fluids, for such patients causes no pain and results in death in two weeks or less, making it unnecessary to kill them. We put this proposal forward here because we think that its adoption significantly reduces the temptation to change the definition of death from its ordinary biological sense to that of an organism which has ceased to be a person.[24]

The Criterion of Death

We have argued that the correct definition of death is the *permanent cessation of all clinically observable functioning of the organism as a whole and the permanent absence of consciousness in the organism as a whole and in any part of that organism.* In order for this definition to be applied to actual cases of death, there must be a criterion that is taken as establishing with complete certainty that the definition has been satisfied. Four criteria of death have been put forward: (1) the permanent loss of cardiopulmonary functioning, (2) the total and permanent loss of functioning of the cortex, (3) the total and permanent loss of functioning of the brain stem, and (4) the total and permanent loss of functioning of the whole brain. Only one of these four proposed criteria is completely compatible with the above definition of death: (4) the total and permanent loss of functioning of the whole brain. Thus it is the only acceptable criterion of death. In the following sections we point out the inadequacies of the other three proposed criteria.

Characteristics of optimum criteria and tests. A criterion of death yields a false-positive if it is satisfied, and yet it is still possible for that organism to function as a whole, or for any part of it to be conscious. An essential requirement for a criterion of death is that it yield no false-positives. Indeed, since the criterion of death serves as the legal definition of death, it cannot have any exceptions. It is not sufficient that the criterion be correct 99.99% of the time. This means that not only can the criterion yield no false-positives, it should also yield no false-negatives. A criterion of death yields a false-negative if it is not satisfied and yet the organism as a whole has permanently ceased to function and there is a permanent absence of consciousness in every part of the organism.

Of course, physicians may sometimes determine death without using the criterion, but it can never be that the criterion is satisfied and yet the person is not dead, or that the criterion is not satisfied and the person is dead. This is why it is so easy to mistakenly regard the criterion as a real definition, rather than solely the legal definition. The criterion serves as the legal definition because it is what is used by the medical profession in declaring death whenever there is any doubt about the matter. Often, however, it is not necessary to directly establish that the criterion is satisfied, for in many circumstances it is absolutely certain that the person is dead, as in automobile accidents where the person's head has been crushed. In less clear cases, when there is some doubt about whether the criterion is satisfied, this determination is provided by validated tests.

Permanent loss of cardiopulmonary functioning. Permanent termination of all heart and lung function seems to have been used as a criterion of death throughout history. Even the ancients observed that all other bodily functions ceased shortly after cessation of these vital functions, and the irreversible process of bodily disintegration inevitably followed. Permanent loss of spontaneous cardiopulmonary function was a perfect predictor of permanent nonfunctioning of the organism as a whole, as well as permanent absence of consciousness in all parts of the organism. There were no false positives. Further, if the loss of spontaneous cardiopulmonary function was not permanent, the organism as a whole continued to function, even if that loss caused a permanent absence of consciousness in all parts of the organism. Thus, there were no false negatives. For a very long time, the permanent loss of spontaneous cardiopulmonary function served as an adequate criterion of death.

Times have changed. Current circulatory-ventilatory technology has had the result that permanent loss of spontaneous cardiopulmonary functioning is no longer a perfect predictor of permanent nonfunctioning of the organism as a whole. Even more clearly, it is not predictive of permanent absence of consciousness in all parts of the organism. Consider a conscious, talking patient who is unable to breathe because of poliomyelitis and who requires an iron lung (thus having permanent loss of spontaneous pulmonary function), who has also developed asystole (loss of spontaneous heartbeat) requiring a permanent pacemaker (thus having permanent loss of spontaneous cardiac function). It would be absurd to regard such a person as dead.

It is now quite clear that the permanent loss of *spontaneous* cardiopulmonary function is not the criterion of death. Even though it does not result in any false-negatives, it does what is far worse, it results in false-positives. To eliminate the false positives, it has been proposed to change the cardiopulmonary criterion from the permanent loss of spontaneous cardiopulmonary function to the permanent loss of all cardiopulmonary function, whether spontaneous or artificially supported. However, now that ventilation and circulation can be mechanically maintained, an organism with permanent loss of whole-brain functioning can have permanently ceased to function as a whole, and all parts of the organism may have permanently lost consciousness, weeks before the heart and lungs cease to function with artificial support. Thus, this revised cardiopulmonary criterion is not satisfied, yet the person is dead. The revised cardiopulmonary criterion eliminates the false-positives, but it produces false-negatives.

The cardiopulmonary criterion can continue to be put forward only if the ambiguity involved is not noticed. The cardiopulmonary criterion of death cannot be permanent loss of spontaneous cardiopulmonary functioning nor can it be permanent loss of artificially supported cardiopulmonary functioning. Permanent loss of spontaneous cardiopulmonary functioning is no longer perfectly correlated with death, and continued artificially supported cardiopulmonary function is no longer perfectly correlated with life. Loss of cardiopulmonary functioning now seems to have no straightforward relationship either to the permanent loss of functioning of the organism as a whole or to the permanent absence of consciousness in the organism as a whole and in any part of that organism.

Total and permanent loss of functioning of the cortex. Total and permanent loss of functioning of the cortex does not provide an adequate criterion of death on the definition of death provided above. Even its supporters acknowledge that total and permanent loss of functioning of the higher brain or cortex is an adequate criterion of death only if one defines death as the permanent absence of consciousness in the organism as a whole and in any part of that organism. We have already given our arguments against accepting this definition of death, so there is no need to provide new arguments against accepting loss of all higher brain functions as the criterion of death. Everyone acknowledges that a human organism can continue to function as a whole even if the entire cortex has ceased to function. On the definition of death that we have provided, this proposed criterion of death continually produces false-positives; people would be declared dead who do not satisfy the definition. Nonetheless, because some people have supported permanent loss of consciousness of all parts of the organism as the definition of death, this criterion has many supporters.[25]

Total and permanent loss of functioning of the brain stem. Total and permanent loss of functioning of the brain stem is, except for purely theoretical considerations, a good criterion of death. Permanent loss of functioning of the organism as a whole inevitably accompanies total and permanent loss of functioning of the brain stem. If permanent loss of functioning of the organism as a whole always results in permanent loss of consciousness of all parts of the organism, total and permanent loss of functioning of the brain stem provides an adequate criterion of death. However, it now seems possible, at least theoretically, for there to be total and permanent loss of functioning of the brain stem and yet for consciousness to remain in one part of the body, the cortex.[26] It is not clear that this possibility will ever be realized, but sufficient work has been done with the higher brain to make it seem a genuine possibility. Patients suffering from locked-in syndrome have been able to manipulate electrical devices by pure thought, that is, by increasing or decreasing the amount of electrical energy given off by their brain. If such devices were attached to a person's cortex, and he continued to operate them even after total and permanent loss of functioning of his brain stem, it would clearly be a mistake to declare that patient dead.

As pointed out above, the essential requirement for a criterion of death is that it yield no false-positives. If the brain stem criterion has even a remote possibility of yielding a false-positive, it is not an adequate criterion of death. It does seem possible for someone who is still conscious to have total and permanent loss of brain stem function. Therefore the brain stem criterion cannot be accepted as the criterion of death. Further, there seems to be minimal practical gain in accepting loss of brain stem functioning over loss of whole brain functioning as the criterion. Except in extremely unusual cases, the tests that are adequate to show that the one criterion is satisfied, are also adequate to show that the other criterion is satisfied. Indeed, the cortex is more sensitive to loss of oxygen than is the brain stem. This is why so many patients in a persistent vegetative state are those who have been resuscitated after a period of cerebral anoxia; the brain stem has survived but the cortex has not. The main difference between the brain stem criterion and the whole brain criterion is theoretical. The former allows for the possibility of a part of the organism being conscious even though the organism as a whole has ceased to function, while the latter does not. Loss of brain stem functioning can be accepted as the criterion of death only if there is an argument showing that when it is satisfied, consciousness of part of the organism is impossible.

Total and permanent loss of whole brain functioning. The criterion for the permanent cessation of functioning of the organism as a whole and the permanent absence of consciousness in the organism as a whole and in any part of that organism, is the permanent loss of functioning of the entire brain.[27] This criterion is perfectly correlated with the permanent cessation of all clinically observable functioning of the organism as a whole because it is the brain stem, which is part of the entire brain, that is necessary for all clinically observable functioning of the organism as a whole. The brain stem integrates, generates, interrelates, and controls complex bodily activities. A patient on a ventilator with a totally destroyed brain stem is merely a collection of artificially maintained subsystems, since the organism as a whole has ceased to function. This criterion also correlates perfectly with the permanent absence of consciousness in the organism as a whole and in any part of that organism, for the cortex, which is part of the "entire brain," is the seat of consciousness, and if it has permanently ceased to function, then no part of the organism can be conscious. The permanent loss of whole-brain functioning entails the permanent loss of function of both the brain stem and the cortex. Using the permanent loss of whole brain functioning as a criterion of death yields no false negatives or false positives, and thus is completely adequate as a criterion.

Using permanent loss of functioning of the whole brain as the criterion for death is also consistent with tradition; it is not a new departure. Throughout history, whenever a physician was called to ascertain the occurrence of death, his examination included the following important indicators of permanent loss of functioning of the whole brain: unresponsivity, lack of spontaneous movements including breathing, and absence of pupillary light response. Only one important sign, lack of heartbeat, was not directly indicative of whole brain destruction. But since the heartbeat stops within several minutes of cessation of breathing, permanent absence of the vital signs is an important sign of permanent loss of whole-brain functioning. Thus, in an important sense, permanent loss of whole-brain functioning has always been the underlying criterion of death.

The Tests of Death

Having provided the definition of death, namely, the permanent cessation of all clinically observable functioning of the organism as a whole and the permanent absence of consciousness in the organism as a whole and in any part of that organism, and the criterion of death, the total and irreversible cessation of functioning of the whole brain, we now briefly discuss the available tests of death. The tests must never yield a false-positive, that is, someone who does not meet the definition of death being declared dead. It would be ideal if no test ever yielded a false-negative, that is, someone who meets the definition of death yet is still living. Unlike the criterion of death, however, a test can remain acceptable if it results in a very few and relatively brief false-negatives.

Cessation of heartbeat and ventilation. Although permanent loss of spontaneous cardiopulmonary function is not the criterion of death, in the vast majority of deaths not complicated by artificial ventilation, it is a completely valid test for determining that the criterion is satisfied. The physical findings of permanent absence of heartbeat and respiration show that the criterion of death has been satisfied, since, in the absence of artificial ventilation, they always quickly produce permanent loss of functioning of the whole brain. However, when mechanical ventilation is being used, these tests lose much of their validity due to the production of numerous false-negatives for as long as two weeks or more. It has become almost common for the death of the organism to occur while the circulatory-ventilatory subsystems are still intact. Although the circulatory-ventilatory tests suffice in the overwhelming majority of deaths, if there is artificial maintenance of circulation or ventilation special tests for permanent cessation of whole-brain functioning are needed.

Tests for irreversible cessation of whole-brain functioning. Numerous formalized sets of tests have been established to determine that the criterion of permanent loss of whole-brain functioning has been met.[28] What we call tests have sometimes been called "criteria," but it is important to distinguish these "second-level criteria" or tests from the criterion of death itself. While the criteria for the death of the organism must be understandable by the layman, the (second-level criteria) tests to determine the permanent loss of functioning of the whole brain need not be understandable by anyone except qualified clinicians. To avoid confusion, we prefer to use the designation "tests" for the second-level criteria.

All the proposed tests require total and permanent absence of all functioning of the brain stem and both hemispheres. They vary slightly from one set to another, but all require unresponsivity (deep coma), absent pupillary light reflexes, apnea (inability to breathe), and absent brain stem reflexes. They also require the absence of drug intoxication and low body temperature, and the newer sets require the demonstration that a lesion of the brain exists. Isoelectric (flat) EEGs are generally required, and tests disclosing the absence of cerebral blood flow are of confirmatory value. All tests require the given loss of function to be present for a particular time interval, which in the case of the absence of cerebral blood flow may be as short as 30 minutes.

Current tests of irreversible loss of whole-brain function may produce many false-negatives of a sort during the 30-minute to 24-hour interval between the successive neurologic examinations which different tests require. Certain sets of tests, particularly those requiring electrocerebral silence by EEG, may produce false-negatives if an EEG artifact is present and cannot confidently be distinguished from brain wave activity. Generally, a few brief false-negatives are tolerable and even inevitable, since tests must be delineated conservatively in order to eliminate any possibility of false-positives. When a physician properly performs and interprets the validated tests for loss of whole-brain function outlined in the 1981 report of the medical consultants to the President's Commission (see below), he can be confident that the loss of whole-brain functioning is permanent.[29]

A Legal Definition of Death

In July 1981 the President's Commission for the Study of Ethical Problems in Medicine and Biomedical and Behavioral Research published its report, *'Defining Death': A Report on the Medical, Legal, and Ethical Issues in the Determination of Death*. In this report they proposed a statute, the Uniform Determination of Death Act (UDDA), which provides a criterion of death which is to serve as the legal definition of death.

An individual who has sustained either (1) irreversible cessation of circulatory and respiratory functions, or (2) irreversible cessation of all functions of the entire brain, including the brain stem, is dead. A determination of death must be made in accordance with accepted medical standards.

This statute, which has been adopted by many state legislatures, has given rise to the view that there are two criteria of death, irreversible cessation of circulatory and respiratory functions, and irreversible cessation of all functions of the entire brain, including the brain stem. However, as we pointed out earlier, the first of these supposed criteria, irreversible cessation of circulatory and respiratory functions, is not properly regarded as a criterion at all; it is, at most, a test to show that the second supposed (and actual) criterion, irreversible cessation of all functions of the entire brain, including the brain stem, has been satisfied. The statute has to be interpreted, not as proposing two distinct criteria for death, but rather as proposing a complex two-part criterion. Otherwise, it is subject to the criticism that we pointed out earlier, that the first supposed criterion, irreversible cessation of circulatory and respiratory functions, is ambiguous, not distinguishing between spontaneous and artificially supported circulatory and respiratory functions.

The wording of the UDDA statute of death promotes the idea that there are two kinds of death, heart death and brain death. Since heart death is what is most well known, and most easily determined, brain death is thought of as a new form of death, one that applies only to those who are on some form of artificial life support. Some have considered that brain death is not really death at all, but merely a legal maneuver to stop life-support systems. Hans Jonas (1974) has asked: "Why are they alive if the heart, etc., works naturally but not alive when it works artificially?" We think that it reduces confusion to make clear that there is only one criterion of death, the irreversible cessation of all functions of the entire brain, including the brain stem. That should be the legal definition of death, and it should be made clear that the other part of the proposed criterion of death, irreversible cessation of *spontaneous* (our addition) circulatory and respiratory functions, is only a test that the real criterion has been satisfied.

We have revised the UDDA statute of death with these points in mind:

An individual who has sustained irreversible cessation of all functions of the entire brain, including the brain stem, is dead.

(a) In the absence of artificial means of cardiopulmonary support, death (the irreversible cessation of all brain functions) can be determined by the prolonged absence of spontaneous circulatory and respiratory functions.

(b) In the presence of artificial means of cardiopulmonary support, death must be determined by tests of brain function.

In both situations, the determination of death must be made in accordance with accepted medical standards.[30]

By using the irreversible cessation of spontaneous circulatory and respiratory functions as a test for irreversible loss of whole-brain function, our proposed statute allows us to answer the question raised by Jonas, "Why are they alive if the heart, etc., works naturally but not alive when it works artificially?" Our proposed statute makes clear that spontaneous circulation and ventilation show that at least part of the brain continues to function, whereas artificial support does not show this. Thus, in the latter case one must directly test if the whole brain has permanently ceased to function.

Finally, our statute makes it explicit that it is the brain, not the heart and lungs, which is essential both for any clinically observable functioning of the organism as a whole, and for any part of the organism to be conscious. Our statute allows for new technological advances, such as a totally implantable artificial heart, which may continue to function after the entire brain has permanently ceased to function.

A statutory definition of death should include as a criterion of death only the irreversible cessation of total-brain functions, for only that criterion always satisfies the ordinary definition of death: *the permanent cessation of all clinically observable functioning of the organism as a whole and the permanent absence of consciousness in the organism as a whole and in any part of that organism.* Irreversible cessation of spontaneous ventilation and circulation can continue as the usual method for determining death, but this method should not be elevated to the status of a criterion of death. Rather, it should be explicitly noted that it is only the most common test for determining that the true criterion of death—irreversible, total cessation of whole-brain functioning—has been satisfied.

Conclusion

We have shown that the meaning of a common word like "death," which is an integral part of many social and legal practices, cannot be separated from its use in those practices. Attempts to use a better understanding of the biological facts concerning death to revise what is meant by "death" is based on a misunderstanding of how the meaning of such a word is determined. Although death is a biological phenomenon, it is not an esoteric event but one with which the vast majority of humanity has had experience. From prehistoric times until the end of humankind, death has been and will be a familiar experience. People have killed animals for food, children have seen their pets die, and wars, famine, and maladies have resulted in death for countless people. Throughout all of this time, there have been almost no problems in determining who had died and who was still living. There have been some problems; some people have been buried who were not yet dead, but only in a profound coma. However, these problems have been rare, and with increasing medical sophistication it has become possible to determine who is dead with 100% accuracy.

This increasing medical sophistication, however, has also brought with it pressure to determine the time of death with greater speed. This speed is desired, not merely to prevent pointless use of expensive medical treatment but, most importantly, to allow the harvesting of organs while they are in the best possible condition, thereby improving the chances for a successful transplant. This increasing medical sophistication and these goals also prompted a reconsideration of the concept of death. The medical sophistication made it impossible to determine death in the way that it had been usually determined throughout the history of humankind, by noting when the person stopped breathing and his heart stopped beating. Techniques and machines became available which could keep the person breathing and his heart beating. The goals made it desirable for a person to be declared dead even though these techniques and machines were maintaining breathing and heart function.

A closer examination of the concept of death makes it clear that the absence of breathing and heart function was historically such a reliable test of death because absence of breathing and absence of heart function inevitably lead to the permanent loss of functioning of the entire brain. The complete and permanent loss of whole-brain function inevitably results in the permanent cessation of all clinically observable functioning of the organism as a whole and the permanent absence of consciousness in the organism as a whole and in any part of that organism. It was this permanent cessation of functioning of the organism as a whole and the permanent absence of consciousness that was always understood, although not explicitly, as death. This may be seen by looking at stories in which either functioning of the organism as a whole or consciousness is present. In these cases, it is universally held that the person is not dead.

Not surprisingly, before it became clear what was meant by death, there was some disagreement about what should serve as the criterion of death, and what should serve as appropriate tests to determine that the criterion was satisfied. Prior to the advent of modern medicine, it was not necessary to distinguish clearly between the tests of death, the criterion of death, and the definition of death. If, for a significant period of time, a person stopped breathing and his heart stopped beating he was dead. But with the advent of modern medicine, with so many people dying in the hospital attached to so many machines, it became necessary to be more precise about what was meant by death. What is the medical criterion on the basis of which a person is declared dead? And what are the tests to determine that the criterion is satisfied? When the controversy concerning death started, there was more concentration on the criterion of death than on the definition of death. In fact, since the criterion of death was the legal definition of death, many were not always clear whether they were discussing the medical criterion of death or the definition of death. Thus, for a long time, it seemed as if people thought that providing a definition of death was a matter to be determined on medical grounds.

Only relatively recently was it recognized that an account of the ordinary meaning of the term "death" must be provided before one could settle on the appropriate criterion of death. For the criterion of death is that state of the organism on the basis of which medical personnel determine that the organism satisfies the definition of death, that is, is dead. The two main proposals for a definition of death were that death means the permanent loss of all features of personhood, namely, the permanent loss of consciousness, and that death means the permanent loss of the functioning of the organism as a whole. However, it is now clear that neither of these proposals, by themselves, is adequate and that the loss of both of these features is necessary for death.

Once this has been recognized, it is clear which of the various proposed criteria of death, permanent loss of functioning of (1) the cortex, (2) the brain stem, (3) the whole brain, and (4) heart and lung functioning, is correct. Only (3), the loss of whole-brain functioning, is perfectly correlated both with loss of functioning of the organism as a whole and with absence of consciousness. (4) turns out to be ambiguous, for it can mean either (4a) loss of spontaneous heart and lung functioning or (4b) loss of all heart and lung functioning, either spontaneous or artificially supported. (4a) can be used as a test when the person is not on a heart-lung machine, for then it is clear that the criterion must be satisfied, the whole brain has permanently stopped functioning. (4b) however, can not be used as a test, for even if a person does not meet this criterion, but continues to breathe and his heart continues to beat, but only because he is on a heart-lung machine, the criterion of death might still be satisfied, and he might still be dead.

Notes

1. For similar reasons, some physicians have adopted controversial tests of death in order to facilitate faster harvesting of organs. If there is the slightest chance that these tests would ever yield a false-positive, that is, would result in someone being declared dead who is not dead according to the accepted definition and criteria of death, these tests should not be allowed. We discuss the criterion and tests of death later in this chapter.

2. Linda L. Emmanuel, "Reexamining Death: The Asymptotic Model and a Bounded Zone Definition," *Hastings Center Report,* 25 (1995), p. 27.

3. Ibid.

4. Charles M. Culver and Bernard Gert, *Philosophy in Medicine*, Japanese ed., translated by Masakatsu Okada and eight others (Tokyo: Hokuju Shuppan Co., 1984).

5. Emmanuel, op cit.

6. See Chapter 12, "Euthanasia," for a discussion of a proposal for dealing with those in a persistent vegetative state.

7. "Death" can be applied in a metaphorical way to companies, projects, feelings, and so forth, but almost everyone recognizes that this is not using "dead" in the basic or literal sense.

8. See, R. J. White, L. R. Wolin, L. Masopust, N. Taslitz, and J. Verdura, "Cephalic Exchange Transplantation in the Monkey" *Surgery* 70 (1971), pp. 135–139, and B. O'Shea, "Brain Transplants: Myth or Monster?" *British Journal of Psychiatry,* 157 (1990), p. 302.

9. See Bernard Gert, "Can the Brain Have a Pain?" *Philosophy and Phenomenological Research* 27 (1967), pp. 432–436, and Gert, "Personal Identity and the Body," *Dialogue,* 10 (1971), pp. 458–478.

10. See *Morality,* Chapter 2, pp. 29, 30.

11. Parts of the "Definitions, Criteria, and Tests" section of this chapter are adapted from Bernat, Culver, and Gert (1981).

12. Patients who have been determined by the laboratory to still have some functioning neuroendocrine cells have been declared dead and will continue to be declared dead and this is completely appropriate. It is not necessary to perform tests on patients to see if there are any functioning cells remaining before they are declared dead as long as it is certain that they have permanently ceased all clinically observable functions of the organism as a whole.

13. See Bernard Gert, "Personal Identity and the Body," *Dialogue,* 10 (1971), pp. 458–478.

14. Establishing a criterion for consciousness is very difficult, however normal human social behavior is a paradigm of conscious behavior and any animal behavior that is sufficiently similar is usually regarded as manifesting consciousness, for example, social behavior among mammals. A prototype of consciousness is a display of a learned response to artificial stimuli, such as a dog sitting up in response to the word-sound "beg." An even clearer criterion is the restraining of a natural response because of learning, such as a dog not attacking another dog because of the word-sound "stay."

15. See note 8.

16. This point was anticipated by Stuart J. Youngner and Edward T. Bartlett in two articles "Human Death and High Technology: The Failure of the Whole-Brain Formulations," *Annals of Internal Medicine* 98 (1983), pp. 252–258, and "Human Death and the Destruction of the Neocortex," *Death: Beyond Whole-Brain Criteria,* edited by Richard M. Zaner (Kluwer Academic Publishers: Dordrecht, The Netherlands, 1988), pp. 199–216.

17. *Philosophy in Medicine,* p. 182.

18. Ibid.

19. Ibid.

20. B. Jennett and F. Plum, "Persistent Vegetative State after Brain Damage: A Syndrome in Search of a Name," *Lancet,* 1 (1972), pp. 734–737.

21. "Multi-Society Task Force on PVS: Medical Aspects of the Persistent Vegetative State," Parts 1 and 2, *New England Journal of Medicine,* 330 (1994), pp. 1499–1508 and pp. 1572–1579.

22. See George Orwell, *Animal Farm, 1984,* and "Politics and the English Language."

23. As we understand the concept of a person, it is at least partly historical. If an organism was a person, it remains a person as long as there is any possibility of any future consciousness. This means that any actual consciousness, even if it is only of pain, entails that the patient remains a person and must be treated as such.

24. See Chapter 12, "Euthanasia," for a more detailed account of our proposal for dealing with patients in a persistent vegetative state who have not filled out an Advance Directive.

25. See James L. Bernat, *Ethical Issues in Neurology* (Boston: Butterworth-Heinemann, 1994), pp. 138–139, note 14.

26. See ibid., pp. 121–122.

27. See ibid., p. 118.

28. Report of the Medical Consultants on the Diagnoses of Death to the President's Commission for the Study of Ethical Problems in Medicine and Biomedical and Behavioral Research. "Guidelines for the Determination of Death," *JAMA*, 246 (1981): 2184–2186.

29. Ibid.

30. This statute is similar to one proposed by the Law Reform Commission of Canada (1979).

References

American Bar Association. "House of Delegates Redefines Death, Urges Redefinition of Rape, and Undoes the Houston Amendments," *American Bar Association Journal,* 61 (1975): 463–464.

Beecher, Henry K. "A Definition of Irreversible Coma: Report of the Ad Hoc Committee of the Harvard Medical School to Examine the Definition of Brain Death," *JAMA,* 205 (1968): 337–340.

Beresford, H. Richard. "The Quinlan Decision: Problems and Legislative Alternatives. *Annals of Neurology,*" 2 (1977): 74–81.

Bernat, James L. *Ethical Issues in Neurology* (Newton, Mass.: Butterworth-Heinemann, 1994), esp. pp. 113–143.

Bernat, James L., Culver, Charles M., and Gert, Bernard. "On the Definition and Criterion of Death," *Annals of Internal Medicine,* 94 (1981): 389–394.

Black, Peter M. "Brain Death," *New England Journal of Medicine,* 299 (1978): 338–344, 393–401.

Brierley, J. B., Adams, J. H., Graham, D. I., and Simpson, J. A. Neocortical Death after Cardiac Arrest. *Lancet,* 2 (1971): 560–565.

Capron, Alexander M., and Kass, Leon R. "A Statutory Definition of the Standards for Determining Human Death: An Appraisal and a Proposal," *University of Pennsylvania Law Review,* 121 (1972): 87–118.

Culver, Charles M., and Gert, Bernard. *Philosophy in Medicine* (New York: Oxford University Press), 1982.

Emmanuel, Linda L. "Reexamining Death: The Asymptotic Model and a Bounded Zone Definition," *Hastings Center Report,* Vol. 25, No. 4 (July–August 1995).

Gert, Bernard. "Can the Brain Have a Pain?" *Philosophy and Phenomenological Research,* 27 (1967): 432–436.

Gert, Bernard. "Personal Identity and the Body." *Dialogue,* 10 (1971): 458–478.

Hastings Center Task Force on Death and Dying. "Refinements in Criteria for the Determination of Death: An Appraisal." *JAMA,* 221 (1972): 48–53.

Ingvar, David H., Brun, Arne, Johansson, Lars, and Sammuelsson, Sven M. "Survival after Severe Cerebral Anoxia with Destruction of the Cerebral Cortex: The Apallic Syndrome," *Annals of the New York Academy of Science,* 315 (1978): 184–214.

Jennett, B., and Plum, F. "Persistent Vegetative State after Brain Damage: A Syndrome in Search of a Name," *Lancet,* 1 (1972): 734–737.

Jonas, Hans. *Philosophical Essays: From Ancient Creed to Technological Man* (Englewood Cliffs, N.J.: Prentice-Hall, 1974), pp. 134–140.

Law Reform Commission of Canada. *Criteria for the Determination of Death* (Ottawa: Law Reform Commission of Canada), 1979.

Molinari, Gaetano F. "Review of Clinical Criteria of Brain Death," *Annals of the New York Academy of Science,* 315 (1978): 62–69.

Morison, Robert S. "Death: Process or Event?" *Science,* 173 (1971): 694–698.

NIH Collaborative Study of Cerebral Survival. "An Appraisal of the Criteria of Cerebral Death: A Summary Statement." *JAMA,* 237 (1977): 982–986.

Veatch, Robert M. *Death, Dying and the Biological Revolution: Our Last Quest for Responsibility* (New Haven, Conn.: Yale University Press, 1976).

Veith, Frank J., Fein, Jack M., Tendler, Moses D., Veatch, Robert M., Kleiman, Marc A., and Kalkines, George. "Brain Death I: A Status Report of Medical and Ethical Considerations," *JAMA,* 238 (1977): 1651–1655.

Veith, Frank J., Fein, Jack M., Tendler, Moses D., Veatch, Robert M., Kleiman, Marc A., and Kalkines, George. "Brain Death II. A Status Report of Legal Considerations," *JAMA,* 238 (1977): 1744–1748.

12

Euthanasia

A Moral Dilemma for Physicians

In the developed countries the benefits of public health measures and new drugs had, until the AIDS epidemic, dramatically reduced deaths due to infectious disease. This has resulted in a significant increase in the number of older people suffering from chronic diseases which are often progressive, incapacitating, and terminal. Ironically, AIDS is, in these respects, very similar to the chronic diseases of the elderly, and what we say about elderly patients also applies to patients with AIDS. Patients with terminal illnesses which are accompanied by considerable pain and suffering often do not wish their disease to be treated aggressively. All want the pain and suffering to be minimized, but many, at least at some stage, do not want their life prolonged. In fact, many actually want their life shortened; they want to die sooner than they would if they simply waited for the disease to run its natural course.

This has put a considerable burden on physicians, whose culture, tradition, and instincts are devoted to the prolonging of life, not to the shortening of it. Of course, physicians also consider their profession to be devoted to the relieving of pain and suffering, but in the past these two goals were not usually seen as conflicting with each other; treatments that relieved pain and suffering were also generally life preserving. The increase in the number of elderly patients with chronic diseases, for whom death is the only way to avoid significant pain and suffering, has increased the frequency of conflict between two of the acknowledged goals of medicine, prolonging life and relieving pain and suffering. Physicians faced with this conflict are often unsure how to respond in a morally acceptable way. If they stop treating a patient, they fear not only that they may be violating the rule against killing, but also that they will be violating what many take to be the most important duty of a physician, to preserve life. On the other hand, if they do not abide by the patient's wish to die, not only may they be depriving the patient of the freedom to make his own decision, they may also be violating another important duty of physicians, to relieve pain and suffering. This has created for many physicians what seems like an unresolvable moral dilemma.

In actual practice, far too many physicians do not provide sufficient relief for the pain and suffering of those who are suffering from chronic diseases or are terminally ill. Inadequate palliative care is one of the significant causes of patients seeking to die. We do not discuss the providing of adequate palliative care to those terminally ill patients who could benefit from it, for no philosophical discussion is necessary. Everyone agrees that such care should be provided, the only questions are practical ones, such as how one trains physicians to take the pain and suffering of terminally ill patients more seriously and to provide adequate palliative care. We think that if such care were universally provided, the question of euthanasia would be a far less pressing problem.[1] Further, we are concerned that some proposals under discussion, such as legalizing physician-assisted suicide and even active euthanasia, are likely to perpetuate the failure to provide adequate palliative care. Nonetheless, there still are some situations where palliative care is not sufficient and patients want to die sooner than they would if life-prolonging treatment were continued, or even sooner than they would if they simply waited for the disease to run its natural course. In these situations, providing palliative care does not resolve the doctor's dilemma.

Active and Passive Euthanasia

In order to help resolve this dilemma, a distinction has traditionally been made between active and passive euthanasia. Active euthanasia is considered killing and, even if requested by the patient, is prohibited by the American Medical Association. Passive euthanasia is considered "allowing to die" and, if requested by the patient, is permitted. The following are the standard ways of making the distinction between active and passive euthanasia: (1) acts versus omissions, (2) stopping treatment (withdrawing) versus not starting treatment (withholding), (3) ordinary care versus extraordinary care, and (4) whether the death is due to natural causes. However, none of these ways of making the distinction has any clear moral significance. It is worthwhile to show their inadequacies before presenting a morally significant way of distinguishing between active and passive euthanasia.

Our concern in this chapter is only with voluntary euthanasia, those cases in which a competent patient has explicitly expressed his rational desire to die. Euthanasia with regard to incompetent patients presents even more difficult problems, but we believe that until it is completely clear what to say about competent patients it will be impossible to become clear about incompetent patients. A clear example of euthanasia for incompetent patients being parasitic on euthanasia for competent patients is when the incompetent patient has an Advance Directive. Insofar as possible, the Advance Directive of the formerly competent patient should be followed just as if the patient were still competent. The most difficult cases are those of nonvoluntary euthanasia, in which the patient is permanently incompetent and has never expressed his desires on the matter. Later in this chapter, we suggest how to avoid some of these difficulties, and we propose a long-term procedure for dealing with the remaining problems.

The point of distinguishing between active and passive euthanasia is to help physicians resolve the moral dilemma caused by caring for patients for whom death seems the best way to relieve their pain and suffering. Many physicians believe it is morally unacceptable to kill a patient, even at a competent patient's rational request, and yet they recognize the futility of keeping a patient alive when the main result is pointless pain and suffering. They hope to resolve the dilemma by distinguishing between active and passive euthanasia, counting only the former as killing and the latter as only allowing to die. This distinction is intended to allow them to continue to hold that it is morally unacceptable to kill a patient, but at the same time to maintain that it may sometimes be morally acceptable to allow a patient to die. Immediately the question arises, is there a morally relevant distinction between killing and allowing to die, and if so, how should it be made?[2] Our examination of four standard ways of making this distinction: acts versus omissions, stopping versus not starting, ordinary care versus extraordinary care, and whether the death is due to natural causes, will show that none of them provide a way of making a morally relevant distinction between killing and allowing to die.

Acts versus Omissions

The philosophical distinction between acts and omissions initially seems a natural way to distinguish between killing and allowing to die. According to this approach, if a physician *does* something, that is, performs an action, such as injecting an overdose of morphine or turning off the respirator, that counts as active euthanasia; it is considered killing, and is prohibited. If the physician does nothing, but rather simply fails to do something—he does not turn on the respirator or does not provide essential antibiotics or does not do CPR—that is an omission; it counts as passive euthanasia, and is considered allowing to die, and is permitted. This way of distinguishing between killing and letting die requires that there be a significant moral distinction between a physician turning off an intravenous solution container (an act) and not replacing it when it is empty (an omission). Since it has not been shown that there is such a moral distinction (that is, that the act is morally prohibited, but omission is morally allowed), some have claimed that the standard medical and legal practice, which permits allowing to die and does not permit killing, should be given up.[3]

Further, the distinction between acts and omissions is a difficult one to make. Some acts do not even require any bodily movement at all—standing at attention, for example. How could such a subtle philosophical distinction be essential for making a fairly common moral decision? The discussion in Chapter 2 showed that morality is a public system that applies to all rational persons and hence must be understandable to all of them. The subtle distinction between acts and omissions is not well understood even by philosophers, hence it cannot be an essential feature of morality. Moreover, a physician has a duty to aid her patients, so that when prolonging life is at issue, the distinction between acts and omissions may not have any moral significance. If a physician has a duty to preserve her patient's life, then her failing to do so is clearly morally unacceptable, even if that failing is an omission on any plausible account of acts and omissions. No one would hold that a physician is morally allowed to neglect her duty if she does so by omissions rather than acts.[4]

Not Starting versus Stopping

Another proposal that has great appeal for some doctors is the distinction between not starting a treatment and stopping it (withholding a treatment and withdrawing it). These doctors maintain that if the patient does not want treatment, they do not have a duty to start it. But once treatment is started they have a duty to continue it if discontinuing it would lead to the patient's death. They are not required to force a patient to go on the respirator if the patient refuses, but once the patient has gone on the respirator, doctors have a duty to keep him on, even contrary to the patient's wishes, if taking him off would result in his death.

Accepting this way of making the distinction between active and passive euthanasia creates serious practical problems. Some physicians are hesitant to put seriously ill patients on the respirator if they think the patient has a poor prognosis and is likely to become respirator dependent. This hesitancy may be due to the prospect of being required to continue a pointless treatment which only prolongs the pain and suffering of the patient. One result is that a patient who has a very small but finite chance of recovering may sometimes not be put on the respirator because once put on he cannot be taken off. Thus this attempt to resolve the moral dilemma creates additional problems of its own.[5]

Further, it has not been shown that there is any morally significant difference between stopping a treatment and not starting it. Consider two patients who have been in an accident, identical twins with identical presenting diagnoses and prognoses. When they arrive at the hospital, everyone agrees that they are unlikely to survive. One twin is conscious and refuses to be put on the respirator, the other twin is put on the respirator while still unconscious. If one were to use the distinction between not starting and stopping to make the distinction between active and passive euthanasia, the second twin, if he becomes conscious several minutes after he is put on the respirator, cannot be taken off even if he requests it. This follows, even though, except for the fact that he is already on the respirator, he is identical to the twin who has refused to be put on. Both patients want to die and without the respirator both would die. Why should the fact that treatment has been started, perhaps mistakenly, make it morally wrong to stop it, when it would have been morally acceptable not to start it? It clearly is psychologically harder for a physician to withdraw treatment than withhold it, but recognition that there is no moral difference between withholding and withdrawing may help to ease the physician's psychological burden.

Ordinary Care versus Extraordinary Care

The next ad hoc attempt to explain the distinction between active and passive euthanasia employs the distinction between ordinary care and extraordinary care. If, given the condition of the patient and the facilities and resources available, the care counts as ordinary, according to this way of making the distinction, not only is a physician required to continue it, she is required to start it, as is the case of a course of antibiotics for an easily curable infection. However, if the care counts as extraordinary (difficult to obtain or very expensive), she is neither morally required to start it, nor is she morally required to continue it. A significant implication of this way of making the active-passive distinction is that it is almost always morally wrong not to provide food and fluids; providing food and fluids, in all normal situations, counts as ordinary care. On this account, the line between ordinary and extraordinary care not only changes over time, but may also be different in different places. Whether a treatment is ordinary or extraordinary is a function of the available level of technology, such as changes in the availability of dialysis machines and improvements in transplant surgery. Although it may have some moral significance, this way of distinguishing between ordinary and extraordinary treatment does not seem to distinguish between killing and allowing to die.[6]

The original way of making the ordinary and extraordinary distinction, namely, comparing the burden imposed on the patient with the benefit to be gained by him, has clear moral significance. If this comparison shows the burden to be "extraordinary," that is, much greater than the likely benefit, treatment can be stopped, or not started; if the burden is "ordinary," that is, small relative to the likely benefit, it cannot be. This interpretation raises the question: who determines if the burden is ordinary or extraordinary, the physician or the patient? If it is the physician, there is a great danger of unjustified paternalism. If it is the patient, then (as we argue below) when he is competent and his decision is not irrational, what he says determines the matter. If he chooses to die rather than continue with treatment, it is morally unacceptable to continue whether the burden is ordinary or extraordinary. However, suppose the patient determines that simply continuing to live is an extraordinary burden and requests the physician to shorten his time of living, what should the physician do? The ordinary-extraordinary distinction, no matter how it is made, does not provide an answer to this question.

Whether Death Is Due to Natural Causes

Euthanasia is sometimes regarded as passive if death is due to natural causes. Thus stopping or not starting a course of antibiotics is often regarded as passive euthanasia, because the patient's death is due to his infection, a natural cause. On the other hand, providing a patient with pills that will kill him, or more clearly, injecting the patient with some drug that kills him, is active euthanasia, for the patient's death is not due to natural causes, but rather to the physician injecting a drug. Because in stopping or not starting a course of antibiotics, the death is caused by the disease process, no person is assigned responsibility for the death. This freedom from responsibility for the patient's death is psychologically helpful for the physician. To make some state laws authorizing Advance Directives more acceptable to the public and to physicians they have even been labeled "natural death acts."

When death results from lack of food and fluids, however, it is less plausible to say that the death is due to natural causes. Thus, someone must be assigned responsibility for the patient's death, and many physicians wish to avoid this responsibility. A partial explanation for the overuse of technology to unjustifiably prolong dying may be an attempt by physicians to avoid responsibility for a patient's death. But if the refusal of food and fluids is rational and made by a competent patient, then the patient is responsible for his own death. Physicians who recognize that patients have the authority to refuse any treatment, including hydration and nutrition, are more likely to avoid unjustified feelings of responsibility for their deaths.[7] However, even holding a patient responsible for his own death is more troubling than assigning the responsibility to natural causes such as the underlying disease process. It is far easier to view stopping or not starting the respirator as allowing the underlying disease process to take its course. Withholding or withdrawing food and fluids creates a new malady, malnutrition, which becomes the cause of death. Thus, withholding or with-drawing food and fluids has been regarded by some as more like killing than stopping or not starting a specific life-prolonging treatment.[8]

If one accepts the view that passive euthanasia requires that the death be due to natural causes, but nevertheless regards allowing patients to refuse food and fluids as morally acceptable, one must take advantage of the fact that the term "natural" is open to many interpretations. To reconcile these two positions one must hold the view that patients can refuse intravenous feeding tubes because they are not natural, and the patient is dying from his inability to eat or drink in a natural way. However, this interpretation has the disturbing implication that patients who can eat and drink in the natural way are not allowed to refuse food and fluids, even if they are competent and their refusals are rational.

"Natural" is often used as a word of praise, or more generally, as a way of condoning something that otherwise might be considered unacceptable.[9] How-ever, the condoning or condemning of something is not, in fact, determined by whether it is natural; rather, if it is condemned it is often called unnatural, and if it is condoned, it is labeled natural. But, just as it is erroneous to think that the distinction between acts and omissions has any moral relevance, it is also erroneous to think that anything morally significant turns on the use of the term "natural" or the phrase "due to natural causes." If a competent patient has rationally refused food and fluids, we will argue below that it is morally and legally unacceptable to overrule that refusal, whether or not the food and fluids is administered in a natural way, or only intravenously.

Using the Common Moral System

The above four ad hoc distinctions mistakenly focus on what the physician does or does not do, or with the medical context in which the physician acts or does not act, but they do not adequately consider the decisions of the patient. It is the failure to appreciate the moral significance of the kind of decision the patient makes (that is, whether it is a request or a refusal) that leads to the mistaken conclusion that there is no morally significant distinction between active and passive euthanasia. A careful investigation of the duties of physicians is neces-sary before one can resolve the moral dilemma caused by patients who believe that death is the best way to relieve their pain and suffering. Clarifying the duties of physicians requires using the standard medical distinction between requests and refusals. Overlooking this distinction makes it impossible to solve this dilemma.

First, a terminological matter needs to be clarified. In the earlier sections of this chapter, we ourselves have used the term "request" when we were talking about refusals. It is perfectly standard English to say, as we did, that a patient requests that a treatment be stopped (for example, that she be taken off of a respirator), when one is actually talking about refusals (the patient is in fact refusing continued use of the respirator). Unfortunately, this perfectly correct and common way of talking obscures the crucial distinction between refusals and requests. When combined with the use of the terms "choice" and "decision" to cover both requests and refusals, it fosters the false conclusion that all patient decisions or choices, whether refusals or requests, generate the same obligation on physicians.

This confusion is compounded because the most common use of the terms "decision" and "choice" with regard to a patient involves neither refusals nor requests, but rather the patient's picking one of the options that her physician has presented to her. However, when dealing with patients who want to die, this most common use of "decision" or "choice" is not relevant. Rather a patient is either (1) refusing treatment, or (2) requesting the physician to kill her (voluntary active euthanasia), or (3) requesting the physician to provide the medical means for the patient to kill herself (physician-assisted suicide). Thus talking of a patient's decision or choice to die can be extremely misleading. Refusals of treatment and requests for treatment, whether or not death is a foreseeable result, are very different in their moral and legal implications.[10]

Physicians, as mentioned above, are troubled because they seem to have two irreconcilable duties, (1) to prolong the lives of their patients and (2) to relieve their pain and suffering. Further, even if they do not believe that they always have a duty to prolong the lives of their patients, they still have a dilemma, for it seems to some physicians that the only way to relieve the pain and suffering of some of their patients is to kill them; but many of these physicians think that it is completely inappropriate for physicians to kill. In order to resolve this dilemma the duties of physicians must first be determined. Then a morally significant way to make the distinction between active and passive euthanasia, or between killing and allowing to die, must be provided. The moral acceptability of helping to die (physician-assisted suicide), a practice which is more controversial than allowing to die, but less controversial than killing, must also be considered.

The Duties of Physicians

It is important to determine what the duties of physicians are, because, since there is a moral rule which requires doing one's duty, neglecting one's duties needs to be morally justified. How does one determine what the duties of physicians are? Partly by sociological investigation of the society in which the physicians are practicing their profession. It cannot be assumed that physicians in every country have exactly the same duties, though substantial similarities should be expected. The duties that are involved in any job or profession are largely determined by the function of that job or profession in the society. The function of medicine is similar in every society, so one would expect physicians in all societies to have similar duties. Some differences in the relative importance of different duties, however, should also be expected; for example, some societies place greater weight on duties to the individual patient while others place greater weight on duties to protect the health of the society as a whole.

However, the concept of duty is not completely equivalent to "what one is required to do by one's job or profession," so that sociological investigation of a society does not completely determine what one's duties are. Duties must be compatible with what an impartial rational person can publicly allow. If no impartial rational person can advocate that a given kind of violation be publicly allowed, having a job or belonging to a profession cannot provide a duty to perform that violation. A "professional" pickpocket does not have a duty to steal, even if he is being paid to do so by his employer. Indeed, it is hard even to imagine a profession in which there is a duty to do what is morally unacceptable, although there are some who mistakenly view lawyers as sometimes having a duty to act in a morally unacceptable way if it is necessary to defend their clients. Showing that what some have claimed that doctors have a duty to do is a kind of action that involves an unjustified violation of a moral rule, shows that physicians do not have a duty to do that kind of action. Thus, it may be possible to rule out as mistaken some claims about the duties of physicians without even doing any sociological investigations. (See Chapter 3, "Application," for further discussion.)

Paternalism and Patient Refusal

Physicians often violate the moral rule against causing pain with regard to their patients, for many treatments involve causing some pain. In most of these cases, however, the physicians are not only acting so as to prevent greater pain, or to prevent death, they are doing so with the valid consent of their patients. The patient usually has a rational desire that the physician cause him pain, for he prefers to have that pain inflicted rather than suffer the harms that he would suffer if the doctor did not administer the painful treatment. Causing pain to a patient with his valid consent in order to prevent greater harms or to promote compensating benefits is strongly justified; all impartial rational persons would advocate that such violations be publicly allowed. This explains why it is morally significant to obtain valid consent, that is, uncoerced consent by a competent patient who has been given adequate information. Having valid consent makes most medical treatments morally unproblematic (see Chapter 7, "Consent," for further discussion.)

Some patients prefer to suffer the harms that are likely to come from not being treated to the harms of being treated. If they do not fully understand the extent of the harms that they will suffer without treatment, then, of course, the physician has a duty to inform them of the consequences of not being treated. Sometimes, however, a patient, who does fully understand, ranks the harms of treatment as worse than the harms of not being treated, and so does not want to be treated.[11] Suppose the physician who has suggested the treatment ranks the harms differently. Whose ranking should determine whether the patient should be treated? Assuming that the physician's rankings are rational, there are two possibilities: (1) the patient's rankings are also rational, and (2) the patient's rankings are irrational. We have already pointed out that rational persons can rank the harms differently, so it should not be surprising that two rational persons can disagree on whether to undergo a given treatment.

Suppose the patient's rankings are both informed and rational. Would any rational person publicly allow a violation of the moral rule against causing pain when the person toward whom the rule is being violated rationally desires that it not be violated? Does it make any difference that the person doing the violating would want the rule violated with regard to herself, given the same harms being caused, avoided, and prevented? An indication of the morally misleading character of the Golden Rule, "Do unto others as you would have them do unto you," is that it allows an interpretation that advises violating a moral rule in these circumstances. If a patient is fully informed, and it is rational, that is, rationally allowed, to prefer the harms of not being treated to the harms of being treated, then in all normal cases, it is irrelevant what anyone else's preferences are, including those of family members or the physician; the patient's refusal should not be overruled. However, if it is clear that, given the values of the person refusing the treatment, it would be unreasonable for him to prefer no treatment to forced treatment, then rational persons may favor publicly allowing that kind of violation. No impartial rational person would advocate that the violation of a moral rule be publicly allowed when the victim of the violation has a rational desire that it not be violated and there are no other countervailing morally relevant facts. This was shown in more detail in Chapter 9, "Justification."

If the rankings of the patient are irrational, is it still true that all impartial rational persons would advocate that physicians be prohibited from forcing treatment? This depends upon how seriously irrational the rankings are. If the balance of the harms of not being treated versus the harms of being treated is such that if the loss of freedom is added to the harms of being treated it would no longer be irrational to prefer not being treated, it still seems as if no impartial rational persons would advocate that such a violation be publicly allowed. (Especially when it is appreciated that the harms of treatment are certain, whereas the benefits of treatment are usually only probable.) To allow such a violation would be to advocate that a violation of the rules be publicly allowed without the consent of the person, when the harm to be avoided or prevented by the violation is no greater than the harm to be caused. No impartial rational person would favor publicly allowing overruling an irrational treatment refusal in those cases in which, when the deprivation of freedom is added to the harms of treatment, it would be rational to rank the total harm as worse than the harms of nontreatment. Publicly allowing such overruling would increase the chances of people suffering unwanted violations of the rules without any decrease in the amount of harm being suffered.

Finally, let us suppose that the rankings of the patient are so seriously irrational that even if one adds the loss of freedom that results from having one's decision overruled it would still be irrational to prefer the harms of not being treated to the harms of being treated. Then, at least some impartial rational persons would favor that kind of violation being publicly allowed, and so it would be at least weakly justified. It may not be strongly justified, for if the difference between the harms caused and the harms prevented is not great, then one might hold that publicly allowing such violations would result in enough mistakes and abuses that more overall harm would be suffered if that kind of violation were publicly allowed. However, if the harms prevented are serious enough and the harms caused trivial enough, all rational persons would favor that kind of violation being publicly allowed, and it would be strongly justified. In these kinds of cases, not only is the desire not to have treatment irrational, there is also no doubt that less harm will be suffered because of the violation, even if everyone knows such violations are allowed.

For the overruling of a refusal to be even weakly justified, the harms to be avoided or prevented by the violation must be serious. If the loss of freedom suffered from having one's refusal overruled counts as a greater harm than the harm that would be prevented or relieved, then that harm is a minor harm and forcing treatment to prevent this kind of minor harm would never be publicly allowed. However, often there is disagreement about the seriousness of the harms caused and the harms prevented, even when all agree the patient's refusal is irrational. When there is disagreement over whether, on the patient's rational rankings, the harms caused to him by overruling are greater then the harms that would be prevented by the treatment, it seems that overruling the refusal cannot be justified. It should be noted that the conclusions reached in this section simply exemplify the points made in our earlier general discussion of the justification of paternalism. Contrary to the popular practice, we are not presenting an ad hoc discussion of when one should abide by a patient's refusal of treatment, including life-sustaining treatment, but rather are showing how our systematic account of rationality and morality informs and clarifies this discussion.

Refusal of Treatment and the Duties of a Physician

Overruling a competent informed patient's rational refusal of treatment, including life-preserving treatment, always involves depriving the patient of freedom, and usually involves causing him pain. We have just shown that no impartial person would advocate that these kinds of paternalistic violations of moral rules be publicly allowed. Since it is morally prohibited to overrule the rational refusal of a competent informed patient, it cannot be the duty of a physician to do so, for no one can have a duty to do what is morally unacceptable. Theoretically, the situation does not change when lack of treatment will result in the patient's death, but as a practical matter, it does make a difference. Death is such a serious harm that it is never irrational to choose any other harm in order to avoid death. Even though it is sometimes rational to choose death over other harms, choosing death may be, and often is, irrational. People are usually ambivalent about choosing death, often changing their minds several times, but death is permanent, and once it occurs no further change of mind is possible.

The seriousness of death requires physicians to make certain that patients recognize that death will result from lack of treatment. It also requires physicians to make sure that the harms patients are suffering cannot be relieved by adequate palliative care and that a patient's continuing suffering is sufficient to make it rational for him to prefer death to continuing to live. The physician also must make sure that patients' desires to die, and hence their requests to die, are not merely the result of a treatable depression. When patients are suffering from terminal diseases, however, it is generally the case that when they want to die, it is rational for them to choose death.[12] Further, although there is often some ambivalence, in our experience their desire to die usually remains their dominant desire. When a competent informed patient makes a rational decision to stop life-prolonging treatment, a physician cannot have a duty to overrule his refusal of treatment, even though treating him counts as trying to prevent his death.

We have shown that physicians cannot have a duty to preserve the lives of their competent patients when those patients want to die and their desires are informed and rational. When following the moral ideal of preserving life requires unjustifiably violating a moral rule, following the ideal is not only not morally good, it is morally unacceptable to do so. We have thus established that physicians do not and cannot have a duty to prolong the lives of their patients when their patients have a rational desire to die. We are not suggesting that whenever a patient with a terminal disease makes any tentative suggestion that treatment be stopped, the physician should, with no question, immediately do so. It is part of the duty of a physician to make sure both that the refusal is rational and that it is the informed and considered preference of the patient. When, however, it is clear that a patient really does want to die and the refusal is rational, then the physician is morally prohibited from treating him.

Killing versus Allowing to Die

Having shown that a physician does not have a duty to prolong the lives of patients who rationally prefer to die, the next issue to be settled is whether not treating such patients counts as killing them. If it does count as killing them, then the conclusions of the previous section may have to be revised. In the previous section not treating was taken as simply failing to follow the moral ideal of prolonging life in the circumstances of a competent patient's rational refusal. Following this moral ideal in these circumstances does not justify breaking the moral rule against depriving of freedom. However, if not treating is killing, then not treating must itself be justified, for it involves killing, perhaps the most serious violation of a moral rule.

Not treating is sometimes correctly regarded as killing. If a physician turns off the respirator of a competent patient who does not want to die, with the result that the patient dies, the physician has killed him. The same is true if the physician discontinues antibiotics or food and fluids, and it may sometimes count as killing if the physician refuses to start any of these treatments for his patient, when the patient wants the treatment and there is no medical reason for not starting it. Just as parents whose children die because of not being fed can be regarded as having killed their children, physicians who have a duty to provide life-saving treatment for their patients can be regarded as killing them if they do not provide that treatment. However, we have shown that a physician does not have a duty to provide life-saving treatment when a competent patient rationally refuses such treatment. Not treating counts as killing only when there is a duty to treat; in the absence of such a duty, not treating does not count as killing.[13]

If the patient refuses treatment and there is no duty to treat, then it does not make any moral difference whether the physician stops treating by an act, such as turning off the respirator, or an omission, such as not giving antibiotics. It also makes no moral difference whether the physician stops some treatment that has already started, like turning off the respirator or discontinuing antibiotics, or simply does not start such treatment. Granted that it may be psychologically easier to omit rather than act, and not to start than to stop, nevertheless there is no moral difference between these different ways of abiding by a patient's refusal. Similarly, it makes no moral difference whether the treatment is extraordinary, involving some elaborate technology, say, or is quite ordinary, like simply providing food and fluids; nor does it make a moral difference whether the death is due to natural causes. If there is no duty to treat, not treating is not killing. If a competent patient rationally refuses treatment, there is no duty to treat. Therefore, if a competent patient rationally refuses treatment, abiding by that refusal is not killing. Further, since the refusal is rational, it is, in fact, morally prohibited to override the patient's refusal by treating, and to do so is an unjustified deprivation of the patient's freedom.

Stopping Food and Fluids

It might be objected that the analysis given above does not apply to providing food and fluids, because providing food and fluids is not a treatment, so failing to provide food and fluids is not merely not treating, it is killing. As noted before, children who die because their parents did not feed them are correctly regarded as having been killed by their parents. Similarly, it may be objected, patients who die because their physicians do not provide them with food and fluids are killed by them. This objection is based on the mistaken view that anything in the above analysis depends upon the concept of treatment. Parents have a duty to feed their children, that is why it counts as killing if they do not feed them. Physicians have no duty to overrule rational refusals by competent patients, so their not doing anything to prolong the life of these patients, including providing them with food and fluids, does not count as killing. When a patient wants not to be kept alive and it is rational to want not to be kept alive, then it is morally required that his physician not force him to keep living, but his physician should continue to provide comfort and palliative care.

Since the point of dying sooner is to avoid the pain and suffering of a terminal illness, stopping only food and continuing fluids is not a good method of dying because it takes a long time, sometimes a month or more. However, when fluids are also stopped, dying is much quicker, usually unconsciousness occurs within a week, and death about a week later. Further, contrary to what is widely assumed, dying because of lack of food and fluids is not painful, if there is even minimal palliative care.[14] When there is no medical treatment which is keeping the patient alive, stopping food and fluids may sometimes be the only way of allowing a patient to die. It is usually painless; it takes long enough for the patient to have the opportunity to change his mind, but is short enough that significant relief from pain and suffering is gained. Recognition that abiding by the rational refusal of treatment, or even of food and fluids, is not killing, but, at most, allowing to die, solves most of the practical problems with passive euthanasia that have led many to recommend legalizing physician-assisted suicide or active euthanasia.

Analysis of Killing

It may be thought that, if abiding by a competent patient's rational refusal of treatment requires the physician to perform some identifiable act, like turning off a respirator, which is the act that causes the patient's death, then regardless of what was said before, the doctor has killed the patient. This seems to have the support of the Oxford English Dictionary, which says that to kill is simply to deprive of life. That the doctor is morally and legally required to turn off the respirator, one could argue, may justify her killing the patient, but it does not mean that she has not killed him. Even those who accept the death penalty, and hold that some prison official is morally and legally required to execute the prisoner, do not deny that the official has killed the prisoner. Killing in self defense is both morally and legally allowed, yet no one denies that it is still killing. Similarly, one could agree that the doctor is doing nothing morally or legally unacceptable by turning off the respirator, even that the doctor is morally and legally required to turn off the respirator, yet claim that in doing so the doctor is killing the patient.

If one accepts this analysis, then it might also seem plausible to say that an identifiable decision to omit a life-prolonging treatment, even if such an omission is morally and legally required, also counts as killing the patient. Why not simply stipulate that doctors are sometimes morally and legally required to kill their patients, namely, when their action or omission is the result of a competent patient rationally refusing to start or to continue a life-prolonging treatment? Isn't the important point that the doctor is morally and legally required to act as she does, not whether what she does is appropriately called killing? However, having a too simple account of killing could cause numerous problems. Although whether a doctor's abiding by a rational refusal counts as killing is not as important as whether she is morally and legally required to so abide, it is still significant whether such an action should be regarded as killing.

Many doctors do not want to regard themselves as killing their patients, even justifiably killing them. More important, all killing requires a justification or an excuse and, if all the morally relevant features are the same, the justification or excuse that is adequate for one way of killing will be adequate for all other ways of killing as well.[15] Thus, if that justification is not publicly allowed by all for other ways of killing (for example, injecting a lethal dose of morphine), then it will not be publicly allowed by all for this way of killing (disconnecting the patient from the respirator). This means that it might be justifiable to prohibit physicians from abiding by the rational refusals of life-sustaining treatments of competent patients. Since even advocates of active euthanasia do not propose that doctors should ever be morally and legally required to kill their patients, even justifiably, doctors would not be required to abide by rational refusals of treatment by competent patients. Unless one favors such restrictions on patients' ability to hasten their death by refusing, changing the way killing is understood (that is, counting abiding by a patient's rational refusal as killing) would have significant risks.

Those who favor legalizing active euthanasia do not want to require doctors to kill their patients; they merely want to allow those doctors who are willing to kill, to do so. Similarly for physician-assisted suicide; no one suggests that a doctor be required to comply with a patient's request for a prescription for lethal pills. Since doctors are morally and legally required to abide by a competent patient's rational refusal of life-sustaining treatment, abiding by such a refusal is not regarded as killing. Providing a patient who refuses life-sustaining treatment with palliative care is not controversial either. Although some physicians feel uncomfortable doing so, no one wants to prohibit such palliative care. Neither killing a competent patient on his rational request nor assisting him to commit suicide are morally uncontroversial, and no one claims that doctors are morally and legally required to do either. Thus it is clear that abiding by a competent patient's rational refusal of treatment is not normally regarded as killing, nor does providing palliative care to such a patient count as assisting suicide.

Part of the problem is that insufficient attention is paid to the way in which the term "kill" is actually used. Killing is not as simple a concept as it is often taken to be. Killing is causing death, but what counts as causing any harm is a complex matter.[16] If the harm that results from one's action, or omission, needs to be justified or excused, then one is regarded as having caused that harm. Of course, causing harm often can be completely justified or excused, so that one can cause a harm and be completely free of any unfavorable moral judgment. So killing, taken as causing death, may be completely justified, perhaps even morally required. Nonetheless, it is important to distinguish these morally justifiable acts of killing from those acts that need no justification or excuse although they result in a person's death, that is, from acts that are not acts which kill the person or cause his death.

Of course, if one intends one's act to result in someone's death, then performing the act which has this result is to cause the person's death or to kill him, for such acts need justification. Also, if the act which results in death is also a violation of one of the second five moral rules, knowingly performing the act, or omission, needs justification and so counts as killing. That is why when a child dies because her parents did not feed her, they have killed her, for parents have a duty to feed their children. This is also why it was important to make clear that doctors have no duty to treat, or even feed, patients who refuse treatment. However, if one does not intend, but only knows, that one's act will result in someone's death, and the act is not a violation of one of the other moral rules, then performing the act which has this result may not be to cause the person's death or to kill him.[17]

When a doctor abides by the rational refusal of a competent patient, she is normally not only not violating any of the second five moral rules, she is not intentionally violating any moral rule. The doctor's intention is to abide by the patient's refusal, even though she knows that the result of her doing so will be that the patient dies. Even if the doctor agrees that it is best for the patient to die, her abiding by that refusal does not count as intentionally causing his death. Of course, an individual doctor can want the patient to die, but one's intention in these circumstances is not determined by what is going on in the doctor's head. Rather, the intention is determined by what facts account for the doctor's action. If she would cease treatment even if she did not want the patient to die, and would not cease it if the patient had not refused such treatment, then her intention is not to kill the patient but to abide by the patient's refusal. Most doctors do not want to kill their patients, even if such an action were morally and legally justified, and so their intention is not to kill the patient, but simply to abide by their patient's rational refusals.[18]

Whether or not an act or omission which, not intentionally but only knowingly, results in someone's death, and does not involve a violation of one of the second five moral rules, counts as killing depends on whether those in the society regard such acts as needing a justification or an excuse.[19] In our society at the present time, doctors do not need a justification or excuse to abide by a competent patient's rational refusal even if everyone knows that such an act will result in the patient's death. It is sufficient for a doctor to say that he was abiding by a competent patient's rational refusal, thus it is not usually considered killing for a doctor to abide by such a refusal.[20] In our society at the present time, it is considered killing for a doctor to grant a competent patient's rational request to do something which will immediately result in the patient's death. Few who favor active euthanasia argue that such actions are not killings; rather, many argue that passive euthanasia, abiding by patients' refusals, is also killing, and since it is allowed, active euthanasia should also be allowed. Thus they accuse, as philosophers are wont to do, people of being inconsistent in allowing, or even requiring passive euthanasia, but not allowing active euthanasia or even assisting suicide.[21]

That our society does not regard the death resulting from abiding by a competent patient's rational refusal, even a refusal of food and fluids, as killing, is shown by the fact that almost all states have Advance Directives that explicitly require a physician to stop treatment, even food and fluids, if the patient has the appropriate Advance Directive. All of them also allow a presently competent patient to refuse treatment and food and fluids. None of these states allow a physician to kill a patient, no matter what the circumstances. Most of these states do not even allow physicians to assist suicide, which strongly suggests that turning off a respirator is not regarded as killing or even as assisting suicide, when doing so is required by the rational refusal of a competent patient.

Abiding by a competent patient's rational refusal of treatment is not killing or assisting suicide, and it may even be misleading to say that the physician allows the patient to die. To talk of the physician allowing the patient to die suggests that the physician has a choice, that it is up to her to decide whether or not to save the patient's life. When a competent patient has rationally refused treatment, however, the physician has no choice. She is morally and legally prohibited from overruling the patient's refusal. She allows the patient to die only in the sense that it is physically possible for her to save the patient and she does not. Abiding by the rational refusal of lifesaving treatment by a competent patient does not violate any moral rule. Overruling such a refusal is itself an unjustified violation of the moral rule against depriving of freedom. Thus it is not merely morally acceptable to abide by such a refusal, it is morally required. It does not make any moral difference whether abiding by that refusal involves an act or an omission, stopping treatment or not starting it, whether the treatment is ordinary or extraordinary, or whether it results in a death from natural causes. If abiding by a competent patient's rational refusal of treatment, or of food and fluids, were all that was involved there would be no further problems to resolve. However, it is normally the case that the doctor must also provide palliative care at the same time, and this creates a new problem.

Physician Assisted Suicide

Showing that it is morally and legally prohibited to overrule competent patients' rational refusals of treatment, or even of food and fluids, does not solve the practical problem that doctors often face. For almost always, refusal of treatment, including refusal of food and fluids, involves some pain and suffering if it is not accompanied by appropriate palliative care. Doctors are not morally and legally required to provide that palliative care. If a doctor does not wish to provide palliative care to a patient who has refused life-prolonging treatment, she is not required to do so. This distinction, that doctors are required to abide by a competent patient's refusal but are not required to provide palliative care, was made quite clearly in the Elizabeth Bouvia case. This woman, who was suffering from a severe case of cerebral palsy and very crippling degenerative arthritis, wanted to stay in the hospital and be given palliative treatment while she was refusing food and fluids. Her doctors wanted to force her to take food and fluids. The court decided, correctly, that her doctors could not force her to take food and fluids, but that she could not force her doctors to keep her in the hospital and provide palliative care.

We believe that if the patient is competent and the request is rational, it would be justifiably acting on a moral ideal to help relieve the preventable pain and suffering of a patient who is refusing life-prolonging treatment. Providing such palliative care is neither killing, nor even assisting suicide, but acting on one of the primary goals of medicine, to relieve pain and suffering. Thus, we strongly support doctors providing psychological support and appropriate palliative care to competent patients who have made rational decisions to discontinue life-prolonging treatment, including refusing food and fluids. We claim that providing palliative care to competent patients who are rationally refusing treatment, or refusing food and fluids, does not count as assisting suicide. However, if the patients' refusals of treatment, especially refusal of food and fluids, do count as suicide, then it seems, at least initially, that providing palliative care to these patients should count as assisting suicide.

There are two questions here. The first is whether a patient's refusal of treatment, including refusing food and fluids, counts as suicide. The second is whether a physician who provides palliative care for such a patient is assisting suicide. Indeed, usually a patient will not refuse treatment if the doctor will not provide the appropriate palliative care. If the answer to the first question is that the patient's refusal does not count as suicide, then there is no need to be concerned with the second question, for providing palliative care to such a patient cannot be assisting suicide. However, if the answer to the first question is that a patient's refusal does count as suicide, then it is still an open question whether providing palliative care to such a patient counts as assisting suicide.

Does the Refusal of Life-Sustaining Treatment Count as Suicide?

That patients' refusals are rational does not show that their action does not count as suicide, for there can be rational suicide. However, if the refusal is irrational, it is more likely to be regarded as suicide. If suicide is regarded simply as killing oneself, then the analysis of killing should apply to it in a fairly straightforward fashion. An action, or omission, intended to result in the death of a patient, and which does result in his death, counts as killing. Therefore, one might argue that the refusal of treatment or food and fluids that is intended by the patient to result in his own death and which does result in his death, should count as suicide. And if "assisting suicide" is not an idiomatic phrase, but simply means doing those acts which help the person commit suicide, then physicians who provide palliative care to patients who are refusing life-sustaining treatments, are assisting suicide. Accepting this analysis would make providing palliative care to a patient refusing life-preserving treatment a kind of assisted suicide.

This conclusion would place physician-assisted suicide much closer to passive euthanasia than to active euthanasia, and so allowing physician-assisted suicide, one could argue, need not lead to allowing active euthanasia. We agree with this aspect of the conclusion, for we believe that physician-assisted suicide does not violate the rule against killing, as active euthanasia does. We believe that the major argument against physician-assisted suicide is that legalizing it will have worse consequences than not legalizing it. Many also hold that doctors should not participate in that practice, that it is inconsistent with their role as physicians, and that it will adversely affect the way in which they are viewed by the public. But unless this change in the view of physicians has overall bad consequences, it is not clear that it is a morally significant point.

It is compatible with our analyses so far that a rational person can either be for or be against legalizing physician-assisted suicide. We agree that one's view on this matter should be determined by the consequences of publicly allowing physician-assisted suicide. But we are also aware that different people can rank these consequences differently. How much additional unwanted pressure to commit suicide would legalizing physician-assisted suicide result in? How much pain and anxiety would be relieved by legalizing physician-assisted suicide? Even if one could answer these questions with any precision, which is extremely unlikely, it is still not clear that everyone would agree that the amount of pain and anxiety relieved outweighs the increase in the number of unwanted deaths, or vice versa.

However, it is not clear that the view that suicide is simply killing oneself should be accepted. Partly, this may be because "killing oneself" does not seem to need a justification or excuse as much as killing another person. This may be because our society, with some limitations, regards each person as allowed to do anything they want to themselves, as long as no one else is harmed. Indeed, it seems that any act which one does not intend but only knows will result in one's own death does not count as suicide, except in the extended sense that someone who continues to smoke or drink or eat too much, when they know that it may result in their death is said to be committing (slow) suicide.[22] It also seems that our society does not count as suicide any death that results from omissions, at least rational decisions to omit or to stop treatment, but only counts as suicide those positive acts that are done in order to bring about one's own death immediately, for these acts so closely resemble the paradigms of killing. The act-omission distinction that was incorrectly applied to killing, may be correctly applied when talking about suicide. Patients who take some pills to bring about their own death are committing suicide, but those who have the respirator removed, or who refuse food and fluids, are not regarded as committing suicide.[23]

This more complex analysis of suicide explains why the law has, never regarded providing palliative care to those who are refusing treatment as assisting suicide. Even those states which explicitly forbid assisting suicide do not prohibit providing palliative care to those who are refusing treatment or food and fluids. Of course, as with killing, those who favor physician-assisted suicide favor the simpler account of suicide, claiming that some physician-assisted suicide is already allowed, so it is simply inconsistent not to allow other quicker and less painful suicides. That our society does not count refusals of treatment as suicide, and hence does not count palliative care for patients who refuse treatment as assisting suicide, is not intended as an argument against allowing physician-assisted suicide. However, it does show that one argument for physician-assisted suicide, namely, that physician-assisted suicide is already allowed by providing palliative care for those who are refusing life-prolonging treatment, is based on a misunderstanding of how our society regards providing such palliative care.

Although our argument against physician-assisted suicide is not based on the use of the term "suicide," we are aware that calling a death a suicide has a negative connotation, even though suicide is no longer illegal. Whether one uses the term "suicide" depends, in part, on one's attitude toward the kind of act or omission by the person that results in his own death. Further, "assisting suicide" also has a negative connotation, and many physicians would refuse to carry out an act so named. We are concerned that describing providing palliative care to those who refuse life-sustaining treatment as assisting suicide may discourage some physicians from providing that palliative care. We want to encourage physicians to provide palliative care to patients who refuse life-sustaining treatment; we are against terminology that may discourage them from doing so. Thus, we advocate not counting as suicide any rational refusal of treatment, including food and fluids, and so do not count providing palliative care to patients who are refusing such treatment as assisting suicide.

We believe that the strongest argument against physician-assisted suicide is that, given the alternatives available, it does not provide sufficient benefit to patients to justify the risks that it poses. Patients already have the alternative of refusing treatment and food and fluids, and of being provided with palliative care while they are refusing that treatment. If physicians were to educate patients about these matters, and to make clear that they will support their choice and continue to care for them if they choose to refuse treatment, there would be little, if any, call for physician-assisted suicide. Patients are far less likely to be pressured into refusing treatment than they are to avail themselves of physician-assisted suicide. There are also far less opportunities for abuse. Physician-assisted suicide provides less incentive to be concerned with palliative care. And finally, given the bureacratic safeguards that most regard as necessary with physician-assisted suicide, death would come as soon or sooner with refusal of treatment, including refusal of food and fluids, than it would with physician-assisted suicide.[24]

In order to clarify this point and to provide a preferable alternative to physician-assisted suicide as a method for allowing seriously ill patients to determine the timing of their death, we think that states should consider passing legislation such as the following:

If a competent patient is terminally ill or suffering from a condition involving severe chronic pain or serious permanent disability, that patient's refusal of treatment, including refusal of food and fluids, shall not count as suicide, even though the patient knows that death will result from not starting or from stopping that treatment. All physicians and other health care workers shall be informed that they are legally prohibited from overruling any rational refusal of a competent patient, including refusal of food and fluids, even though it is known that death will result. All patients will be informed that they are allowed to refuse any treatment, including food and fluids, even though it is known that death will result, and that physicians and other health care workers are legally prohibited from overruling any such rational refusal by a competent patient.

Further, there shall be no prohibition placed upon any physician who provides pain relief in any form, in order to relieve the pain and suffering of the patient who has refused treatment, including food and fluids. In particular, providing pain medication shall not be considered as assisting suicide, and there shall be no liability for the physician who provides such pain medication for the purpose of relieving pain and suffering.

The physician shall not provide such medication for the purpose of hastening the time of death, but is not prohibited from providing medication which is consistent with adequate pain relief even if he knows that such medication will hasten the time of death. Physicians are required to follow rigorously the accepted standards of medical practice in determining the competence of patients who refuse any treatment, including food and fluids, when they know that death will result from abiding by that refusal.

Recent Court Decisions on Physician-Assisted Suicide

Unfortunately, in a recent decision (*Vacco v Quill*), the United States Court of Appeals for the Second Circuit does adopt an overly simple account of assisted suicide:

Moreover, the writing of a prescription to hasten death, after consultation with a patient, involves a far less active role for the physician than is required in bringing about death through asphyxiation, starvation and/or dehydration. Withdrawal of life support requires physicians or those acting at their direction physically to remove equipment and, often, to administer palliative drugs which themselves may contribute to death. The ending of life by these means is nothing more nor less than assisted suicide. It simply cannot be said that those mentally competent, terminally-ill persons who seek to hasten death but whose treatment does not include life support are treated equally.

The court is simply wrong in saying that providing palliative care to those who are refusing life-saving treatment is assisting suicide.[25] It seems to have been seduced by overly simple accounts of suicide and assisted suicide. If withdrawing treatment and providing prescription for pills with which to commit suicide were both assisting suicide, then not merely should laws prohibiting assisting suicide be rendered unconstitutional, doctors should be legally required to prescribe such pills. For doctors are now legally required to withdraw treatment when mentally competent, terminally ill persons refuse further treatment.

The quoted paragraph contains another serious error, in denying that "mentally competent, terminally-ill persons who seek to hasten death but whose treatment does not include life support are treated equally." This error is one that we discussed earlier, namely, that patients can refuse food and fluids only when these are provided intravenously. Any patient can refuse food and fluids and can be given palliative care while he is refusing, whether or not he is on life support.[26] So it is false that those mentally competent, terminally ill persons who seek to hasten death but whose treatment does not include life support, cannot be treated in exactly the same way as those who are on life support.

Thus the court is at least misleading when it concludes:

New York does not treat similarly circumstanced persons alike; those in the final stages of terminal illness who are on life-support systems are allowed to hasten their deaths by directing the removal of such systems; but those who are similarly situated, except for the previous attachment of life-sustaining equipment, are not allowed to hasten death by self-administering prescribed drugs.

It is true that those who are not on life-sustaining equipment "are not allowed to hasten death by self-administering prescribed drugs," but they are allowed to hasten death by refusing food and fluids and being given palliative care while they are refusing food and fluids. Thus they are not being denied equal treatment under the law. Since, as we have argued, there is a difference between actively committing suicide and refusing treatment, permitting palliative care for all refusals of treatment and not permitting assisting suicide is not treating people unequally.[27]

The court is correct in refusing to use whether death is due to natural causes as a way of distinguishing between morally acceptable and moral unacceptable ways of dying.

The district judge [whom this court is reversing] has identified 'a difference between allowing nature to take its course, even in the most severe situations, and intentionally using an artificial death-producing device.' But Justice Scalia, for one, has remarked upon "the irrelevance of the action-inaction distinction," noting that "the cause of death in both cases is the suicide's conscious decision to put an end to his own existence."

However, although the action-inaction or act-omission distinction does not distinguish killing from allowing to die, it may, as we pointed out earlier, distinguish suicide from deciding to die by refusing treatment or food and fluids. To talk as if any "conscious decision to put an end to [one's] own existence" is to commit suicide, is to impose an oversimplification on the concept of suicide. It is clear that in the normal understanding of suicide, a rational refusal of life-sustaining treatment by a competent patient is not a suicide.

Given that the court seems to realize that whether or not the death is due to natural causes is irrelevant, it is not clear why they then try to show that refusal of treatment is not natural.

Indeed, there is nothing "natural" about causing death by means other than the original illness or its complications. The withdrawal of nutrition brings on death by starvation, the withdrawal of hydration brings on death by dehydration, and the withdrawal of ventilation brings about respiratory failure. By ordering the discontinuance of these artificial life-sustaining processes or refusing to accept them in the first place, a patient hastens his death by means that are not natural in any sense. It certainly cannot be said that the death that immediately ensues is the natural result of the progression of the disease or condition from which the patient suffers.

The important point, however, is that physicians are not allowed to overrule a rational refusal of treatment by an informed competent patient. Physicians are allowed not to grant a request for a prescription for lethal drugs. Thus there is clearly a difference between these two acts, and to equate them for moral or legal purposes is a mistake. Further, as we have pointed out, a realization of the complexity of the concepts of killing and suicide makes it clear that not over-ruling the rational refusal of life-sustaining treatment is not killing, and rationally refusing life-sustaining treatment is not suicide. Given this latter point, providing palliative care to those who are refusing treatment cannot be assisting suicide.[28]

Recognition of the moral significance of the standard medical distinction between requests and refusals is essential for resolving the situation in which some competent patients with terminal illnesses want to hasten their death.[29] Failure to appreciate this distinction has also caused significant problems in the decision of the Ninth Circuit court of Appeals (*Washington v Glucksberg*). This court correctly notes that refusal of treatment does not count as suicide, and that helping the patient carry out that refusal does not count as assisting suicide. It also correctly notes that a competent adult has a "liberty interest" in refusing to be connected to a respirator or in being disconnected from one, even if he is terminally ill and cannot live without mechanical assistance."[30] However, it then mistakenly characterizes the liberty interest of the patient, which is the liberty to refuse treatment, as if it were better described as "the right to die," "controlling the time and manner of one's death," and "hastening one's death." These overbroad phrases apply to active euthanasia as well as to assisted suicide, and it seems extremely unlikely that one has a constitutional liberty interest in having someone kill him.

Later the majority writes about "[t]he debate over whether terminally ill patients should have the right to reject medical treatment or to receive aid from their physicians in hastening their deaths," as if this were a single debate. But the debate about the right to reject treatment has already been settled, the only debate now is a debate about the right to receive aid in committing suicide. This confusion is explicitly stated in their conclusion "that Cruzan, [referring to the case of *Cruzan v Director, Missouri Department of Health,* 497 U.S. 261 (199)] by recognizing a liberty interest that includes the refusal of artificial provision of life-sustaining food and water, necessarily recognizes a liberty interest in hastening one's own death." The court correctly rejects the four ad hoc ways of making the distinction between active and passive euthanasia, that we discussed earlier, however it does not discuss what we regard as the only morally significant way to make this distinction, namely, by distinguishing between requests and refusals. It is interesting and significant that the dissenting opinion agrees completely with our view.[31]

Is Killing Patients Ever Justified?

Stopping food and fluids is often the very best way of allowing a patient to die, but it may be claimed that killing is sometimes better. Given present knowledge and technology, one can kill a patient absolutely painlessly within a matter of minutes. If patients have a rational desire to die, why wait several days or weeks for them to die, why not kill them quickly and painlessly in a matter of minutes? We have provided no argument against killing patients who want to die that applies to an ideal world where there are never any misunderstandings between people and everyone is completely moral and trustworthy. In such a world, if one can inject the appropriate drugs and kill the patient painlessly and almost instantaneously, there is no need to worry about the distinction between killing and allowing to die, or between active and passive euthanasia. But in the real world, there are misunderstandings and not everyone is completely moral and trustworthy, so that in this world no one even proposes that killing patients be allowed without elaborate procedural safeguards, which almost always require at least two weeks. So, on a practical level, legalizing physician-assisted suicide or killing would not result in a quicker death than stopping food and fluids.[32]

On our account, passive euthanasia is abiding by the rational refusal of life-saving treatment (or food and fluids) by a competent patient. Since there is no duty to overrule a rational refusal by a competent patient, abiding by this refusal does not count as killing. Further, failing to abide by such a refusal is itself morally prohibited, for it is an unjustified deprivation of the freedom of the patient. Also, in some newer codes of medical ethics, for example, that of the American Academy of Physicians, respecting patients' refusals is now listed as a duty. Physicians are not merely morally allowed to practice passive euthanasia, they are morally required to do so. Active euthanasia is killing; it is complying with the rational request of a competent patient to be killed. It involves active intervention by a physician, which is more than merely stopping treatment. It is not simply abiding by the patient's desire to be left alone, it is, say, injecting some substance that causes his death, when one has no duty to do so.

Since active euthanasia is killing, it is a violation of a moral rule and so needs to be justified. This contrasts quite sharply with passive euthanasia, and even physician-assisted suicide, which need not violate any moral rule, and hence may not even need to be morally justified. It is the overruling of a patient's refusal that involves the violation of a moral rule and hence needs to be justified. But, as noted earlier, physicians often break the moral rule against causing pain with regard to their patients and are completely justified, because they do so at their patients' request, or at least with their consent, and do it in order to prevent what the patient takes to be a greater harm, greater future pain or death. Why should active euthanasia be regarded as anything different from any other instance of a doctor breaking a moral rule with regard to a patient, at the patient's request, in order to prevent what the patient takes to be a greater harm? In active euthanasia, the patient takes death to be a lesser harm than suffering pain and requests that the moral rule prohibiting killing be violated.

If causing pain can be justified, why is killing not justified when all of the other morally relevant features are the same? Because of a special feature of death that distinguishes it from all of the other serious harms, killing needs a stronger justification than violations of the other moral rules. The special feature is that after death, the person killed no longer exists, and so cannot protest that he did not want to be killed. All impartial rational persons would advocate that violations against causing pain be publicly allowed when the person toward whom the rule is being violated rationally prefers to suffer that pain rather than suffer some other harm such as greater pain or death. It is uncertain how many impartial rational persons would advocate that killing be publicly allowed when the person being killed rationally prefers to be killed rather than to continue to suffer pain. This uncertainty stems from taking seriously the two features that make moral rules central to morality, the public character of morality and the fallibility of persons.

Violations, with valid consent, of the rule against causing pain can be publicly allowed without any significant anxiety being caused thereby. Patients need have no anxiety that the rule will be mistakenly violated and that they will suffer serious unwanted pain for a prolonged period, for they can usually correct the mistake rather quickly by ordering a stop to the painful treatment. Also physicians have a strong incentive to be careful not to violate the rule by mistake, for patients will complain if they did not really want the rule violated. Violations of the rule against killing, even with valid consent, being publicly allowed may create significant anxiety. Patients may fear that the rule will be mistakenly violated and that they will have no opportunity to correct that mistake. That a patient will not be around to complain if the rule is mistakenly violated removes a strong safeguard against mistaken violations. It is not merely mistakes about which a patient would not be able to complain. If a physician tries to take advantage of this kind of violation being publicly allowed and intentionally killed a patient, complaint would also not be possible. Taking advantage of violations of the rule against causing pain being publicly allowed, does not pose similar problems.

Although voluntary active euthanasia, killing a patient painlessly and quickly when requested by that patient, would, if publicly allowed, prevent a significant amount of pain and suffering, it would also be likely to create significant anxiety and some unwanted deaths. Impartial rational persons can therefore disagree on whether or not they would advocate that such violations of the rule against killing be publicly allowed. There should be no disagreement among impartial rational persons about passive euthanasia, for no moral rule is even being violated. Further, once it is recognized that withholding of food and fluids (1) can be painless, (2) usually results in unconsciousness in one week and death in two weeks, (3) allows for patients to change their minds, and (4) is not killing at all, the need for active euthanasia or killing of patients, and even for physician-assisted suicide, significantly diminishes, even if it is not completely eliminated.

Unlike others who argue against active euthanasia, we do not claim that physician-assisted suicide or active euthanasia is morally unjustified, only that they are not strongly justified. Since they are only weakly justified, they are controversial. If the goal is to allow a patient to choose her own time of dying and also to allow dying to be accomplished relatively painlessly, there seems to be little need for active euthanasia or physician-assisted suicide. If patient refusal of treatment, including refusal of food and fluids, were not sufficient for a relatively quick and painless death for the overwhelming number of terminally ill patients, then we would favor physician-assisted suicide, although we would still have serious reservations about active euthanasia. However, since passive euthanasia, especially when this includes refusing food and fluids, is available together with appropriate palliative care, it seems far more difficult to justify controversial methods like physician-assisted suicide or active euthanasia. The harms prevented by physician-assisted suicide or active euthanasia are no longer the long-term suffering of patients who have no other way to die, they are only the one week of suffering that may be present while the patient is refusing food and fluids, and this suffering can be almost completely controlled by appropriate palliative care. This is an excellent example of why the presence of an alternative is a morally relevant feature (see Chapter 2).

Given the alternative of refusing food and fluids, very little harm seems to be prevented by physician-assisted suicide or active euthanasia. The presence of an alternative which does not violate any moral rule is a morally relevant feature and makes it far more difficult to justify violating a moral rule. Thus it seems far more difficult to justify active euthanasia. Physician-assisted suicide, if legalized, would not violate a moral rule, but it is questionable whether it provides sufficient benefits to justify the risks involved in legalizing it.[33] There are good reasons for believing that the advantages of refusing food and fluids, while receiving adequate palliative care, make it preferable to legalizing physician-assisted suicide. This is especially true in a multicultural society where doctors and patients sometimes do not even speak the same language. There are a small number of cases in which refusal of food and fluids might be difficult, but it is necessary to weigh the benefit of physician-assisted suicide to this relatively small number of people against the harm that might be suffered by a great number of people by the legalizing of physician-assisted suicide.[34]

There are several morally significant disadvantages that are shared by physician-assisted suicide and active euthanasia that are not shared by the refusing of food and fluids. Physician-assisted suicide and active euthanasia, although they would usually require a two-week waiting period, allow for almost instantaneous death. This makes it less likely that their legalization will support the use of palliative care. The refusal of food and fluids takes a week before the patient is unconscious, thus it is clear that palliative care must be practiced. The relative speed and ease with which physician-assisted suicide and active euthanasia can bring about death, makes it more likely that patients will be pressured to hasten their death when they would prefer not to do so. Because of the time it takes, it is much less likely that patients will be pressured to refuse food and fluids. This time also permits patients to change their mind, and for friends and family to be confident that the patient was firm in his decision to die. Indeed, for patients not on life-sustaining treatments, refusing food and fluids seems to have more overall benefits than any other method of hastening death.[35] There are three major drawbacks: physician ignorance that it need not be painful for terminal patients to do without food and fluids, the association of feeding with caring, and some patients' dislike of the idea of refusing food and fluids.

Since both physician-assisted suicide and active euthanasia are morally controversial, physicians cannot be required to practice them. This means that physicians would always have to take full personal responsibility for assisting suicide or performing active euthanasia. Like physicians performing abortions, they are likely to be subject to criticism from those opposed to such practices. Physicians are morally required to practice passive euthanasia, that is, they are not allowed to overrule a competent patient's refusal of treatment, so in such cases they do not have to bear this burden. Patients cannot require someone to kill them; they can require others to leave them alone, even if that requires physicians to discontinue their treatment. Thus, from the point of view of physicians, providing their terminally ill patients with adequate palliative care and informing them that they may refuse any life-preserving treatment, including food and fluids, together with assuring them that palliative care will continue for as long as necessary during their refusal, seems, on balance, a safer and more desirable option than the legalization of physician-assisted suicide.

Advance Directives

Since a person often loses competence in the latter stages of a terminal illness, all that has been said above may seem to be of limited practical value. However, abiding by the Advance Directives of a formerly competent patient, after that patient becomes incompetent, is similar in all moral respects to abiding by the directives of a currently competent patient. This means that if competent patients explicitly state in an Advance Directive (either a Living Will or Durable Power of Attorney for Health Care) that if they reach a hopeless stage, they want food and fluids to be withheld, then the physician is morally required to abide by that refusal. Advance Directives avoid the very troubling matter of dealing with gravely ill, permanently incompetent patients who have not expressed their wishes about whether they would wish life-prolonging treatment to be discontinued, and in particular whether they would want food and fluids withdrawn or withheld.

We have not discussed the questions of nonvoluntary euthanasia, since morality does not provide as clear an answer to the questions it raises as it does to the questions raised by voluntary euthanasia. Recognizing that voluntary passive euthanasia is not merely morally allowed, but is morally required, whereas nonvoluntary passive euthanasia is at most morally allowed and that some impartial rational persons would not advocate publicly allowing it, is itself of moral significance. Physicians should make every effort to have patients, when competent, express their desires about what they would want to be done if they should become permanently incompetent and appoint someone to determine when it is appropriate to have those desires acted on. In particular patients should be told the facts about the withholding of food and fluids—that it is not a painful way to die.

If competent patients explicitly state in an Advance Directive that, if they become permanently incompetent, they want life-prolonging treatments to be discontinued, then physicians are morally required to abide by those refusals. This view has been challenged by those claiming that the views of the competent person who filled out the Advance Directive are not always the same as the views of the incompetent person to whom they are being applied.[36] They hold that Advance Directives need not be followed if the physician believes that the incompetent person would not choose to have life-prolonging treatment withdrawn. One must judge a public policy, however, in terms of the effects that this policy would have on all of the people involved if all of them knew about the policy. Competent persons who fill out Advance Directives refusing life-prolonging treatment if they become permanently incompetent consider it very distasteful and devoid of dignity to live as a permanently incompetent person. The now incompetent person, however, having no sense of dignity, does not view her life with distaste.

If everyone knew that Advance Directives need not be honored in these cases, some permanently incompetent persons would live longer than they would if such Advance Directives were honored. This might be viewed by some as a positive result, but it is not clear whether the incompetent person views it in that way. It is clear, however, that another result of everyone knowing that their Advance Directives might not be honored, would be anxiety, anger, and other unpleasant feelings by those competent persons who had made out such Advance Directives. This could result in an increase in such competent persons taking their own lives while they were competent, as was the case with Janet Adkins, the first client of Dr. Kevorkian, in order to avoid the unwanted prolongation of their lives as incompetent persons. The consequences of a public policy of not honoring such Advance Directives seems likely to have worse consequences than the present policy of honoring them.

Hospitals are now required to ask patients if they have filled out an Advance Directive. It would be even better if they made filling out an Advance Directive a standard part of their admitting procedure. Persuading patients to express their desires on these matters and to appoint someone to determine how best to satisfy their desires when they become incompetent, could, if properly implemented, give patients a genuine sense of being able to control their own death. We realize, however, that at present Advance Directives seem to have little or no effect on the treatment of seriously ill patients in the hospital. (See the SUPPORT studies by Joanne Lynne and Joan Teno.[37]) We regard this as unfortunate and know that much more work must be done in order for physicians and patients to see Advance Directives as an appropriate and desirable opportunity to allow patients greater control over the time of their death.

Gravely Ill Patients without Advance Directives

Even with aggressive attempts to have large numbers of persons fill out Advance Directives, there will inevitably be, in the foreseeable future, many incompetent and gravely ill patients who have not done so. How should such patients be treated? The current procedure frequently seems to be to continue treatment and life support until the patient dies or until the probability that the patient will die very soon becomes essentially 100%. One reason this is done is because it is assumed that, unless otherwise stated, persons would want to be treated until their situations became hopeless. This assumption is mistaken in most cases.

Our experience, for example, suggests that essentially no one would want to be kept alive if he were in a persistent vegetative state or any other state in which there was no chance of his becoming conscious again. Our experience also suggests that almost no one would want to be kept alive even if there were a chance of his becoming conscious, if there were not also a chance of significant interaction with others. Almost no one wants to be kept alive while in a coma when the best they can expect if they come out of the coma does not include recognition of family and friends. In fact, we believe that only a small minority of gravely ill patients would want to be kept alive if their chances of completely recovering from a coma were less than 5% and they would still be gravely ill after their recovery.[38]

Our experience is limited, however, and we would not want to base any public policy upon it. Rather, we propose that over a several-year period there be a very large survey of suitably constructed Advance Directives. If the overwhelming majority (at least 90%) of those filling out Advance Directives state that they would not want treatment to be continued in a particular clinical state, we propose that in the absence of an Advance Directive requesting treatment in that clinical state, that treatment be discontinued. These data would rebut the presumption that most persons want to be kept alive in that situation. Of course, if a patient had completed an Advance Directive requesting that treatment be continued, this should be honored. Further, this policy would not be implemented until it had been given sufficiently wide publicity that essentially every-one had heard of it, so that those who did not wish treatment to be stopped would have had an opportunity to fill out a suitable Advance Directive.

We do not propose that people vote on whether or not people without Advance Directives should be kept alive or allowed to die. We are not concerned with whether other people want a patient in a particular clinical state to be kept alive or allowed to die. This is not a decision that people should make for others. Rather, we want to know what people choose for themselves when they fill out Advance Directives. It is what people choose for themselves that is the best guide for determining what would be chosen by someone who has not made an explicit choice. That is why we want a very large survey of actual Advance Directives, not a vote, to determine what should be done in particular clinical situations.

Another reason sometimes given for continued treatment is that since death is irreversible, if doctors err they should err on the side of life. We agree that normally doctors should err on the side of life and that is why we state that treatment should be discontinued only when the overwhelming majority (at least 90%, and not a mere majority of 51%) would choose to have treatment and life-support stopped in particular circumstances. Given the great costs, emotional as well as financial, as well as the minimal benefits of any kind that are involved in continuing treatment in situations where the overwhelming majority of persons would want it discontinued, we believe it is harder to justify continuing treatment than to justify discontinuing it.

Summary

The examination of four standard ways of making the distinction between active and passive euthanasia—acts versus omissions; stopping versus not starting; ordinary care versus extraordinary care; and whether death is due to natural causes—shows that they cannot provide a way of making a morally relevant distinction between killing and allowing to die. Using the distinction between patient requests and patient refusals, however, does provide such a way. Our moral analysis of the distinction between active and passive euthanasia reaches some different conclusions than all of the ad hoc ways of making the distinction. On the four standard ways of making the distinction, active euthanasia is morally prohibited and passive euthanasia is morally allowed. We claim only that active euthanasia is morally controversial, not that it is morally prohibited and for us, voluntary passive euthanasia is morally required, not merely morally allowed.

Physician-assisted suicide was seen to be neither active euthanasia nor passive euthanasia. It resembles active euthanasia in that it is a request for an action by the physician, prescribing lethal drugs that will result in the patient's death, but it does not violate the rule against killing as active euthanasia does. It is not passive euthanasia, for it is not based on a refusal of treatment that a physician is morally required to abide by. However, it partly resembles providing palliative care to those who are refusing life-prolonging treatment, or food and fluids. It differs from providing such palliative care in that those who refuse life-prolonging treatment, or food and fluids, are not committing suicide, and those for whom the lethal drugs are prescribed are committing suicide. Since physician-assisted suicide does not violate the rule against killing, the only moral argument against legalizing it is that it will lead to overall worse consequences. Whether or not this is true is an empirical matter. Since physician-assisted suicide does not violate the rule against killing, its legalization is not a reason for legalizing active euthanasia, which does violate this rule.

The moral system thus makes clear the moral significance of the distinction between refusals and requests and allows for a meaningful distinction between active and passive euthanasia. There is no need to make an ad hoc distinction that applies only to dying patients, as the standard discussions do; rather the moral significance of a commonly used distinction in medical practice, between requests and refusals, is acknowledged and applied to the question of euthanasia. The medical facts about the consequences of refusing food and fluids, that it normally causes no additional suffering, makes clear that there is a viable alternative, open to all patients, whether or not they are on life support, to hasten the time of their death. Our explicit account of morality is not only helpful in showing the inadequacy of accepting the standard ad hoc, unsystematic attempts to distinguish between active and passive euthanasia, it also shows how a commonly applied medical distinction, between requests and refusals, can be used to make this distinction.

Notes

1. See Kathleen M. Foley, "The Relationship of Pain and Symptom Management to Patient Requests for Physician-Assisted Suicide," *Journal of Pain and Symptom Management,* 6 (1991), pp. 289–297.
2. See K. Danner Clouser, "Allowing or Causing: Another Look," *Annals of Internal Medicine,* 87 (1977), pp. 622–624.
3. J. Rachels, "Active and Passive Euthanasia," *New England Journal of Medicine,* 292 (1975): 78–80. D. W. Brock, "Voluntary Active Euthanasia," *Hastings Center Report,* 22 (1992), pp. 10–12.
4. See United States Court of Appeals for the Ninth Circuit, no. 94-35534, March 6, 1996.
5. Ibid.
6. Ibid.
7. "Nutrition" and "hydration" are the terms normally used when food and fluids are being supplied by medical means; it is considered a medical treatment. Since patients can refuse any medical treatment, they are the terms used by those who hold that a

patient can refuse food and fluids. Since we hold that patients are not limited to refusing medical treatments, we generally use the simpler phrase, "food and fluids."

8. United States Court of Appeals for the Ninth Circuit, no. 94-35534, March 6, 1996.

9. This is true not only of a "natural death," but also of "natural ingredients," "natural behavior," etc.

10. See Bernard Gert, James L. Bernat, and R. Peter Mogielnicki, "Distinguishing between Patients' Refusals and Requests," *Hastings Center Report,* 24 (1994), pp. 13–15.

11. Sometimes the patient has a rationally allowed belief, for instance a religious belief, that is not shared by the doctor, and this difference in belief accounts for his refusal to consent to the suggested treatment.

12. Of course, sometimes it is rational because they have not been provided with adequate palliative care and do not know that such care is available. That this happens so often is another reason that many are reluctant to make physician-assisted suicide or active euthanasia legal.

13. See K. Danner Clouser, "Allowing or Causing: Another Look."

14. See Kathleen M. Foley, "The Relationship of Pain and Symptom Management to Patient Requests for Physician-Assisted Suicide." A reply to that line of reasoning is Gregg A. Kasting, "The Nonnecessity of Euthanasia" from Humber, et al., eds. *Physician-Assisted Death* (Totowa, N.J.: Humana, 1994), pp. 25–45. See also James L. Bernat, Bernard Gert, and R. Peter Mogielnicki, "Patient Refusal of Hydration and Nutrition: An Alternative to Physician Assisted Suicide or Voluntary Euthanasia," *Archives of Internal Medicine,* 153 (1993), pp. 2723–2728.

15. It may be that "killing" that is the result of abiding by a refusal never would have the same morally relevant features as killing that is done at the request of a patient. However, killing is such a serious violation of a moral rule, that the morally relevant features would have to be dramatically different for one way of killing to be justified and the other not.

16. Contrary to one's initial inclination, what counts as "causing harm" is not determined by some scientific analysis, but rather by whether it is held that a justification or excuse is needed for such behavior. See *Morality,* pp. 111–113.

17. But one can also kill a person unintentionally, even when one is not negligent, as when one's car skids on some black ice and hits a person, resulting in his death. Such a killing may be completely excusable, but it is still killing.

18. Given that it is not only morally but also legally required to abide by a patient's rational refusal of treatment, legally abiding by such refusals cannot be treated as intentionally killing the patient.

19. Some who are involved in cognitive science suggest that people do not operate on the basis of rules, but rather of paradigms or prototypes. But as this discussion makes clear, there is no conflict between using both rules and prototypes in moral reasoning. Indeed, the proper role of paradigms or prototypes is to determine whether an act should be considered as an act of a certain kind, such as killing, and hence needs a justification or excuse. See Larry May, Marilyn Friedman, and Andy Clark, eds., *Mind and Morals,* (Cambridge, Mass.: MIT Press, 1996). See especially Chapters 5, "The Neural Representation of the Social World" by Paul M. Churchland, and 6, "Connectionism, Moral Cognition, and Collaborative Problem Solving," by Andy Clark.

20. In our society not everyone uses or extends the paradigms or prototypes in the same way, and so there will be disagreements on whether a given act counts as killing. Nonetheless, there is usually substantial agreement on most cases. However, in trying to

change a longstanding practice, it is not uncommon for people, especially philosophers, to try to change the ways of extending the paradigms, so as to justify the change they are promoting. And sometimes these efforts are successful; what counts as killing does change.

21. See D. W. Brock, "Voluntary Active Euthanasia." People would be inconsistent if such concepts as "killing" were as simple as some philosophers claim them to be. However, some philosophers confuse complexity with inconsistency.

22. That this is an extended sense is shown by the fact that life insurance policies that exclude payment if death is due to suicide, cannot refuse to pay if death is due to these kinds of causes.

23. This view is not held by all. Some, especially those with religious views, regard refusing treatment, and especially refusing food and fluids, as committing suicide. They may not regard such refusals as suicide if death is imminent with or without treatment, but they would regard all refusals of treatment as suicide when treatment would sustain life for a long time.

24. See K. Danner Clouser, "The Challenge for Future Debate on Euthanasia," *Journal of Pain and Symptom Management,* 6 (1991), pp. 306–311.

25. This is also the view of the United States Court of Appeals for the Ninth Circuit, no. 94-35534, March 6, 1996: "The law does not classify the death of a patient that results from the granting of his wish to decline or discontinue treatment as 'suicide.' Nor does the law label the acts of those who help the patient carry out that wish, whether by physically disconnecting the respirator or by removing an intravenous tube, as assistance in suicide."

26. See David M. Eddy's article "A Conversation with My Mother" about his mother refusing food and fluids. *JAMA* 272 (1994), pp. 179–181.

27. New York Attorney General Dennis Vacco makes exactly the same point in his argument to the Supreme Court in appealing the decision of the Second Circuit Court of Appeals.

28. The court may have been mistakenly persuaded by the claim of Timothy Quinn: "It is legally and ethically permitted for physicians to actively assist patients to die who are dependent on life-sustaining treatments. . . . Unfortunately, some dying patients who are in agony that can no longer be relieved, yet are not dependent on life-sustaining treatment, have no such options under current legal restrictions. It seems unfair, discriminatory, and inhumane to deprive some dying patients of such vital choices because of arbitrary elements of their condition which determine whether they are on life-sustaining treatment which can be stopped." The errors in this paragraph have already been pointed out. It wrongly claims that patients who are not on life-sustaining treatments cannot refuse food and fluids and be provided with appropriate palliative care, thereby hastening their time of death.

29. Bernard Gert, James L. Bernat, and R. Peter Mogielnicki, "Distinguishing between Patients' Refusals and Requests," *Hastings Center Report,* 24 (1994), pp. 13–15,

30. United States Court of Appeals for the Ninth Circuit, no. 94-35534, March 6, 1996.

31. In a "Sounding Board" article in the *New England Journal of Medicine*, 335 (1996), "The Legalization of Physician-Assisted Suicide") discussing these Appeals Court decisions, David Orentlicher also fails to appreciate the moral importance of the distinction between refusals and requests and completely ignores the feasibility of patient refusal of food and fluids as an alternative to physician-assisted suicide.

32. This is not an argument against killing someone in an emergency situation, for example, someone who has been captured by a sadistic enemy, or an unrescuable person in an accident who is about to be burned to death. This shows the importance of the morally relevant feature concerning emergency situations. (See Chapter 2 for further discussion of morally relevant features.)

33. Many people claim to prefer physician-assisted suicide, or even active euthanasia, to discontinuing food and fluids. However, this may be due to their focus on their own particular cases, namely, they see only the ease and quickness of the former two methods, and fail to appreciate their far greater potential for abuse. Also, there is so much misinformation about the pain and suffering involved in discontinuing food and fluids, that it is unlikely that their preferences count as informed preferences. However, even with accurate information and the support of their physicians, some patients may still prefer physician-assisted suicide to discontinuing food and fluids. How much importance should be given to these preferences is a matter of dispute, even among the authors of this book.

34. This is an argument against legalizing physician-assisted suicide. It is not an argument against using it if it were legalized.

35. However, for some the personal benefits of knowing that they can die quickly and painlessly may outweigh all of the benefits of discontinuing food and fluids. This is not an irrational ranking.

36. See Rebecca S. Dresser and John A. Robertson, " Quality of Life and Non-treatment Decisions for Incompetent Patients," *Law, Medicine & Health Care,* 17 (1989), pp. 234–244.

37. The SUPPORT Principal Investigators. "A Controlled Trial to Improve Care for Seriously Ill Hospitalized Patients." *JAMA* 274 (1995), pp. 1591–1598.

38. Charles M. Culver and Bernard Gert, "Beyond the Living Will: Making Advance Directives More Useful," *Omega,* 21 (1990), pp. 253–258.

Index